OXFORD PROFESSIONAL PRACTICE

Handbook of Management for Hospital Dentistry

W0114064

OXFORD PROFESSIONAL PRACTICE

Handbook of Management for Hospital Dentistry

EDITED BY

Clara Gibson

Consultant Orthodontist, UK
Private Practice, Singapore

Suhaym Mubeen

Consultant Orthodontist
Great Ormond Street Hospital, London

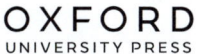

OXFORD
UNIVERSITY PRESS

OXFORD
UNIVERSITY PRESS

Great Clarendon Street, Oxford, OX2 6DP,
United Kingdom

Oxford University Press is a department of the University of Oxford.
It furthers the University's objective of excellence in research, scholarship,
and education by publishing worldwide. Oxford is a registered trade mark of
Oxford University Press in the UK and in certain other countries

Published in the United States of America by Oxford University Press
198 Madison Avenue, New York, NY 10016, United States of America

British Library Cataloguing in Publication Data
Data available

Library of Congress Control Number: 2024948806

ISBN 978–0–19–889090–4

DOI: 10.1093/med/9780198890904.001.0001

Printed in the UK by
Bell & Bain Ltd., Glasgow

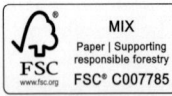

Contents

Contents

Detailed Contents

Scenarios

Contributors

Farooq Ahmed
Consultant Orthodontist, Guy's and St Thomas' NHS Foundation Trust. Treehouse Dental Practice, Crouch End, London, UK

Elizabeth Akers
Head of Education for Patient Safety, Great Ormond Street Hospital, London

David Bailey
NHS finance trainer and author

Edmund Bailey
Clinical Reader/Honorary Consultant in Oral Surgery, Institute of Dentistry, Queen Mary University of London

Alan Bray
Accredited Specialist & Consultant Occupational Physician, SWIMS Ltd, West Midlands

Simon Critchlow
Consultant in Restorative Dentistry, Clinical Lead for Maxillofacial and Dental, Great Ormond Street Hospital, London

Andrew Dickenson
Chief Dental Officer, Wales

Brett Duane
Associate Professor Dental Public Health, Trinity College Dublin, Ireland

Peter Duffy
Ex-Consultant Urological Surgeon and Whistleblower. Chair of Healthcare Group, Whistleblowers, UK

Mohammed Dungarwalla
Clinical Lecturer/Specialist in Oral Surgery, Institute of Dentistry, Barts and The London School of Medicine & Dentistry & The Royal London Hospital, Barts Health NHS Trust, London, UK

Tom Ferris
Chief Dental Officer, Scotland

Clara Gibson
Consultant Orthodontist, UK. Private Practice, Singapore

James I. J. Green
Maxillofacial and Dental Laboratory Manager, Great Ormond Street Hospital for Children NHS Foundation Trust, London/ Broomfield Hospital, Mid and South Essex NHS Foundation Trust, Chelmsford, UK

Janak Gunatilleke
Medical Doctor, Using data and technology to improve healthcare

Priya Haria
Consultant Orthodontist, Great Ormond Street Hospital, London

Norman Hay
Consultant Orthodontist, Great Ormond Street Hospital, London

Nicola Holland
Clinical Dental Fellow, Department of Health, Northern Ireland

Neil Hubbard
Interim Head of Research Governance & Clinical Trials, Great Ormond Street Hospital, London

Ama Johal
Professor & Consultant Orthodontist, Institute of Dentistry, Barts and The London School of Medicine and Dentistry

Anup Karki
Consultant in Dental Public Health, Primary Care Division, Public Health Wales

Caroline Lappin
Chief Dental Officer, Northern Ireland

Simon J. Littlewood
Consultant Orthodontist, Department of Orthodontics, St Luke's Hospital, Bradford, UK

Gerry McKenna
Chair of Oral Health Services Research and Gerodontology, Consultant in Restorative Dentistry, Centre for Public Health, Queens University Belfast

Suhaym Mubeen
Consultant Orthodontist, Great Ormond Street Hospital, London

Lucy H. H. Parker
Royal Free London NHS Foundation Trust, London

Brijesh Patel
Consultant Orthodontist, Great Ormond Street Hospital, London

Kunal Patel
Paediatric Dentistry Consultant, Great Ormond Street Hospital, London

Raj Rattan
Dental Director, Dental Protection Ltd.

Mariam Shahid Noorani
Consultant Orthodontist, Clinical Lead in Orthodontics Kings College Hospital, NHS Foundation Trust

Yvonne Shaw
Deputy Dental Director/ Underwriting Policy Lead, Dental Protection

Kyle Squire
Trust Barrister, Great Ormond Street Hospital, London

Helen Tippett
Consultant Orthodontist, King's College Hospital NHS Foundation Trust, Regional Associate Postgraduate Dental Dean, NHS England (London and Kent, Surrey and Sussex)

Abbreviations

AAC	Advisory appointments committee
ACAS	Advisory, conciliation, and arbitration service
ACE	Adverse childhood experiences
ACF	Academic clinical fellowship
AD	Associate dean
AE	Adverse events
AES	Assigned educational supervisor
AGP	Aerosol-generating procedures
ALB	Arm's length bodies
AMRC	Association of Medical Research Charities
ARSAC	Administration of Radioactive Substances Advisory Committee
BADN	British Association of Dental Nurses
BBV	Blood-borne viruses
BCP	Business continuity plan
BF	Bradford factor
BFE	Bacterial filtration efficiency
BNF	British National Formulary
BSA	Business Services Authority
BSB	Bar Standards Board
BSO	Business services organization
CAF	Common assessment framework
CAG	Confidentiality advisory group
CBCT	Cone-beam computed tomography
CBD	Case-based discussion
CBT	Cognitive behavioural therapy
CC&C	Confirmation of capacity and capability
CCG	Clinical commissioning groups
CCST	Certificate of completion of specialist training
CDO	Chief dental officer
CDS	Community dental service
CEO	Chief executive officer
CI	Chief investigator
CIN	Child in need
CIW	Care Inspectorate Wales
CJD	Creutzfeldt–Jakob disease
COI	Conflicts of interest
COSHH	Control of Substances Hazardous to Health
COT	Course of treatment
CPC	Child Protection Conference
CPD	Continuing professional development
CPP	Child protection plan
CQC	Care Quality Commission
CRE	Clinical radiation expert
CRES	Cash releasing efficiency savings
CRF	Case report form
CRN	Clinical research nurse
CS	Clinical supervisor
CSCDFT	Certificate of Satisfactory Completion of Dental Foundation Training
CSSD	Central Sterile Services Department
CTA	Clinical trial authorization
CTIMP	Clinical trial of investigational medicinal products
CTP	Clinical trial practitioners
CV	Curriculum vitae
DBS	Disclosure and Barring Service
DCC	Direct clinical care
DCP	Dental care professionals
DCS	Dental Complaints Service
DCT	Dental core training
DCTAG	Dental Core Training Advisory Group
DDRB	Doctors' and Dentists' Review Body
DFT	Dental foundation training
DFTAG	Dental Foundation Advisory Group
DHCW	Digital health and care Wales
DHSC	Department of Health and Social Care
DMBC	Decision-making business case
DME	Director of Medical Education
DNA	Did not attend

DoLS	Deprivation of Liberty Safeguards
DPA	Data protection agreement
DPIA	Data protection impact assessment
DPMD	Defence Postgraduate Medical Deanery
DPO	Data protection officer
DSA	Data sharing agreement
DSPI	Department of Social Policy and Intervention
DSPT	Data Security and Protection Toolkit
DSS	Data security standards
DST	Dental Speciality Training
DVT	Dental Vocational Training
DWSI	Dentist with special interest
EAP	Employee assistance programme
EEA	European Economic Area
EHIC	European health insurance card
ENT	Ear, nose and throat
EPP	Exposure prone procedures
EPR	Electronic Patient Record
ES	Educational supervisor
FCA	Financial Conduct Authority
FFT	Friends and family test
FGM	Female genital mutilation
FOI	Freedom of Information
FOIA	Freedom of Information Act
FTSU	Freedom to Speak Up
GA	General anaesthetic
GCP	Good clinical practice
GDC	General Dental Council
GDP	General dental practitioner
GDPR	General Data Protection Regulation
GDS	General Dental Services
GHIC	Global Health Insurance Card
GIRFT	Getting it Right First Time
GMC	General Medical Council
GPA	Government Procurement Agreement
HDS	Hospital Dental Services
HEE	Health Education England
HEI	Health Education Institute
HEIW	Health Education and Improvement Wales
HIS	Healthcare Improvement Scotland
HIW	Healthcare Inspectorate Wales
HR	Human resources
HRA	Health research authority
HRG	Healthcare resource groups
HSC	Health and social care
HSCB	Health and social care board
HSE	Health and Safety Executive
HSS	Highly specialized services
HSWPG	Health, Safety and Well-being Partnership Group
HTLV	Human T-cell lymphotropic virus
HWB	Health and well-being boards
IAO	Information asset owner
IAR	Information asset register
IC	Investigating committee
ICB	Integrated care boards
ICO	Information Commissioner's Office
ICP	Integrated care partnership
ICS	Integrated care systems
ICT	Immediate care team
ICT	Information and communications technology
IDC	Individual duty of candour
IDT	Inter-deanery transfer
IELTS	International English Language Testing System
IG	Information governance (also Integrated governance)
IMCA	Independent Mental Capacity Advocate
IMSAFE	Illness medication stress alcohol fatigue emotions
IOC	Interim orders committee
IRAS	Integrated research application system
ISF	Investigator site folder
ISRCTN	International Standard Randomized Controlled Trial Number
JCPTD	Joint Committee for Postgraduate Training in Dentistry
JD	Job description
JDFCT	Joint Dental Foundation Core Training
JSNA	Joint strategic needs assessment

KLOE	Key lines of enquiry	NI	Northern Ireland
KPI	Key performance indicator	NIHR	National Institute for Health and Care Research
LAC	Looked after child		
LDC	Local dental committee	NIHR	National Institute of Health Research
LDN	Local dental network		
LDS	Licence in dental surgery	NIMDTA	Northern Ireland Medical and Dental Training Agency
LEP	Lead education provider		
LFPSE	Learning from patient safety events	NIS	Network and information systems
LIP	Local information pack	NOTSS	Non-technical skills for surgeons
LocSSIPs	Local Safety Standards for Invasive Procedures		
		NRLS	National reporting and learning system
LPN	Local professional network	NSS	NHS staff survey
LRMC	Local risk management committee	NTN	National training number
		ODN	Operational delivery network
LTFT	Less than full-time training	OECD	Organisation for Economic Co-operation and Development
LTPS	Liabilities to third parties scheme		
M&M	Morbidity and mortality	OH	Occupational health
MAPPA	Multi-agency public protection arrangements	OHD	Occupational health department
MARS	Medical appraisal and revalidation system	OHID	Office for Health Improvement and Disparities
MCA	Mental Capacity Act	OHWB	Occupational health and well-being
MCN	Managed clinical network		
MD	Medical director	OMFS	Oral and maxillofacial surgery
METIP	Multiprofessional education and investment plan	OoH	Out-of-hours
		OOP	Out of programme
MHRA	Medicines and Healthcare Regulatory Agency	OPCS	Office of Population Censuses and Surveys—Classification of Interventions and Procedures
ML	Machine learning		
MPE	Medical physics expert	OPG	Office of the Public Guardian
MPTS	Medical Practitioners Tribunal Service	ORE	Overseas Registration Examination
NACPDE	National Advice Centre for Postgraduate Dental Education	PA	Programmed activities
		PALS	Patient advice and liaison service
NatSSIP	National Safety Standards for Invasive Procedures		
		PbR	Payment by results
NCDCE	National Certificate of Dental Core Equivalence	PCN	Primary care network
		PDP	Personal development plan
NCSC	National Cyber Security Centre	PDS	Personal Dental Services
		PDS	Public Dental Service
NDG	National Data Guardian	PDSA	Plan, do, study, act
NDOO	National Data Opt-Out	PGD	Patient group directions
NDPB	Non-departmental public bodies	PHA	Public Health Agency
		PHW	Public Health Wales
NES	NHS Education for Scotland	PI	Principal investigator
NHS	National Health Service	PO	Purchase order
NHSE	National Health Service England	POD	Pharmaceutical, ophthalmic, and dental
NHSR	NHS Resolution		

PPE	Personal protective equipment
PPI	Patient and public involvement
PPIE	Patient and public involvement and engagement
PR	Parental responsibility
PREM	Patient-reported experience measure
PROM	Patient-reported outcome measure
PS	Person specification
PSA	Professional Standards Authority
PSI	Patient safety incidents
PSIRF	Patient Safety Incident Response Framework
PVG	Protecting Vulnerable Groups
QIP	Quality improvement programme
RAG	Risk action group
RCA	Root cause analysis
RCP	Review of competency progression
RCS Eng	Royal College of Surgeons, England
RDN	Research delivery network
RDS	Research Data Scotland
REC	Research ethics committee
RFI	Request for further information
RO	Responsible officer
ROBRICES	Reasons, Options, Benefits, Risks, Income, Cost, Evaluation, and Stakeholder
RPA	Review of Public Administration
RQIA	Regulation and Quality Improvement Authority
RTT	Referral-to-treatment
SAAR	Safeguarding adults at risk referral
SAC	Specialist advisory committee
SAE	Serious adverse event
SAR	Subject access request

SAS	Staff, Associate Specialist, and Speciality doctor
SCR	Serious case review
SEND	Special educational needs and disabilities
SEPA	Scottish Environment Protection Agency
SHO	Senior house officer
SI	Serious incident
SIGN	Scottish Intercollegiate Guidelines Network
SIRO	Senior information risk owner
SLE	Supervised Learning Event
SOAR	Scottish online appraisal resource
SOP	Standard Operating Procedure
SOSR	Some other substantial reason
SPA	Supporting professional activities
SPPG	Strategic Planning and Performance Group
SRA	Solicitors Regulation Authority
STC	Speciality Training Committee
StEIS	Strategic executive information system
SUI	Serious Untoward Incident
SWOT	Strengths, Weaknesses, Opportunities, and Threats
TAC	Team Around the Child
TOOT	Time out of training
TPD	Training Programme Director
UCEA	Universities and Colleges Employers Association
UTI	Urinary tract infection
VCSE	Voluntary, community, and social enterprise
VL	Vicarious liability
WBA	Workplace Based Assessment
WG	Welsh Government
WHO	World Health Organization
WMA	World Medical Association
WNB	Was Not Brought
WTE	Whole time equivalent

Chapter 1

History of the NHS

Establishment of the NHS

The NHS was founded as one component of a series of welfare measures following the end of the Second World War. The 'post-war consensus' between the major political parties was that, in addition to post-war recovery, public healthcare and welfare would be a priority. When a Labour government came into power in 1945, Aneurin Bevan was the Minister of Health and thus he was tasked with introducing this new healthcare system. The NHS Act of 1946 aimed to provide free healthcare for all in need. The focus of the post-war government was for a healthcare system with access based on need rather than ability to pay. Thus, the NHS began on the 5th July 1948, at Park Hospital, near Manchester. During the subsequent 70 years, the structure of the NHS and manner in which it is run has continued to evolve. The NHS has undergone almost continuous change and restructuring from its inception to date, in response to challenges and changes in the health and resource landscape, underpinned by variations in political priorities.

Current NHS

The NHS currently comprises of:

- 42 Integrated Care Boards
- 229 trusts, of which 154 are foundation trusts
- 50 mental health trusts
- 10 ambulance trusts
- 124 acute trusts
- 220 general acute hospitals, 49 specialist hospitals, 245 community hospitals
- 826 community providers
- 6,925 GP practices
- Employs approximately 140,000 doctors, 350,000 nurses, 160,000 scientific and technical staff

Legislation, reforms, and reports

The NHS Reorganization Act 1973

This Act introduced the first major reform in the structure of the NHS and marked a shift towards the government taking a more direct role in setting its strategic goals. This Act aimed to break down the separation and boundaries that existed between GPs, hospitals, local authority public health services and teaching hospitals. It aimed to integrate them into one structure and tackle previous poor service coordination. Thus, NHS bodies responsible for managing all health services in their area (including primary, hospital and community) were established. They reported to the government through the Secretary of State for Health. Prior to 1973, regional boards managed hospital services and reported to the government while local authorities were responsible for managing primary care services and social care. In England, the recent Health and Care Act 2022 has now returned some of the responsibilities for healthcare back to local authorities. The 1973 Act (and subsequent changes implemented from 1974) was widely disliked, due to the excess degree of bureaucracy it created, in particular, the rigid organizational structure it produced with too many layers of decision making.

The Black report 1980

The Black report, or 'inequalities in health: report of a research working group' highlighted the link between social class and life expectancy. It argued for action to be taken to reduce health inequalities. Many of these inequalities still persist and their reduction continues to be a theme in the modern NHS.

The Griffiths report 1983

The Griffiths report identified a lack of general management in NHS structures. It resulted in a strengthening of the role of general managers within hospitals. The report recommended that doctors were also placed into positions of managerial leadership. Clinical budgeting systems were introduced, enabling each speciality to become its own unit of management (the beginning of clinical directorates), directly responsible for managing their own resources and funds.

Working for patients 1989

Despite changes in the 1980s, demand for healthcare services was steadily increasing and the pressure on resources was mounting. A 'business-like' approach was devised for the provision of hospital services. The Working for Patients White Paper led this change. Trusts were created and a business ethos with the promotion of competition encouraged. The concept of an 'internal market' was devised, through the separation of providing services from the purchasing of them (commissioning) i.e. the provider-purchaser split. This would create competition, reward efficient providers, and ultimately improve overall service standards. This reflects the modern-day NHS structure, where hospitals are self-governing trusts, while service planners have a range of care providers to choose from (the NHS internal market). The intention was to ensure a focus on improving patient choice, experience, and satisfaction.

The NHS Plan 2000

In 1997, 'The new NHS. Modern. Dependable' was published. This maintained the provider-purchaser split but reinforced that a move towards a primary care led NHS was intended. Thus, Primary Care Groups were established for this role, to both provide primary care and purchase secondary care. Clinical Governance was introduced and the National Institute for Clinical Excellence (NICE) was developed (see page 39).

The 2000 NHS Plan (see Box 1.1) was designed to modernize the NHS by launching the next set of reforms, both structurally and target-based. NHS foundation trusts were created, to provide hospitals with greater independence from the government and accountability over their own self-governance. There was a notable increase in funding and investment for the NHS. Targets were also introduced for all hospitals, to address waiting times for treatment—an increasing concern at the time. For example, the four-hour A&E waiting time target and the 18-week referral to hospital treatment were introduced, both of which remain key features of the current NHS landscape (see page 83).

Box 1.1 Changes implemented by the NHS Plan 2000

- Established a mandatory reporting scheme for adverse healthcare events
- Established a requirement for all doctors to engage in annual appraisal and audit
- Established the National Clinical Assessment Authority to provide expert assessment of a doctor's performance
- Established the UK Council of Health Regulators

The NHS Constitution 2009

Background

The Constitution (see Box 1.2) brought together for the first time all the principles, values, and responsibilities that underpin the NHS. It was designed to ensure that patients, the public and NHS staff are aware of their rights and responsibilities with the ultimate aim of improving service and care. Lord Darzi's NHS Next Stage Review was instrumental in development of the NHS Constitution.

Box 1.2 Core parts of the NHS Constitution 2009

Part I: NHS Values
- Working together for patients
- Respect and dignity
- Commitment to quality of care
- Compassion
- Improving lives
- Everyone counts

Part II: Principles that guide the NHS
- The NHS provides a comprehensive service, available to all
- Access based on clinical need, not an individual's ability to pay
- Highest standards of excellence and professionalism
- Patients at the heart of everything it does
- In partnership across boundaries with other organizations in the interest of patients, local communities, and the wider population
- Best value for taxpayers' money and the most effective, fair, and sustainable use of finite resources
- Accountable to the public, communities, and patients

Part III: Patients and the public
Rights and pledges are outlined, covering the seven key areas of the Constitution:
- Access to health services
- Quality of care and environment
- Nationally approved treatments, drugs, programmes
- Respect, consent, and confidentiality
- Informed choice
- Involvement in your healthcare and in the NHS
- Complaints and redress

Part IV: Staff
The Constitution outlines staff rights, pledges, legal duties and expectations.

The Francis and Berwick reports

The Francis and Berwick reports were pivotal documents in NHS history. The Francis report evolved from an inquiry of the same name while the Berwick report was commissioned to outline required changes, arising from findings in the Francis and other similar reports.

The Francis report

In 2007, the Healthcare Commission (HCC) – an NHS care regulator- became concerned about unusually high mortality rates at Mid Staffordshire NHS Foundation Trust. The hospital cited 'coding errors' for this but the HCC was not satisfied and opted to investigate further. The same year, Julie Bailey, the daughter of a Mid Staffordshire hospital patient, formed the 'Cure the NHS' campaign group, to highlight failings at Mid Staffordshire NHS Foundation Trust by demanding a public enquiry. The campaign led to the exposure of significant ongoing failures at the hospital. Although a number of investigative reports were subsequently commissioned, the two led by Sir Robert Francis QC led to significant notable changes in the NHS. His public enquiry was focused on how poor care at Mid Staffordshire Foundation Trust was allowed to happen and why no regulators or monitoring bodies identified the issues.

The first enquiry

- An independent enquiry, held behind closed doors
- Published in 2010 and focused on the trust itself and what failings occurred internally, rather than failings in the wider NHS
- Notably poor standards of care in the trust were exposed, in addition to a failure of leadership and a culture of fear and bullying which prevented staff from speaking up
- 'Cure the NHS' called for a second, public enquiry into the trust, within the broader context of the NHS

The second enquiry

The second public enquiry 'the Francis Report' examined the wider NHS system, focusing on the commissioning, supervisory and regulatory bodies involved in monitoring at Mid Staffordshire NHS Foundation Trust, in order to examine why problems at the trust were not identified sooner and relevant appropriate action taken.

The report made 290 recommendations, focused on five themes of fundamental care standards:

1. Openness
2. Transparency and candour
3. Nursing standards—compassionate, caring, committed nursing
4. Patient-centred leadership
5. Information about performance against service standards

Duty of candour

One of the more significant proposals of the Francis report was the introduction of a statutory duty of candour (see Box 1.3). This places a legal obligation on health providers to discuss with the patient and relatives any incidents of harm or mistake. The purpose is to encourage a culture of openness and transparency (see also Chapter 6).

> **Box 1.3 Principles of duty of candour**
> - Patients should be informed of a 'notifiable safety incident' as soon as is practical
> - The health service provider must explain what is known at that time and what further enquiries are planned
> - An apology must be offered
> - Reasonable support should be provided to the patient, e.g. counselling
> - A written record must be kept of the notification to the patient
> - A written record of the initial discussion, notification, and an apology must be provided to the patient

There is an ethical duty of candour for low threshold notifications (any harm or distress to patients) and a statutory duty for higher threshold incidents. Higher threshold incidents are anything unintended or unexpected in the patient's care that, in the reasonable opinion of a healthcare professional, could or has resulted in:
- The death of the patient
- The patient suffering severe or moderate harm, or prolonged psychological harm

Freedom to Speak Up

Two years after the final report on the Mid Staffordshire failings, Sir Robert Francis published an independent review 'Freedom to Speak Up'. This detailed cases of bullying and harassment towards staff, discrimination, and a culture in which it was difficult to raise patient concerns. This was impacting on patient safety. Thus, the report outlined ways to create an open and honest reporting culture in the NHS including:
- Appointment of a Freedom to Speak Up Guardian in every trust
- All trusts to establish processes to ensure concerns are raised, listened to, and investigated
- A national independent officer to support the guardians
- A support scheme for NHS staff who raised concerns

The Berwick report

After receiving the 2013 Francis report, the UK Government commissioned Professor Don Berwick of the Institute for Healthcare Improvement in Boston, USA, to specify changes needed based on the Francis report and other related reports. A report with four key principles was produced 'A Promise to Learn–a Commitment to Act. Improving the Safety of Patients in England'.

1. Patient safety and quality of patient care is the most important aim.
2. Engage, empower, and hear patients and carers.
3. Fostering growth and development of staff, in particular with regard to their ability and opportunity to improve the processes within which they work.
4. Embracing transparency, accountability, trust, and growth of knowledge.

In 2014, the Sign up to Safety campaign was launched, which formed part of the response to the Berwick report. It encouraged healthcare organizations to sign up to safety pledges to help prevent avoidable harm and improve patient safety.

Health and Social Care Act 2012

The main focus of the 2012 Act (see Box 1.4) was to increase competition to drive improvement and modernize the NHS. This Act put clinicians at the centre of commissioning.

> ### Box 1.4 Key changes from the Health and Social Care Act 2012
>
> #### Clinically led commissioning
> New clinical commissioning groups (CCGs) would directly commission services for their populations. CCGs took over this role from primary care trusts (PCTs), in response to feedback from clinicians about the previous process of negotiating with PCTs. CCGs were comprised of local GP practices.
>
> #### Provider regulation to support innovative services
> Patients can choose services that best suit their needs, even from independent sector providers. Healthcare providers, including foundation trusts, are given the freedom to innovate in order to deliver high quality services. Monitor was established to act as a regulator, to protect patients.
>
> #### Greater voice for patients
> Healthwatch was established to encourage patient involvement across the NHS and strengthen the voice of patients.
>
> #### New focus for public health
> The Act provides the underpinning for Public Health England, a new body to drive improvements in the public's health.
>
> #### Greater accountability locally and nationally
> Although government ministers retain ultimate responsibility for the NHS, the Act aims to limit political micro-management. It gives more responsibilities and roles to local authorities and local service providers.
>
> #### Streamlined arms-length bodies
> The Act removed additional unnecessary tiers of management and gave NICE a statutory frontline role.

NHS Five Year Forward View 2014

This outlined a consensus about why and how the NHS should continue to change, in particular, improvements in overall health, quality, and financial sustainability. The plan outlined the ambition for greater partnership within the NHS to deliver care due to the changing healthcare environment:

- An increase in demand for care as life expectancy increases and patients with chronic conditions live for longer
- Changes in personal care preferences, with patients wishing to be more involved and informed about their own care
- Technological advancements in the diagnosis and management of conditions
- Financial pressures from a mismatch between resources and patient needs

In 2016, NHS England divided the country into 44 footprints to form these new models of care. These were known as Sustainability and Transformation Partnerships (STPs) and brought together the NHS, local authorities, and other health and care organizations. STPs subsequently evolved into integrated care systems (ICS).

NHS Long Term Plan 2019

This plan built on the policies and goals laid out in the Five-Year Forward View, in particular, integrated care models to adapt to changing and increasing health needs of the population. It outlined how the NHS will continue developing over the next ten years to make it 'fit for the future'. Specific focus was given to certain clinical conditions which are seen as priorities due to the extent of their impact on the populations health (cancer, cardiovascular disease, maternity, neonatal, mental health, stroke, diabetes, respiratory). Key features included:

- Integrated care systems (ICSs) models of care delivery: collaboration between GPs, their teams, communities, local partners, and patients to reduce the number of hospital outpatient appointments
- Emphasis on public health prevention to reduce avoidable health issues (obesity, alcohol reduction, smoking cessation, etc.)
- Making better use of data and digital technology, such as the new NHS app, and virtual appointments
- Getting the most out of the taxpayers' investment in the NHS by ensuring efficiency, reduce duplication in clinical service delivery, and reduce spending on administration
- Increase the NHS workforce by increasing undergraduate training places, new routes into healthcare such as apprenticeships, better retention of staff through flexible working patterns etc. The NHS People Plan takes a more comprehensive view of this strategy

Dentistry and NHS strategy plans

Little mention was made of dentistry or oral health in the Five-Year Forward View 2014 or the Next Steps on the NHS Five-Year Forward View. This is surprising given the emphasis on prevention. Public health measures aimed at reducing rates of childhood obesity and diabetes may have had an indirect benefit on oral health.

The NHS Long-Term Plan does mention dental services (see Box 1.5); dissolving the divide between primary and community dental services and redesigning health services for children and young people.

Box 1.5 Dental strategy within the NHS Long Term Plan

Special needs dentistry

Increasing accessibility of dental care for children and young people with a learning disability, autism, or those in special residential schools. Ensuring there is ease of access for ongoing care.

Enhanced Health in Care Homes (EHCH)

This strategy ensures individuals in care homes are supported by care home staff to have good oral health and access to both routine and specialized dental care.

Local area holistic care

Local areas will design and implement holistic models of care for children and young people. This will bring together primary care, community services, speech and language therapy, school nursing, and oral healthcare.

Starting well core initiative

This is a prevention framework which aims to support 24,000 dentists across England to see more children from a young age to establish effective oral health habits.

HPV vaccine

This was extended to boys aged 12 and 13 years to reduce oral and throat cancer risk.

Health and Care Act 2022

This Act builds on the proposal brought forward by the NHS in the Long-Term Plan 2019 and the 2021 White Paper—Integration and Innovation: Working Together to Improve Health and Social Care for All. It aims to improve health outcomes through collaboration between the NHS, social care and public health services at a local level, in order to provide everyone with the best start in life, deliver world-class care for major health conditions, and help people age well.

There are three core themes:

1. The Act removes barriers which are preventing different parts of the healthcare system from being fully integrated.
2. Bureaucracy across the system is reduced, in order to facilitate easier decision making.
3. Appropriate accountability arrangements are in place so that responsiveness to patients and staff is prioritized.

The Long-Term Plan 2019 established and strengthened the role of ICSs. The Health and Care Act (HCA) 2022 builds on this by putting them on a statutory footing through the creation of integrated care boards (ICBs). Prior to 2022, STPs and ICSs were voluntary partnerships. From the HCA 2022, ICS were given legal entity status. The Act had a 'triple aim' duty: health and wellbeing, quality of services and efficiency and sustainability (see Box 1.6). The Health and Care Act 2022 replaced clinical commissioning groups (formerly PCTs) with ICSs, leading to the merger of CCGs with acute hospitals, mental health hospitals, community trusts, and general practices. Within ICSs, commissioning powers lie with the ICBs.

Integrated care boards (ICBs)

ICBs will now take on the commissioning role of CCGs and some of NHS England's commissioning roles (see page 26).

- ICBs are comprised of a chair, chief executive officer and representatives from NHS trust/foundation trust, general practice, and the local authority
- Local areas have flexibility to decide any further representation in their area
- ICBs need to ensure that they have acquired the appropriate clinical advice before making decisions

---

Box 1.6 Key features of Health and Care Act 2022

- CCGs abolished and absorbed into their local ICSs
- Within ICS, commissioning functions lie with the ICB
- Collaboration instead of competitive rendering
- NHS England and NHS Improvement merged
- The national tariff is replaced with a new NHS payment scheme
- Care Quality Commission (CQC) will oversee and assess ICBs
- Health Services Safety Investigations Body (HSSIB) given statutory power

- ICBs and their foundation trusts must prepare their own five-year forward plan focused on meeting the local population's health needs
  They must establish an integrated care partnership (ICP) which outlines a strategy for addressing combined health, social care, and public health needs
- They must aim to break even financially each year

Dentistry and the Health and Care Act (HCA) 2022

Following implementation of the HCA 2022, all ICBs will commission dental services. The funding for this is ringfenced i.e. set aside for dentistry and cannot be used for other purposes. ICBs took over this dental commissioning role from NHS England.

See Chapter 3 for further information on commissioning of dental services.

NHS Long Term Workforce Plan 2023

This was the first time that the government tasked the NHS with devising a comprehensive workforce plan for the long term. Published in June 2023 it outlined expected demand and supply for NHS healthcare services over the next 15 years and action plans to meet this. The Plan highlighted that, without focused action, the NHS will face a workforce gap of more than 260,000–360,000 staff by 2036–2037. The plan has the triple aim to train, retain and reform. There is a plan to increase training places for dental therapists and hygienists and a 40% increase in training places for dentists. It focuses on developing career paths, to improve professional development and fulfilment with a view to helping with retention of staff in the NHS.

Pragmatic action plans were outlined on a national, regional, and local level to address workforce challenges in the short to medium term.

NHS England 2025

As of March 2025, NHS England is being abolished and its functions will be returned back into the Department of Health and Social Care. Given the lack of detail at the time of the announcement and publication of this book, 'NHS England' has been maintained in the text.

Further reading

Berwick review into patient safety 2015. Available at: ℘ https://www.gov.uk/government/publicati ons/berwick-review-into-patient-safety

Freedom to Speak Up Report 2015. Available at: ℘ http://freedomtospeakup.org.uk/wp-content/ uploads/2014/07/F2SU_web.pdf

Health and Care Act 2022. Available at: ℘ https://www.legislation.gov.uk/ukpga/2022/31/conte nts/enacted

Health and Social Care Act 2012. Available at: ℘ https://www.legislation.gov.uk/ukpga/2012/7/ contents/enacted

NHS Five-Year Forward View. Available at: ℘ https://www.england.nhs.uk/wp-content/uploads/ 2016/05/fyfv-tech-note-090516.pdf

NHS Long Term Plan 2019. Available at: ℘ https://www.longtermplan.nhs.uk/publication/ nhs-long-term-plan/

NHS Long-Term Workforce Plan June 2023. Available at: ℘ https://www.england.nhs.uk/wp-cont ent/uploads/2023/06/nhs-long-term-workforce-plan-v1.2.pdf

NHS Next Stage Review. High Quality Care for All. Available at: ℘ https://assets.publishing.service. gov.uk/media/5a7c3a5b40f0b67d0b11fbaf/7432.pdf

NHS Reorganization Act 1973. Available at: ℘ https://www.legislation.gov.uk/ukpga/1973/32/ enacted

Report of the Mid Staffordshire NHS Foundation Trust Public Inquiry. Available at: ℘ https://www. gov.uk/government/publications/report-of-the-mid-staffordshire-nhs-foundation-trust-public- inquiry

The Black Report 1980. Available at: ℘ https://sochealth.co.uk/national-health-service/public-hea lth-and-wellbeing/poverty-and-inequality/the-black-report-1980/

The Griffiths Report on NHS 1983. Available at: ℘ https://sochealth.co.uk/national-health-serv ice/griffiths-report-october-1983/

The NHS Constitution 2009. Available at: ℘ https://www.gov.uk/government/publications/the- nhs-constitution-for-england

The NHS Plan 2000. Available at: ℘ https://webarchive.nationalarchives.gov.uk/ukgwa/+/ www.dh.gov.uk/en/publicationsandstatistics/publications/publicationspolicyandguidance/ dh_4002960

Working for patients white paper. *Department of Health. CM 555.* London: HMSO; 1989.

Chapter 2

Current structure of the NHS and commissioning

Essential facts about the UK healthcare system

1. The UK Treasury calculates the annual block grants for the Scottish government, Welsh Government, and Northern Ireland. Health is a fully devolved matter, and each UK nation decides how much of the funding available to them is spent on National Health Services (NHS).

2. Responsibility for health policy rests with the Secretary of State for Health and Social Care in England and their equivalent in the devolved governments. They may also have junior ministers who lead on a certain area within health and care and are supported by their respective Department of Health and Social Care (Civil Service) and advisors or advisory bodies.

3. The UK has a publicly funded healthcare system. The UK national health system differs from healthcare systems in many other countries as it is largely funded through general taxation rather than health insurance or out-of-pocket systems.

4. Most NHS services are provided free of charge to UK residents. However, there are contribution charges for dental treatment and prescription charges, which vary across the devolved nations.

5. Children, pensioners and those receiving certain benefits are entitled to an exemption or a reduction of the NHS charges. This applies to both dental charges and prescription costs.

6. The NHS provides healthcare services to over one million patients every 24 hours.

7. Annual spending on public healthcare in the UK is approximately 11% of gross national product.

8. There is also a smaller private healthcare sector that people can self-fund or use insurance policies.

The Department of Health and Social Care

The UK Department of Health and Social Care (DHSC) is responsible for government policy on health and adult social care matters in England, along with any UK wide functions that are not devolved. The department is led by the Secretary of State for Health and Social Care, with three ministers of state and three parliamentary under-secretaries of state.

The role of the DHSC

- The DHSC and the Secretary of State for Health and Social Care are responsible for meeting the health and healthcare needs of the population in England
- The DHSC receives funding directly from the Treasury (see Box 2.1)
- It develops policies and allocates funding to NHS England and other relevant organizations to meet the population's healthcare needs
- It conducts its work through various arms-length bodies, including executive non-departmental public bodies such as NHS England, and executive agencies such as the UK Health Security Agency and the Medicines and Healthcare Regulatory Agency (MHRA) (see Table 2.1)

The largest body to receive DHSC funding is NHS England, which legally merged with NHS Improvement, NHS Digital and Health Education England (HEE) under the 2022 Health and Care Bill.

The work of the DHSC is scrutinized by the Health and Social Care Select Committee (HSC). HSC is a Departmental Select Committee of the House of Commons, which examines the policy, administration, and expenditure of the DHSC, associated agencies, and public bodies. As a select committee it has the authority to initiate inquiries into government and the policies of the DHSC's agencies.

Table 2.1 Structure of the DHSC

Arm's length bodies (ALBs)	Executive agencies (EAs)	Non-departmental public bodies (NDPBs)
Public bodies established with a degree of autonomy from the Secretary of State and play important advisory, regulatory, and/or public health functions for supporting the health and care system. Their role and function are set out in law, giving each organization a clearly defined role. Healthcare ALBs are subdivided into executive agencies and non-departmental public bodies.	Clearly designated and financially viable business units within departments and are responsible for undertaking the executive functions of that department, as distinct from giving policy advice, e.g. MHRA, UKHPA.	Play a role in the process of national government but are not part of a government department. They operate at arm's length from ministers, though a minister will be responsible to Parliament for the administration and performance of the NDPBs in their departments.

Arm's length bodies (ALBs)

The DHSC acts as a steward for the health and adult social care system in England and it oversees 12 ALBs, each having a governance framework that aligns their working and financial accountability to the DHSC:

- Medicines and Healthcare Products Regulatory Agency (MHRA)
- UK Health Security Agency (formerly Public Health England)
- Care Quality Commission (CQC)
- National Institute for Health and Care Excellence (NICE)
- NHS Business Services Authority (NHSBSA)
- NHS Resolution
- NHS Counter Fraud Authority
- Human Fertilisation and Embryology Authority
- Human Tissue Authority
- NHS Blood and Transplant
- Health Research Authority
- NHS England

There is alignment of specific ALB functions across the UK, but some ALBs only support NHS England (see Table 2.2):

Table 2.2 Scope of executive non-departmental public bodies across UK, England, and Wales

Country	Executive non-departmental public bodies
United Kingdom	Human Tissue Authority
	Human Fertilisation and Embryology Authority
England and Wales	NHS Blood and Transplant
	National Institute for Health and Care Excellence (NICE)
	NHS Business Services Authority
England only	Care Quality Commission (CQC)
	NHS England
	Health Research Authority
	NHS Resolution
	NHS Counter Fraud Authority

Advisory non-departmental public bodies

DHSC also works with advisory non-departmental public bodies, such as the NHS Pay Review Body and the Review Body on Doctors' and Dentists' Remuneration. More commonly known as the Doctors' and Dentists' Review Body (DDRB), this body considers the remuneration for NHS doctors and dentists.

The Review Body takes evidence from a range of stakeholders, including trade unions and government, then provides a recommendation to the government on annual pay uplifts. The recommendation is taken under advisement, allowing the government to set the pay rise through the NHS Employers organization. The pay rises are published, with the implementation schedules, in the NHS Medical and Dental Pay Circular (hosted on the NHS Employers website and published every year on 1st April).

> **Box 2.1 Key points**
>
> Spending on health per person in the UK is slightly above the OECD (Organisation for Economic Co-operation and Development) average but significantly less than G7 and western European countries.
>
> The government and HM Treasury determine how much money each government department receives based on spending reviews.
>
> Money is allocated for both day-to-day (revenue) and capital spending.
>
> The Department of Health and Social Care (DHSC) decides how the budget is used in England with over 80% of the revenue budget going to NHS England.

- In principle, the DDRB matches doctors' pay with others doing similar jobs in the public and private sector and ensures that doctors' pay continues to match that of others doing comparable jobs, and on comparable incomes
- Primary care services are provided predominantly by independent contractors who receive income via contracts agreed with ICBs or NHS England
- While the DHSC determines how the funding it receives from HM Treasury is allocated in England, health and social services in Northern Ireland, Scotland, and Wales are the responsibility of the devolved administrations

Health and care policy

What is a policy?

A policy is a system of evidence-based guidelines to assist decision making and achieve rational outcomes to the challenges of real-world issues (see Further reading). Public policy influences all aspects of people's lives.

Who decides on healthcare policies?

Health policy in the UK is a devolved function, with the UK Parliament legislating for England's NHS, and the Welsh Parliament (Senedd), Scottish Parliament, and Northern Ireland Assembly responsible for health legislation within their own country. Policymakers draft policy under direction from the government of the day, so neither the DHSC nor the NHS are responsible for setting their own healthcare policies.

The main purpose of government is to have lawmakers set policy and instruct civil servants to identify solutions that enact those policies. While policies are important because they assist subjective and objective decision making, they differ from rules or law. While laws compel or prohibit behaviours, policy only guides actions that are likely to achieve a positive outcome for the population.

How does UK healthcare compare to other countries?

Although the United Kingdom excels in terms of access to health services, it is a middling performer relative to OECD peers in the domains of health status, risk factors, and quality. The Organisation for Economic Co-operation and Development (OECD) is an international organization comprising 38 member countries that promotes policies to improve the economic and social well-being of people around the world. UK investment is required to improve acute care and primary care services, prevent obesity and harmful use of alcohol, and expand coverage of long-term care.

Successful integration involves the planning, commissioning, and delivery of coordinated, joined up and seamless services to support people to live healthy, independent, and dignified lives, which improve outcomes for the entire population. Everyone should receive the right care, in the right place, at the right time. The UK Government's health and social care integration white paper (2022) laid out measures to make integrated health and social care a universal reality for everyone in England.

NHS England

NHS England (see page 14) is the largest executive non-departmental public body of the DHSC. It oversees the budget, planning, delivery, and day-to-day operation of the commissioning of healthcare services across England. As the DHSC is responsible for the NHS, it is ultimately accountable to Parliament and the Chancellor of the Exchequer. As UK healthcare is a devolved function, funding is only allocated for NHS England, with social care being separately funded by local authorities.

NHS Constitution

The NHS is founded on a common set of principles and values that bind together the people it serves and the staff who work for it. The Constitution (see Box 1.2) establishes:

- Principles and values of the NHS in England
- The rights to which patients, public, and staff are entitled
- Pledges to which the NHS is committed to achieve
- Responsibilities needed to ensure that the NHS operates fairly and effectively
- There is a legally binding requirement for the Constitution to be renewed every 10 years. This guarantees that the principles and values are reviewed and that any government wishing to amend the NHS principles are required to consult with the public, patients, and staff

Funding

The DHSC receives funding from HM Treasury through the government's spending review, which occurs every 3 years, and is amended annually through the chancellor's budget report. The spending review sets firm expenditure limits and, through public service agreements, defines the key improvements that the public can expect from these resources. The expenditure, administration, and policy of the department is scrutinized by the Health and Social Care Select Committee. The DHSC publishes consolidated accounts for the whole of the NHS in England each year.

Funding for health services in England comes from the Department for Health and Social Care's budget (see Figure 2.1). The government decides the NHS budget and sets top-level priority targets. Determining the correct health allocation is crucial for the resilience of a country's healthcare

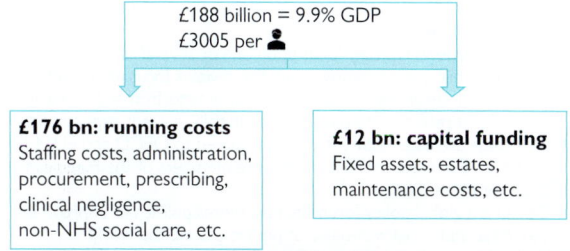

Figure 2.1 Breakdown of NHS healthcare budget 2023/2024.

provision, workforce stability and preparedness for future surges in demand (expected and unexpected).

Funding for public services, such as health, in the devolved nations is through a block grant from the UK Government. Since 1978, any changes to the block grant made by the UK Government for spending levels on health or education in England, requires a proportionate adjustment to the funding to the devolved nations. The Barnett formula (see Box 2.2) is the accepted policy which the Treasury has chosen to apply to calculate the contribution. The devolved governments have flexibility to apportion any extra funding on priority services which doesn't need to reflect how England use its funding.

Box 2.2 Barnett formula calculation

Extra funding for devolved nations = Change to UK budget × comparability percentage × population proportion (compared to England)

The DHSC passes on the majority of the funding to NHS England but holds back some funding for central services and arms' length bodies, such as the Office for Health Improvement and Disparities.

NHS England allocates the bulk of the money it receives to integrated care boards (ICBs) but retains some to fund its own direct commissioning functions and running costs. NHS trusts and foundation trusts receive the bulk of their income via contracts with ICBs and NHS England, while other revenue sources are generated through research and development income.

- Total expenditure 2023/24 across the DHSC group was £194.9bn, of which £175.8bn was allocated to NHS England and subsequently approximately £129.5bn to NHS Providers
- Staff costs accounted for approximately 65% of NHS provider expenditure
- NHS England's operating expenditure 2023/24 (excluding funding of group bodies) totalled £174.8bn. Of this, approximately 70% of commissioners' expenditure was on secondary care, while 18% was spent on primary care

Health spending in the UK has increased over the decades due to increasing population size, an ageing population with increasingly complex healthcare needs, and increases in treatment, and drug costs. After adjusting for population growth and demographic changes though, health spending has however remained constant over the past 15 years (see Box 2.3).

Box 2.3 Key facts

- Spending reviews typically focus upon one or several aspects of public spending while comprehensive spending reviews focus upon each government department's spending requirements from a zero base (i.e. without reference to past plans or, initially, current expenditure)
- UK healthcare expenditure is often compared to OECD and EU14 countries. EU14 are countries who were members of the European Union prior to 2004
- OECD is a global policy forum that promotes policies to improve the economic and social well-being of people around the world
- UK health spending was 12% GDP in 2021, compared to OECD average (9.7%) and EU14 average (10.2%)

Structure

In 2018 it was announced that NHS England, while maintaining its statutory independence, would merge with NHS Improvement to create seven 'single integrated regional teams'. Regional teams are responsible for the quality, financial, and operational performance of all NHS organizations in their region, adopting a corporate approach to service improvement and local transformation (Figure 2.2). The Health and Care Act 2022 builds on the NHS Long Term Plan to support health integration.

NHS Operating Framework

The NHS Operating Framework sets out the parameters on how service delivery is achieved in England. There are four core foundations to the framework.

- Purpose: To lead the NHS in England to deliver high-quality services for all
- Areas of value: Focus activities on eight key ways that uniquely add value. This can be summarized as:
  - Set direction
  - Allocate resources
  - Ensure accountability
  - Support and develop people
  - Mobilize expert networks
  - Enable improvement
  - Deliver services
  - Drive transformation
- Leadership behaviours and accountabilities: Twelve leadership behaviours, aligned to the six values within the NHS Constitution have been defined
- Medium-term priorities and long-term aims: In order to deliver value, five transformational medium-term priorities have been agreed. This focuses on specific interim objectives that will deliver longer term goals but will help to address the immediate challenges faced by the current system

Functions

NHS England is responsible for using the funding it receives from the DHSC to deliver against the NHS mandate priorities (see Further reading).

NHS England's allocation fund is divided between its services:

- Directly commissioning activities: For the 2023/24 fiscal year:
  - £160bn was allocated for direct commissioning of services—primary care and public health, military healthcare, health services in the justice system and specialized services
  - £27bn was allocated to 154 specialist services, within six programmes of care: internal medicine, cancer, trauma, women and children, blood and infection, mental health
  - It directly commissions NHS general medical services, dental services, optometry, and some specialist services through delegated responsibility to local commissioners

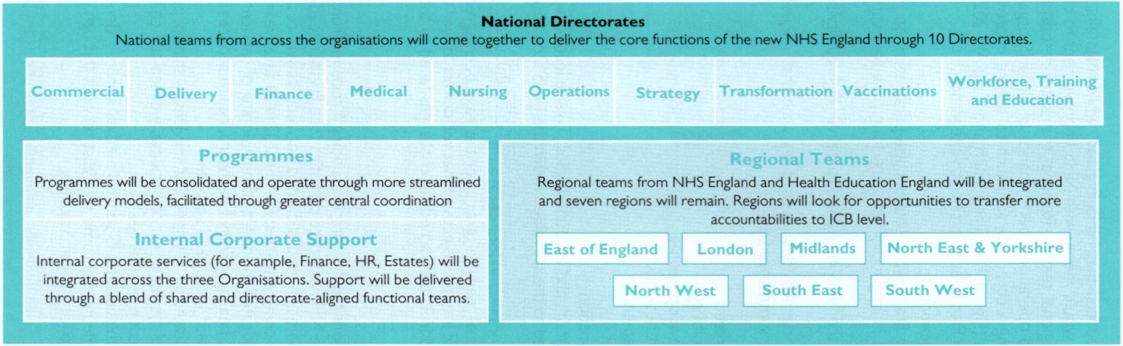

Figure 2.2 NHS England structure.

Reproduced from Operating Framework for NHS England, 2023, p26. Contains public sector information licensed under the Open Government Licence v3.0

- Integrated care board (ICB) allocations fund the services they commission including elective and emergency hospital care, community care, and mental health services
- The running costs for NHS England itself, its regional teams, local professional networks, clinical senates, and networks
- Running cost allowance of the ICBs
- Some services that are commissioned by local authorities

Operating model

Nine regional committees (see Figure 2.2) commission specialized services, jointly between the NHS and integrated care systems (ICS), commencing from April 2023. Partnerships between ICBs, NHS Providers, local authorities and other partner agencies are now a core component of the NHS's operating framework and ways of working.

Integrated care systems (ICSs)

The 42 ICSs were formed on a statutory basis under the Health and Care Act 2022. They are partnerships that bring together NHS organizations, local councils, and others to take collective responsibility for managing resources, delivering NHS standards, and improving population health. They are the commissioners of local NHS services to:

- Improve population outcomes
- Tackle inequalities, outcomes, and access
- Productivity and value for money
- Social and economic development

Healthcare organizations will be expected to jointly plan services at a system level (ICSs), nationally (NHS England), and through care providers (NHS trusts and foundation trusts) to achieve the 'triple aim' of:

- Better health and well-being for everyone
- Better quality of health services for all individuals
- Sustainable use of NHS resources (see Box 2.4)

Box 2.4 Learning points

- Each ICS is made up of an ICB and an ICP
- The ICB is responsible for planning and funding NHS services, including ambulances, primary care, mental healthcare, hospital (acute), community, and specialist care
- They have both a chief executive and a chair, and they are accountable to NHS England for NHS spending and performance within their boundaries
- The ICP develops health strategy. It has a broader focus, covering public health, social care, and wider issues impacting the health and well-being of their local populations. It operates as a statutory committee between the ICB and each of the local authorities in the ICS's geography, as well as voluntary, community and social enterprise (VCSE) organizations, care providers, and other key partners. Exact membership is determined locally

Integrated care boards (ICBs)

ICBs are the component of ICSs which are given the responsibility for commissioning NHS services and hold accountability for population health planning and budgetary management. Thus, CCGs (Clinical Commissioning Groups) have been absorbed into their local ICS, with the CCG's commissioning role now carried out by the ICB. Each ICB has a chair, CEO, and stakeholder engagement from NHS Providers, general practice, and local authorities. Of the £160bn DHSC allocation, ICBs have £107.8bn for commissioning local health services, including community health services, mental health, learning disability services, GP services, urgent and emergency care, rehabilitation, and planned hospital care.

Key facts about ICBs

- Each ICB is required to meet performance targets and break even financially each year. They oversee the budget for NHS services in their system
- ICBs must provide effective leadership and balance immediate and longer-term priorities
- An ICB and its foundation trusts/partner trust must prepare their own five-year forward plan focused on meeting the local population's health needs. They must establish an integrated care partnership (ICP) which outlines a strategy for addressing combined health, social care, and public health needs
- They are responsible for overseeing delivery of NHS strategies
- They work with local authorities to act as the stewards of local population health outcomes and equity
- There is a roadmap in place to enable ICBs to take on more commissioning responsibilities, such as the commissioning of some of the 149 specialized services, which are currently commissioned directly by NHS England. ICBs would therefore be the commissioner for primary, community, secondary and tertiary care, enabling them to design care around patients' needs and make decisions to invest upstream in interventions that reduce the demand for more specialized services

Integrated care partnerships (ICPs)

ICPs are statutory organizations formed of an ICS CEO, NHS Providers, local authority, and representation from other bodies (justice, police, housing association, and third sector). ICPs have responsibility for strategic commissioning and creating a collaborative approach to planning care at a regional level. ICPs are able to flexibly manage resources, based on aligned payments and incentive basis (termed flexible commissioning). They oversee the wider public and population health objectives of the ICS.

NHS commissioning

NHS England commissions (see Box 2.5) some services directly but transfers most of its budget to ICSs, each providing subregional levels of NHS administration across England. Geographical boundaries between services have been removed to enable services to be designed as required; this ranges from services for local populations through to rare, highly specialized conditions (less than 500 annually) that are secured on a national basis (e.g. liver transplant services, Beckwith-Wiedemann syndrome, enzyme replacement therapy, and proton beam therapy, which require a small number of centres of excellence).

Box 2.5 Definition of commissioning

Commissioning is the continual process of planning, agreeing, and monitoring services. Commissioning is not one action but many, ranging from the health-needs assessment for a population, through the clinically based design of patient pathways, to service specification and contract negotiation or procurement, with continuous quality assessment.

NHS England commissions a wide range of services across primary, community and secondary care areas:
- Primary care commissioning
- Primary care co-commissioning
- Public health commissioning
- Specialized services
- Armed forces
- Health and justice

Underlying the Long Term Plan 2019, is the transformation of primary care, offering patients with diverse needs a wider choice of personalized, digital-first health services to reduce reliance on specialist services. Primary care commissioning includes general practice, dentistry, pharmacy, and eye health. The full budget for the pharmaceutical, general ophthalmic and dental (POD) functions and the direct commissioning of POD staff has been transferred to ICBs to support the safe delivery of these delegated functions.

General practice commissioning
- The aim is to deliver proactive, integrated, preventative healthcare
- GP practices work with community, mental health, social care, pharmacy, hospital and voluntary services as primary care networks (PCNs)
- There are 1,250 PCNs serving communities of 30,000–50,000 people
- PCNs are small enough to provide personalized care but large enough to have impact and economies of scale through collaboration with the local health and social care systems
- Commissioning has expanded access to a wide range of personalized care services (delivered by clinical pharmacists, physician associates, first contact physiotherapists, community paramedics and social prescribing link workers), releasing GPs to focus on patients with complex needs

Dental commissioning
- A national Dental Commissioning and Policy team supports regional primary care commissioning teams to develop and improve the contractual framework for commissioning of dental services, and

to undertake related national projects to improve the quality and responsiveness of services (see Chapter 3 for more information)
- Primary care commissioning teams hold direct commissioning responsibilities for all dental services including specialist, community, and out-of-hours dental services, with the autonomy for flexible commissioning of locally required services to ensure equitable access to care

Pharmacy commissioning

- The Community Pharmacy Contractual Framework integrates pharmacy into the PCN functions by providing healthy living support, minor illness advice, and reducing demand on general practice and urgent care settings

Optometry commissioning

- Independent optometry providers deliver over 13 million NHS eye health assessments across England per year
- NHS England commissioning teams ensure that patients receive high-quality and clinically robust eye examinations, which has changed the emphasis from dispensing glasses to a clinical eye health assessment

Specialized services

- These are conditions that are rare and complex and thus a smaller amount of the population is affected by them
- Most healthcare services are now planned and provided locally, however, specialized services are still planned nationally and regionally by NHS England
- These services are not available in every hospital as due to their rarity, they require a specialized team of clinicians to deliver the care
- Some of the conditions require cutting-edge treatment or pioneering innovative treatments
- There are 149 of these specialized services directly commissioned by NHS England
- Within these 149 services, 80 are considered 'highly specialized' (see also page 54);
  - Have usually no more than 500 affected patients
  - Are clinically distinct
  - Benefit from national coordination
  - Are delivered in a small number (1–3) of centres
- NHS England decides whether it commissions a service as a prescribed specialized service based on:
  - The number of patients who require it
  - The cost of providing the service
  - The number of available providers of the service
- The 2023–2024 expenditure for providing specialized services was £25 billion. The funding for this area is increasing as the population ages and requires more complex treatment modalities
- Although directly commissioned by NHS England, ICBs will take on a bigger role in commissioning these services going forward, with a roadmap in place to help enable ICBs to take on this commissioning responsibility, to better integrate patient care

NHS trusts

A trust is a public sector body that provides healthcare services on behalf of the NHS in England and Wales.

- Trusts were established under the National Health Service and Community Care Act 1990 to serve either a geographical area or specialized function (e.g. ambulance service)
- Most community, acute (hospitals), specialist, and mental healthcare in England is provided through trusts
- Individual hospitals usually form their own trust or increasingly, merge with nearby hospitals so that a single trust manages multiple hospitals
- A foundation trust is a semi-autonomous organizational unit within the National Health Service in England. They have a degree of independence from the Department of Health and Social Care

Funding of trusts

- Trusts manage the costs of providing healthcare services (of which staff salaries are normally the largest element)
- They receive income from ICBs (or from NHS England for some specific services) via contracts that specify the quantity, quality, and price of services to be provided
- Each ICB (or NHS England) is responsible for meeting the cost of services provided to its population in line with the contract's terms. ICBs, NHS England, and providers are responsible for ensuring that patient treatments are clinically appropriate and provided in a cost-effective way
- Trusts receive additional income from sources such as private patient revenue, hosting services, car park charges, leasing of buildings, teaching, research, and development
- In teaching hospitals, funding is provided to the NHS to specifically deliver undergraduate and postgraduate medical training in an acknowledgement that clinical education is not resource neutral. The undergraduate medical tariff (formerly known as SIFT—service increment for teaching) is set by the Secretary of State for Health. It is not a direct payment for teaching but aims to cover the additional costs incurred by trusts and other placement providers for delivering teaching (see Further reading). Funding is also available to support postgraduate education and training through the multiprofessional education and investment plan (METIP)
- Many trusts also have access to funds donated by members of the public on a charitable basis. However, these can be used only for the purpose for which they were given

Foundation and non-foundation trusts

- NHS trusts are financially accountable and financial surpluses ('underspend') cannot be retained and are returned to HM Treasury
- In contrast, foundation trusts are established in law as independent 'public benefit corporations' with the financial freedom to retain surpluses, borrow, raise capital, and sell assets

- Foundation trusts are not subject to directions from central government, allowing strategic decision making to be more agile and solely focused on population needs. Instead, local managers and staff have the freedom to innovate and develop services tailored to the needs of their patients and local communities
- Reflecting this, local public and staff directly elect representatives to serve on a board of governors. Foundation trusts must still meet national targets and standards like the rest of the NHS, but they are free to decide the manner in which they achieve this

Local authorities and local and regional bodies

Local authorities have a significant role in the provision of public health including preventative healthcare. This includes planning for emergencies, preventative measures such as immunizations and screening, and monitoring the plans that individual providers have in place.

Local authorities are responsible for:

- Providing information and advice, services and facilities designed to promote healthy living
- Services or facilities for the prevention, diagnosis, or treatment of illness such as immunization, screening, and monitoring programmes
- Assistance to help individuals minimize risks to health arising from their accommodation or environment
- Population health advice e.g.; development of joint strategic needs assessments (JSNA)
- Ensuring that there are plans in place to protect the local population from health threats, including emergencies

Local authorities receive ring-fenced funding through Public Health in the form of a public health grant, which was £3.529 billion in 2023–24.

The OHID (Office for Health Improvement and Disparities) produces local authority health profiles, which provide an overview of health for each local authority in England. This collates existing information in one place and contains data on a range of indicators for local populations, highlighting issues that can affect health in each locality. These profiles help local government and health services to plan place-based health improvement and reduce health inequalities.

Under the Health and Care Act (2022), local authorities are a key partner to ICSs. Some ICSs are place-based, aligned to local authority boundaries, while some include several local authorities within their footprints. Equally, a local authority can be part of more than one ICS, cutting across existing boundaries of England.

Local authorities are also involved in the local health and well-being boards and Healthwatch, a body for patient and public voice in England.

Local health and well-being boards

- Health and well-being boards (HWBs) are statutory forums where political, clinical, professional and community leaders from across health and care in a region come together to agree a shared vision and shared strategy to improve the health and well-being of their local population and reduce health inequalities
- HWBs were established in 2013 as committees of local authorities, which are not subject to the extensive restructuring that impacts the NHS
- There are 152 HWBs in England, one for each local authority with adult social care statutory duties

Healthwatch England and local Healthwatch

Healthwatch was established under the Health and Social Care Act 2012 to understand the needs, experiences and concerns of people who use health and social care services and to speak out on their behalf. Healthwatch England is a statutory, operationally independent, committee of the CQC.

Healthwatch England is responsible for:

- Escalating concerns about health and social care services which have been raised by local Healthwatch to the CQC. The CQC is mandated to respond to advice from the Healthwatch England Committee
- Provide advice to the Secretary of State for Health and Social Care, NHS England, and English local authorities, when the quality of services are inadequate. The Secretary of State for Health and Social Care is required to consult Healthwatch England on the NHS mandate, which sets the objectives for the NHS
- Local Healthwatch are funded by and accountable to local authorities. Their statutory function is:
  - Obtain and report the needs and experiences of healthcare users to commissioners and regulators
  - Make recommendations about service improvement
  - Provide information to the public about accessing health and social care services
  - Make recommendations to Healthwatch England to advise the CQC to carry out special reviews or investigations into areas of concern

NHS Regulators

Regulation is an important entity in healthcare and healthcare insurance. The role of regulatory bodies is to:

- Protect healthcare consumers from health risks
- Provide a safe working environment for healthcare professionals
- Ensure that public health and welfare are served by health programmes
- Regulation is required at all levels, and the regulatory standards are developed by government and private organizations. Healthcare is managed and regulated differently in the four UK countries

Proportionate, risk-based regulation plays an important role in building public confidence in the NHS. Regulation requires openness and transparency, in return the regulatory framework ensures that providers can deliver high-quality services, lead their own improvement, innovate and transform (see Further reading).

Regulation in healthcare refers to any law, rule, or standard (see Box 2.6) that relates to the healthcare industry, such as healthcare crimes, testing, manufacture, safety, efficacy, labelling, storage, record keeping, and privacy of patient information. It ensures compliance, quality, and legal accountability of healthcare bodies and facilities. Regulation is applicable at all levels and is developed and enforced by government and private agencies.

Professional regulation

There are ten statutory regulatory bodies for healthcare professionals, regulating 34 professions across the UK (see Table 2.3). Each regulator maintains a register of individuals who meet the required standards set for the specific profession, which includes standards for education, training,

---

Box 2.6 Key terms

Acts: A piece of statutory legislation that has been approved by both the House of Commons and the House of Lords and been given royal assent by the monarch. it is enshrined in statute law, with breaches liable to enforcement by the courts.

Examples of statutory legislation include:

- Health and Care Act 2022
- The Health and Safety at Work Act 1974
- The Human Rights Act 1998

Regulations: These are supplements to an act. They link to existing acts and assist in applying the principles of the primary act. They are formal guidelines, and breaches are not always legally enforceable.

Examples of regulations include:

- The Health and Safety (First Aid) Regulations 1981
- The Management of Health and Safety at Work Regulations 1999

Guidance: These sit below acts and regulations, usually referred to as codes of practice. They are formed from evidence-based recommendations developed by independent professional committees and consulted on by stakeholders. Guidance breaches are not necessarily an offence but should directly link back to the primary act offence.

professional skills, behaviour, and health. The regulatory bodies are over-seen by the Professionals Standards Authority (PSA).

System regulation

Healthcare systems and clinical settings are regulated by eight service regu-lators in England (see Table 2.3). Their scope of function includes:

- Providing standards and guidelines
- Monitoring healthcare providers' safety and performance to establish compliance with policies and quality standards
- They have statutory powers to impose enforcing measures which span from suspension or removal from the registry in case of non-compliance to criminal prosecution and penalties
- The devolved nations (Wales, Scotland, Northern Ireland; see Box 2.7) have their own independent regulatory bodies for specific functions

Table 2.3 UK professional and system regulators

Professional regulators	System regulators
General Chiropractic Council (GCC)	Care Quality Commission (CQC)
General Dental Council (GDC)	United Kingdom Accreditation Service
General Medical Council (GMC)	Human Fertilisation and Embryology Authority
General Optical Council (GOC)	Health and Safety Executive
General Osteopathic Council (GOsC)	Environment Agency
General Pharmaceutical Council (GPhC)	NHS Resolution
Health and Care Professions Council (HCPC)	Human Tissue Authority
Nursing and Midwifery Council (NMC)	Medicines and Healthcare Products Regulatory Agency (MHRA)
Pharmaceutical Society of Northern Ireland (PSNI)	
Social Work England	

Box 2.7 Regulatory agencies in the UK devolved nations

Healthcare services in Wales are inspected and regulated by Healthcare Inspectorate Wales (HIW). Care Inspectorate Wales (CIW) is the regu-lator for social care and social services, from child minders and nurseries to homes for older people.

Health Improvement Scotland supports health and social care, through the regulation of independent hospitals and clinics.

The Regulation and Quality Improvement Authority (RQIA) is the inde-pendent body responsible for monitoring and inspecting the availability and quality of health and social care services in Northern Ireland and encouraging improvements in the quality of those services.

What is the regulation process?

Regulation of healthcare in England comprises two main elements:

- Regulation of the quality and safety of care offered by healthcare providers, currently undertaken by the Care Quality Commission (CQC)
- Regulation of the market in healthcare services (by DHSC)

Some NHS services, for example general medical and general dental services, have always been provided by independent contractors and private sector bodies. There has been an expansion of private provision within hospital and community services, with the aim of creating a mixed economy in which providers can offer services to NHS patients.

Commissioners, on behalf of patients, can contract with private providers, although DHSC sets national tariffs for hospital activity to encourage competition based on quality of service, rather than cost. These arrangements also fall under regulation.

Public trust and legitimacy are integral to effective regulation, which requires openness and independence. Regulatory powers derive from primary and secondary legislation, but it remains essential that regulators are independent to achieve their objectives of data gathering, investigation, or enforcement.

The five key principles of regulation are:

- Identification: early identification of potential risks within a service
- Prevention: provide advice on risk management
- Monitoring and detection: observe and openly report risk
- Resolution: proactive identification and correction of compliance issues
- Advisory: advocate on rules and regulation; education and sharing lessons learned

Who regulates?

Many areas of regulation involve one or more main regulators with specific powers and duties to enforce or otherwise influence compliance with rules and standards. These regulators can be at national and local level, and sometimes there is not a clear boundary between regulators' remits, requiring them to work closely together. Some public bodies that are not generally considered regulators also deliver regulatory functions, such as local authorities and some enforcement bodies.

Regulators often operate within a wider regulatory framework that includes other organizations, such as appeals bodies, advocacy bodies, or complaints services. As public bodies, regulators also typically have responsibilities from general legislation such as the Equality Act, Competition Act, or net zero legislation.

Funding for regulation

Government and parliament expect regulators to have a funding model that is sufficient to regulate effectively, adaptable to changing risks, and fair to citizens and businesses. Where the funding comes from—for example, fees on regulated entities or general taxation—may also affect a regulator's actual or perceived independence from industry or ministers.

NHS regulators

Care Quality Commission (https://www.cqc.org.uk/)

The CQC is the independent regulator of health and social care in England (see also Chapter 5). Care providers must be registered with the CQC:

- Healthcare provided by hospitals, GPs, dentists, clinics (family planning, slimming, substance misuse), ambulances, hospices, and mental health services
- Adult social care in care homes and in people's own homes (both personal and nursing care)
- Services for people whose rights are restricted under the Mental Health Act

The CQC monitors, inspects and rates services, producing and publishing a report with a rating. They have the power to take action to protect service users if they find the service level is below a certain standard.

The CQC uses a single assessment framework, based on five key questions combined with quality statements, to produce the rating:

- Safe—are patients protected from abuse and avoidable harm?
- Effective—does the care, treatment, and support achieve satisfactory results and help maintain quality of life? Is it based on the best available evidence?
- Caring—do staff involve and treat patients with compassion, kindness, dignity, and respect?
- Responsive—are services organized so that they can meet patients' needs?
- Well-led—does the leadership of the organization make sure that it is providing high-quality care that is based around needs. Does it encourage learning and innovation and promote an open and fair culture

The quality statements focus on specific topic areas under each of the key questions. This sets a clear expectation of providers, based on patients' experiences and the standard of care expected. This has replaced the former key lines of enquiry (KLOEs), providing a more structured and consistent report, including the experiences of service users.

The CQC is the key regulator with which a dental hospital or department will interact.

Some organizations, such as dental practices, are not given a rating, only assessed as to whether they meet their obligations.

United Kingdom Accreditation Service (https://www.ukas.com/)

UKAS is appointed by government to assess and accredit organizations that provide services including certification, testing, inspection, and calibration of medical laboratories.

Human Fertilisation and Embryology Authority (https://www.hfea.gov.uk/)

The UK's independent regulator of fertility treatment and research using human embryos.

Health and Safety Executive (HSE) (https://www.hse.gov.uk/)

The HSE is the national regulator for workplace health and safety, where both criminal and civil law applies to the working environment. Employers have a legal obligation to protect their staff against injury or illness in the workplace. HSE provides general guidance on safety in the workplace and areas with specific legal duties: manual handling, personal protective equipment, fire safety, home working, use of display screens.

Environment Agency (https://www.gov.uk/government/organisations/environment-agency)

Responsible for the regulation of clinical waste management facilities in England. In Scotland it is the Scottish Environment Protection Agency (SEPA).

NHS Resolution (https://resolution.nhs.uk/)

Previously known as the NHS Litigation Authority, NHS Resolution manages negligence and other claims against the NHS in England on behalf of its member organizations.

NHS Resolution's main roles are:
- Providing indemnity schemes for the NHS in England and resolving compensation claims
- Resolving concerns about the performance of individual practitioners (National Clinical Assessment Service)—see Chapter 7, Staff management
- Resolving primary care contracting disputes (Family Health Service Appeals Unit)

Human Tissue Authority (HTA) (https://www.hta.gov.uk/)

The HTA is a non-departmental public body of the DHSC, overseen by an authority board of lay and professional members appointed by the government. It is the independent regulator for organizations that remove, store, and use human tissue for research, medical treatment, post-mortem examination, education and training, and display in public. HTA approves organ and bone marrow donations from living people.

Medicines and Healthcare products Regulatory Agency (https://www.gov.uk/government/organisations/medicines-and-healthcare-products-regulatory-agency)

The MHRA regulates medicines, medical devices, and blood components for transfusion in the UK. It has a wide remit that includes responsibility to:
- Ensure medicines, medical devices, and blood components for transfusion meet safety, quality, and effectiveness standards
- Secure safe supply chains for medicines, medical devices, and blood components
- Promote international standardization and harmonization to assure the effectiveness and safety of biological medicines
- Educate the public and healthcare professionals about the risks and benefits of medicines, medical devices, and blood components, leading to safer and more effective use

- Enable innovation and research and development that is beneficial to public health (see Chapter 10, Research governance)
- Collaborate with partners in the UK and internationally to support timely access to safe medicines and medical devices and to protect public health

The MHRA works under a statutory framework to set policy, which ensures public health improvements. The key policy areas are:
- Medicines and vaccines
- Medical devices
- Blood components
- E-cigarettes
- Traditional herbal and homeopathic remedies

The MHRA runs the yellow card scheme, the UK system for collecting and monitoring information on suspected safety concerns or incidents involving medicines and medical devices. It relies on voluntary reporting of suspected adverse reactions by health professionals and patients.

NHS institutions

NHS Employers

NHS Employers is an organization which acts on behalf of NHS trusts in the National Health Service in England and Wales. It was formed in 2004, is part of the NHS Confederation, and negotiates contracts with healthcare staff on behalf of the government.

NHS Providers

The trade body for foundation trusts is NHS Providers, formerly known as the Foundation Trust Network, which has 95% of all acute, ambulance, community, and mental health foundation trusts in its membership. NHS Providers is the membership organization for NHS trusts in England, which takes part in negotiations between the trusts and the Department of Health and provides development support to trust leaders.

NHS Business Services Authority

The BSA is an executive non-departmental public body of the DHSC, responsible for a £35 billion annual budget. BSA delivers a range of services to NHS organizations, NHS contractors, patients, and the public in England and Wales, which includes:

- NHS Help With Health Costs programme that provides free or reduced cost prescriptions through the Low Income Scheme, medical exemption certificates, maternity exemption certificates, NHS Tax Credit Exemption Certificates and prescription prepayment certificates
- Administer the NHS Bursary and Social Work Bursary schemes, including the NHS Learning Support Fund
- NHS Dental Services administers payments to dentists in England and Wales, offers advice and information for dentists, commissioners, and patients
- Administration of the NHS Pension Scheme for England and Wales
- Scanning Services to support digital medical record storage
- NHS Jobs
- Electronic Staff Record
- Overseas Healthcare Services
- NHS Prescription Services, responsible for medical exemption certificates and prescription pre-payment

National Institute of Health and Care Excellence

NICE provides national guidance and advice to improve health and social care. They focus on evidence-based, effective, and financially viable healthcare. NICE guidelines are intended for use by those providing, commissioning, and managing health and social care services.

NICE was established to help reduce variation in the availability and quality of NHS treatments and care, by producing useful and usable guidance for health and care practitioners. Its role is to improve outcomes for people using the NHS by developing recommendations that focus on what matters to patients and drive innovation into the hands of health and care practitioners. NICE provides national guidance and produces quality standards for different diseases and conditions. It also conducts evidence surveillance reviews and rigorous, independent assessment of complex evidence for new health technologies.

The NHS Constitution sets out the right for people to receive drugs and treatments that have been recommended by NICE for use in the NHS, if their healthcare provider indicates that the treatment is clinically appropriate for them.

Scottish Intercollegiate Guidelines Network (SIGN)

The aim of SIGN is to improve the quality of healthcare for patients in Scotland by reducing variation in practice and outcome. Similar to NICE, it develops and disseminates national clinical guidelines containing recommendations for effective practice based on current evidence.

Further reading

Healthcare policy
Available at: ✍ https://www.england.nhs.uk/long-term-plan/
Available at: ✍ https://www.gov.uk/government/publications/the-green-book-appraisal-and-eva
luation-in-central-governent/the-green-book-2020
Available at: ✍ https://www.gov.uk/government/publications/health-and-social-care-integration-
joining-up-care-for-people-places-and-populations
NHS principles and values
Available at: ✍ https://www.gov.uk/government/publications/the-nhs-constitution-for-england/
the-nhs-constitution-for-england
NHS finances
Available at: ✍ The Health Foundation (2022). https://www.health.org.uk/news-and-comment/
charts-and-infographics/how-does-uk-health-spending-compare-across-europe-over-the-past-
decade
NHS operating framework
Available at: ✍ https://www.england.nhs.uk/wp-content/uploads/2022/10/B2068-NHS-England-
Operating-Framework.pdf
NHS mandate
Available at: ✍ https://assets.publishing.service.gov.uk/government/uploads/system/uploads/atta
chment_data/file/1065713/2022-to-2023-nhs-england-mandate.pdf
Integrated care systems
Available at: ✍ https://www.kingsfund.org.uk/audio-video/integrated-care-systems-hea
lth-and-care-act
Direct commissioning of POD
Available at: ✍ https://www.nhsconfed.org/publications/delegation-integration
Education costs
Available at: ✍ https://www.hee.nhs.uk/our-work/education-training-placement-funding
NHS regulation
Available at: ✍ https://www.kingsfund.org.uk/projects/nhs-white-paper/health-care-regulation
ICB specialized services roadmap
Available at: ✍ https://www.england.nhs.uk/wp-content/uploads/2022/05/PAR1440-specialised-
commissioning-roadmap-addendum-may-2022.pdf

Chapter 3

Structure and commissioning of NHS dentistry

Commissioning of NHS dentistry in England

NHS England is responsible for commissioning all dental services: primary, specialist, community, and out-of-hours services. The Primary Care Commissioning team works directly with local commissioning teams for both primary and secondary dental care. The National Dental Commissioning and Policy team helps develop the commissioning contractual framework.

Current priorities include:
- Reduce inequalities in oral health and improve oral health in children under 5 years
- Flexible commissioning and movement towards locally based, clinically-led commissioning
- Overseeing national dental access and improving areas of weakest dental provision
- Dental contract reform

Dental contracting framework

Many organizations are involved in the commissioning and delivery of NHS dentistry (Figure 3.1). Payments for primary contracts are managed by the NHS Business Services Authority via the online Compass system. There are currently two types of contracts.

General dental services contract (GDS)

These form 85% of primary care contracts and are of indefinite duration. The contracts are for general dental treatment that is clinically necessary, 'to meet the reasonable needs of patients' and thus excludes treatment which is only for cosmetic reasons.

Personal dental services agreement (PDS)

These are time-limited contracts, usually lasting five years, pertaining to specialist dental services. A large portion of specialist services are carried out in secondary care settings under local and national tariff arrangements. NHS England is committed to increasing the amount of complex dental treatment which can be carried out in a primary care setting, rather than referring to a secondary hospital setting.

Community dental services may be held as GDS or PDS.

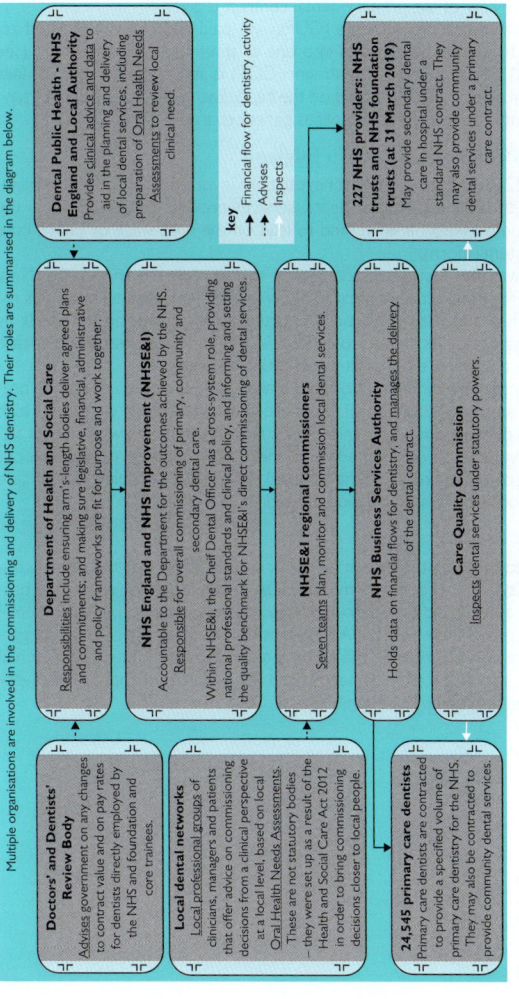

Figure 3.1 Organizations involved in commissioning NHS dentistry. Reproduced from Dentistry in England—National Audit Office. February 2020.

Primary NHS dental contract

The current NHS dental contract was introduced in England in 2006. Although not applicable to a secondary care environment, for context a brief overview of the primary dental contract is given.

General dental practitioners (GDPs) are paid and patients charged according to activity categorized into one of three bands of treatment (see Table 3.1). Each course of treatment (COT) is assigned a number of units of dental activity (UDA), based on the band. Each UDA has an agreed payment amount. This system simplifies patient charges.

Dental contract reform in England

The 2022-2023 dental contract negotiations involved 12 months of engagement with stakeholders and dental services providers, subsequent to the government asking NHS England to lead on the next stage of dental contract system reform.

This was the first significant change to the contract since 2006. New dental pilot contracts and 'prototypes' were implemented to begin this reform. They aimed to focus on supporting patients with higher needs by amending the UDA system to reflect this group and implementing a care pathway approach, emphasizing prevention and self-care.

The remuneration system offered a mix of capitation payment for prevention and a modification of the existing activity system of UDAs, such that the dental team is recognized for supporting patients who need a significant volume of work. In addition, more information is provided about the use of skill mix in a primary dental care setting, enabling dental care professionals (DCPs) to provide more direct access to care.

Dental contract reform in Wales

Similar to England, the Welsh Government identified that the dental contractual system needed reform. The UDA system does not encourage prevention, a needs-led care model, or maximize the skills of the whole dental team. A move away from UDA targets as the sole measure of contract performance was prioritized. The focus is on an increase in the use of dental skill mix, implementation of need-based dental care and improved delivery of evidence-based prevention.

Table 3.1 GDPs and patient charges according to treatment band

Band	UDA	
1	1	Clinical examination, radiographs, scaling and polishing, preventive dental work, such as oral health advice
2a	3	Band 1, plus additional treatment such as fillings, extractions
2b	5	COT involving either non-molar endodontics to permanent teeth or a combined total of three or more teeth requiring permanent fillings or extractions
2c	7	COT involving molar endodontics on permanent teeth
3	12	Complex treatment, which includes a laboratory element, such as bridgework, crowns, and dentures
4	1.2	Urgent treatment including examination, radiographs, dressings, recementing crowns, up to two extractions, one filling

Commissioning of dental specialities

NHS England is responsible for commissioning dental specialities but actions this through a system of local commissioners working closely with managed clinical networks (MCNs), local dental networks (LDNs) and regional public health consultants.

The aim is a smooth patient journey, equitable access to specialist care and fulfilling the population's dental needs while achieving national standards of care. The commissioning aspiration is location-based, clinically-led commissioning: the patient is treated by a clinician with the appropriate skill, ideally in the local setting rather than automatically being referred to a dental hospital.

Clinical and commissioning standards

The standards were previously called the 'commissioning guides for dental specialities'. These are a collection of standardized frameworks (see Box 3.1) produced by dentists, commissioners, chief dental officer, NHS England, Public Health England, Health Education England, specialist societies, patients, and the public.

They aim to:

- Establish a pathway approach to standardize commissioning
- Reduce the divide between primary and secondary care
- Outline mandatory clinical competencies to deliver care, rather than dictating the setting in which to carry it out
- Enable local commissioners to review the current provision of services, assess the level of need and implement these nationally agreed standards

Common commissioning themes

The commissioning standards agree at a national level much of the detail around specialist services commissioning. Each framework outlines:

- Dental care pathways with defined levels of care, complexity, and procedures
- Competencies of each level of care
- Referral criteria and core data set required on referral

Box 3.1 Clinical and commissioning standards

Clinical standard: paediatric dentistry
Clinical standard: oral medicine
Clinical standard: oral surgery
Clinical guide for dental anxiety management
Clinical guide for dentistry
Clinical standard: special care dentistry
Clinical standard for restorative dentistry
Guides for commissioning dental specialities—orthodontics
Clinical standard for dental specialities—orthodontics
Clinical standard for urgent dental care
Commissioning standard for dental care for people with diabetes
Accreditation of performers and providers of level 2 complexity care

---

- Consistent measures of clinical outcomes, quality standards, patient reported outcome/experience measures
- The minimum environment and equipment standards for each level of care
- Consistent approach to coding and costing measures for the care pathway across all settings
- Direction on completing a needs assessment to assess the level and distribution of care in local areas
- Access to services across each pathway to ensure that people with disabilities and other 'hard to reach' groups have equitable access to good oral health outcomes
- Contractual frameworks

Patient care pathways and complexity levels

Patient care pathways

The Independent Review of NHS Dental Services 2009 (Steele Review) suggested a pathway approach to dental care provision, both in the primary dental care setting (see Figure 3.2) and when accessing secondary care (see Figure 3.3).

- Pathways form a network of care
- The patient can move seamlessly through primary, secondary, community or acute care
- This is based on clinical need rather than location/organization

The creation of these networks requires a needs assessment. Tools for each speciality to assist this assessment are provided in each of the speciality commissioning standards as per Box 3.1. The focus is on clinical engagement and commissioning at a local level, through MCNs and LDNs.

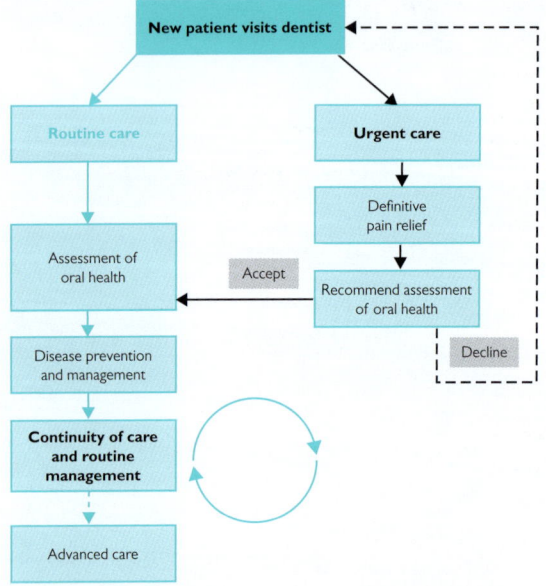

Figure 3.2 Patient care pathway in a primary dental setting. From: NHS dental services in England. An independent review led by Professor Jimmy Steele June 2009.

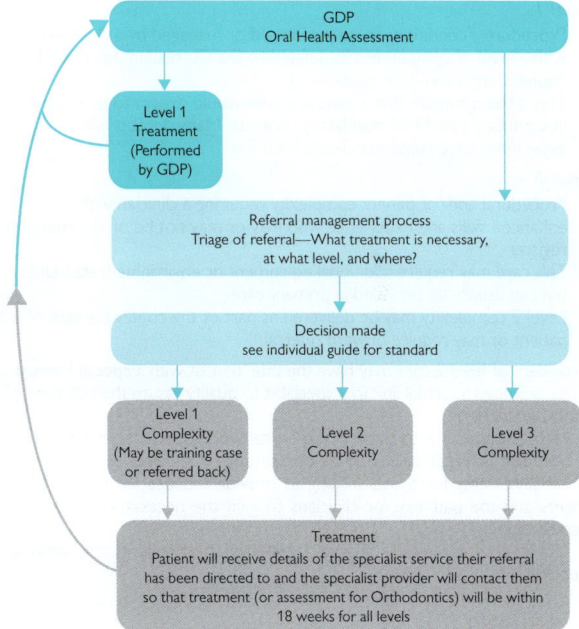

Figure 3.3 Patient care pathway in specialized/secondary care. Adapted from the Dental commissioning guide.

Complexity levels

The commissioning standards identify levels of clinical complexity for dental procedures (see Table 3.2). Figure 3.3 provides an example of a patient pathway through these.

Table 3.2 Treatment complexity providers

Complexity level	Minimum clinical proficiency
1	General dental practitioners (dental foundation training or equivalent)
2	Dentists with enhanced skills, who may or may not be on the specialist register. May be an accredited DwSI
3a	Specialist or consultant
3b	Consultant or consultant-led

Level 1
- Procedures/conditions to be performed or managed by a clinician with a level of competence as defined by the Curriculum for Dental Foundation Training (or equivalent)
- This is the minimum that a commissioner would expect to be delivered in a primary care NHS mandatory contract. Many dentists with experience have competencies beyond this

Level 2
- Procedural and/or patient complexity requiring a clinician with enhanced skills and experience who may or may not be on the specialist register
- This care may require additional equipment or environment standards but can usually be provided in primary care
- Level 2 complexity may be delivered as part of the continuing care of a patient or may require onward referral

Providers of level 2 care may have the title 'dentist with a special interest'. They will need a formal link to a specialist to quality assure the outcome of pathway delivery.

NHS England aims to support the dental workforce in facilitating level 2 procedures taking place in primary care settings. It provides clear guidelines on requirements for those wishing to provide facilities for level 2 treatments and the pathway for clinicians to gain the necessary competency accreditation.

The level of complexity of level 1 and level 2 procedures may vary depending on:
- Medical history
- Social history
- Patient anxiety
- Requirement for skill mix/multidisciplinary team
- Requirement for general anaesthetic
- Other patient-associated modifiers

Level 2 accreditation
Documents are available to guide clinicians in the standardized process to obtaining accreditation for level 2 procedures.
- Provider Assurance Framework for Commissioning of Level 2 Complexity Services—Facilities and Equipment
- Guidance for Commissioners on the Accreditation of Performers of Level 2 Complexity Care
- Accreditation of Performers of Level 2 Complexity Care—Application Bundle

These set out the function and composition of a Local Accreditation Panel (LAP) which will be formed by the appropriate MCN or LDN. They also include application forms, logbook requirements, and the minimum facilities required.

The LAP may award full or partial accreditation, with detailed feedback to the applicant. Dentists who provide level 2 care are titled 'dentist with enhanced skills' or 'dentist with a special interest' (DwSI).

Level 3a

Procedures/conditions to be performed or managed by a clinician recognized as a specialist by the General Dental Council (GDC)-defined criteria and on a specialist list; or by a consultant.

Level 3b

Procedures/conditions to be performed or managed by a clinician recognized as a consultant in the relevant dental speciality, who has received additional training that enables them to deliver more complex care, lead multidisciplinary teams (MDTs), and deliver specialist training.

The consultant team may include trainees and specialists, associate specialists, and Speciality and Associate Specialist (SAS) grades (speciality doctors and specialist-grade doctors with at least four years of postgraduate training, two of which must be in a relevant speciality).

Oral surgery may be delivered by consultants in oral and maxillofacial surgery who have the necessary competencies and are registered with the General Dental Council. Recognition on the General Medical Council specialist list alone is not sufficient.

Complexity assessment

The commissioning guides for each dental speciality provide a complexity assessment flowchart, indicating which treatment procedures correspond to each complexity level. As an example, the orthodontic complexity assessment is shown in Figure 3.4.

Integration of complexity levels and the patient pathway

The commissioning standards aim to outline all the necessary information to ensure a smooth patient journey through NHS dental services. The aim is to reduce the burden of care and waiting lists in hospital dental departments, by signposting patients to appropriately trained clinicians, in a more local setting.

The Five Year Forward View aimed to deconstruct the boundary between primary and secondary care services with the intention of creating networks of care based on patient need rather than organizations.

The clinical standards explain what dental speciality care is, when it is needed, and how to access it. They outline the patient pathway to ensure consistent quality and outcomes. All dental specialities have a coherent patient pathway as exampled by oral surgery in Figure 3.5.

COMPLEXITY ASSESSMENT – ORTHODONTIC TREATMENT

- The benefits of Orthodontic treatment outweigh the risks
- Orthodontic treatment needed and not precluded by either patient co-operation or medical history

Level 1	Level 2	Level 3a	Level 3b
Recognise malocclusion and normal occlusion. Ensure oral health is good prior to referral Perform basic Orthodontic examination, review the level of complexity and be familiar with IOTN, explain to a patient what Orthodontic treatment may involve and make valid and timely referrals Monitor post-Orthodontic care maintenance	Patients with developing dentition requiring straight forward interceptive measures Removable appliances in patients without skeletal discrepancies Non-complex fixed appliance alignment in patients without skeletal discrepancies or significant anchorage demands	Patients requiring Orthodontic treatment for the management of skeletal discrepancies (removable, functional and fixed appliances) Patients with restorative problems, which do not require complex multidisciplinary care with secondary care input Patients with impacted teeth where the Oral Surgery/ Orthodontics liaison can be managed from specialist practice Advice to those providing Level 1 or 2 care	Patients with clefts of the lip and/or palate or craniofacial syndromes Patients with significant skeletal discrepancies requiring combined Orthodontics and Orthognathic surgery Patients who require Orthodontics and complex Oral Surgery input (e.g. multiple impacted teeth) Patients with complex restorative problems requiring secondary care input in a multidisciplinary environment Patients with complex medical issues, including psychological concerns, which require close liaison with medical personnel locally. Patients with medical, developmental or social problems who would not be considered suitable for treatment in specialist practice Complex Orthodontic cases not considered suitable for management in specialist practice Referrals where advice or a second opinion is required from a secondary care Consultant (i.e. to those providing Level 1, 2, 3a care)
Work to be carried out by primary care	**Level 2 care delivery requires a minimum of 50 case starts per year per clinician** Patient modifying factors may result in referral to 3a or 3b	**Work to be referred to Specialist services** Patient-modifying factors may result in referral to 3b 14	**Work to be referred to consultant Specialist Services**

Figure 3.4 Complexity assessment for orthodontic treatment.

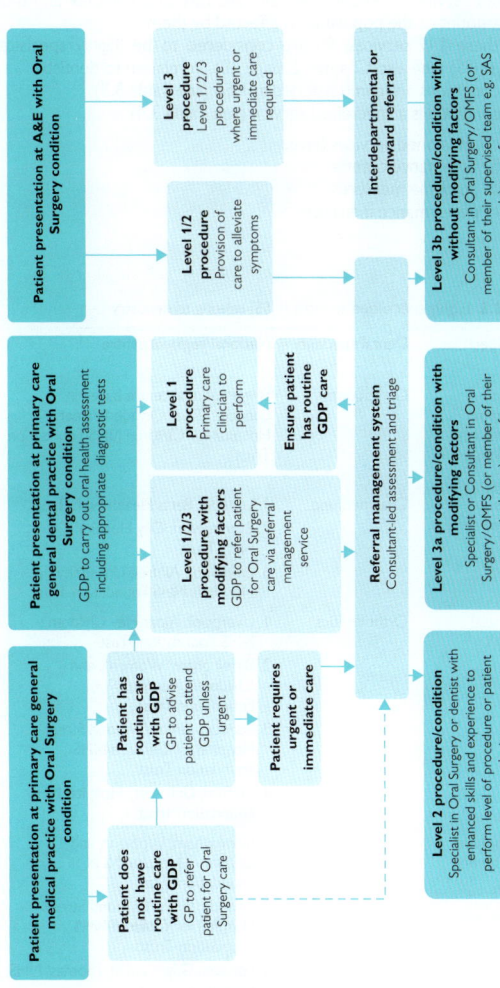

Figure 3.5 Oral surgery patient pathway and complexity of treatment. From: Clinical standard: oral surgery.

Commissioning of dental specialized services

Specialized services are conditions that are rare and complex and thus a smaller amount of the population is affected by them.

Within these 149 services, 80 are considered to be 'highly specialized' services (HSS) (see also Chapter 2, page 28). In relation to dentistry:

• Four conditions are commissioned as HSS (see Table 3.3)
• One condition is a specialized service (see Table 3.4)

These commissioned services have:

• Specific acceptance criteria
• Clinical outcome measures
• Quality performance indicators

Table 3.3 Highly specialized services (HSS) relating to dentistry

Highly specialized service	Dental speciality	National/regional centre
Beckwith-Wiedemann syndrome with macroglossia service	Orthodontics	Single national centre based in London: Great Ormond Street Hospital for Children NHS Foundation Trust
Behçet's syndrome service	Oral medicine	1. London: Barts Health NHS Trust 2. Birmingham: City Hospital NHS Trust 3. Liverpool: Aintree University Hospitals NHS Foundation Trust
Craniofacial service	Orthodontics	1. Liverpool: Alder Hey Children's NHS Foundation Trust 2. Birmingham: Women's and Children's Hospital NHS Foundation Trust 3. London: Great Ormond Street Hospital for Children NHS Foundation Trust 4. Oxford: University Hospital NHS Foundation Trust
Epidermolysis bullosa service	Paediatric and general dentistry	1. Birmingham: Women's and Children's Hospital NHS Foundation Trust 2. London: Great Ormond Street Hospital for Children NHS Foundation Trust 3. London: Guy's and St Thomas' NHS Foundation Trust 4. Birmingham: University Hospitals NHS Foundation Trust

Table 3.4 Specialized services relating to dentistry

Specialized service	Dental speciality	National/regional centre
Cleft lip and palate services	Orthodontics Paediatric dentistry Restorative Oral and maxillofacial surgery	Nine regional UK cleft services that operate a centralized or hub and spoke model. Within these, there are 13 individual specialist cleft units within hospitals. 1. Northern and Yorkshire 2. The North West, Isle of Man, and North Wales Regional Network 3. Trent 4. West Midlands 5. Cleft.Net.East (Cambridge) 6. North Thames 7. The Spires (Oxford and Salisbury) 8. South Wales and South West MCN 9. South Thames

Structure and commissioning of NHS dentistry in Wales

Structure of the Welsh healthcare system

Welsh government

- The Welsh Parliament (Senedd Cymru) makes laws for Wales on devolved matters and can agree Welsh taxes
- The Welsh Parliament, commonly called the Senedd, has powers to make laws on health and healthcare
- The Senedd and its committees (e.g. Health and Social Care Committee, Children, Young People and Education Committee) also hold the Welsh Government to account
- The Cabinet Secretary for Health and Social Services and their respective civil service departments within the Welsh Government set vision and policy for the health and social services and provide national strategy, frameworks, and guidance
- The Welsh Government's national healthcare policies, strategies, and clinical frameworks are implemented by NHS Wales and its partners when planning and delivering services for the people of Wales

NHS Wales

- NHS Wales delivers healthcare services through seven local health boards that provide healthcare for their local population and 3 NHS trusts (Public Health Wales NHS Trust, Velindre University NHS Trust and Welsh Ambulance Services NHS Trust) that provide services for the whole of Wales
- Responsibility for public health is shared among all NHS bodies in Wales, with leadership provided by the Welsh Government's Chief Medical Officer (who is also the Medical Director of NHS Wales), Public Health Wales (PHW) and Director of Public Health in Health Boards
- Velindre University NHS Trust provides Welsh Blood Service and specialist cancer services
- The Welsh Ambulance Services NHS Trust provide Welsh ambulance services, non-emergency patient transport for specific medical need, 111 service, and clinical triage element of the GP out-of-hours service
- Health boards and trusts are supported by the NHS Wales Executive and NHS Wales Shared Services Partnership

NHS Wales also has two special health authorities:

- Health Education and Improvement Wales (HEIW) that provides education and training and carries out workforce planning
- Digital Health Care Wales (DHCW) that is responsible for building and designing digital services for health and care in Wales

Commissioning of healthcare in Wales

The NHS system in Wales focuses on developing services based on co-operation, collaboration, and partnership, working between NHS bodies, other public services, and the wider community. It is not based on the concepts of an internal market nor the division of purchaser and provider of services. At its core, is a planning process that centres on a conversation between the Welsh Government and NHS bodies regarding:

- Using resources to address healthcare needs over a 3-year period
- Working with other public services to improve population health outcomes
- Reducing health inequalities in line with the Social Services and Wellbeing Act and the Well-being of Future Generations Act
- NHS trusts and local health boards then focus on delivering care in light of these targets and longer-term aims

Health boards

Local health boards are responsible for planning and delivering services in their respective areas. This includes primary and community healthcare including mental health, secondary and tertiary healthcare services.

Health boards are also responsible for:

- Improving physical and mental health outcomes
- Promoting well-being
- Reducing health inequalities across their population
- Commissioning services from other organizations to meet the health and care needs of their residents

Other bodies

- Healthcare Inspectorate Wales (HIW) is the independent inspectorate and regulator of healthcare in Wales, for both hospitals and private clinics
- Llais is an independent statutory body that has responsibility for representing public and patient voice in health and social care. It was set up by the Welsh Government (WG) to give the people of Wales more say in the planning and delivery of their health and social care services locally, regionally, and nationally

Commissioning of dental care in Wales

- The chief dental officer for Wales and dental policy team in the WG provide national dental policy and strategy for the health boards and other NHS bodies in Wales
- Health boards receive funding from the WG for delivery of NHS services, including dental services and oral health programmes
- Each health board decides their local oral health plans and what proportion of this healthcare funding will be allocated for delivery of NHS dental care within their area
- Their planning is guided by the WG's policy and guidance on oral health and dentistry
- Each health board then employs the required workforce to deliver:
  - Consultant-led specialist dental services
  - Community Dental Services (CDS), whose role is defined in a Welsh Health Circular by the WG
- Additionally, health boards also commission NHS general dental services (GDS) from independent primary dental care providers that range from large dental corporates to small local dental practices. In some areas, health boards may choose to provide GDS by expanding their Community Dental Service, e.g. a salaried dental service unit within the CDS
- In addition to delivering NHS GDS most independent dental care providers also provide private dentistry under different financial arrangements from dental insurance to patients paying a fee-per-item

Commissioning of specialist services
- Health boards also commission specialist orthodontic services (in line with the national orthodontic contract) from independent orthodontic practices
- They may also commission or provide minor oral surgery, treatment under conscious sedation, dental care to people in prisons, domiciliary dental care, etc.

Table 3.5 outlines the members and responsibilities of key post holders and committees in the Welsh dental network.

Table 3.5 Stakeholder networks in Wales

Post/committee/group	Organization/area	Comment
Clinical director of the service	Health board	Usually a clinical consultant with additional leadership and management role
Medical director	Health board	Responsible for quality and safety
Executive team and board members	Health board	One or more Board members have ultimate responsibility for oral health and dental services in their area
Local dental committee	Statutory committee covering one or more Health boards	Health boards consult with the local dental committee (LDC) on matters relating to dental services including dental service planning, contracts, and commissioning
Dental governance groups within health boards	Health board	Multistakeholder groups to support health board in dental services planning, implementation
Managed clinical network (MCN)	Regional network covering more than one health board	Speciality or clinical area specific
British Dental Association Welsh Council, Wales General Dental Practice Committee and Wales Committee for Community Dentistry	BDA Wales	Trade union representing dentists
Chief dental officer (CDO) for Wales	Welsh Government (WG)	Dental policy and professional lead at the WG
Postgraduate dental dean	Health Education and Improvement Wales (HEIW)	Leads dental section within the HEIW

Table 3.5   (Contd.)

Post/committee/group	Organization/area	Comment
Welsh Dental Committee (WDC)	Statutory committee	Advises WG with representation from Health Board groups HEIW, PHW, dental school, BDA Wales, Welsh General Dental Practice Committee, LDCs across Wales
Dental public health team	Public Health Wales	Advises WG, health boards, HEIW and other organizations in Wales

Structure and commissioning of NHS dentistry in Scotland

Legislative framework

- The NHS (Scotland) Act 1978 is the primary legislation for the NHS in Scotland; it establishes the framework for dental care delivery
- A set of secondary legislation underpins the operational framework for delivery. These regulations cover general dental services, vocational training delivery and equivalence, and patient charges

NHS Scotland structure

NHS Scotland is structured across:
- 14 territorial NHS boards
- 7 national NHS boards with specialist functions (e.g. workforce education, ambulance services, and healthcare regulation)
- Public Health Scotland

Scottish NHS boards

NHS boards are accountable to Scottish Ministers, supported by the Scottish Government Health and Social Care Directorates.

Each territorial NHS board is responsible for the protection and improvement of their population's health and for the delivery of frontline healthcare services. National NHS boards support the territorial NHS boards by providing a range of important specialist and support services.

NHS boards work collectively with their partners, including patients, staff, local authorities and the voluntary sector to deliver effective healthcare services and to safeguard and improve health in line with the Scottish Government's National Performance Framework. The Scottish Government sets the national objectives and priorities for the NHS, agrees delivery plans with each NHS board, monitors performance, and supports boards to ensure they achieve these key objectives. Each NHS board has a director of dentistry.

Since 2016, work has been underway across Scotland to integrate health and social care services in line with the requirements of the Public Bodies (Joint Working) (Scotland) Act 2014.

General dental services (GDS)

- The population of Scotland was 5.5M (mid-2021) and the vast majority (95%) are registered with a high-street dentist who can offer NHS or private services and most often, a combination of both
- Since 2010, once a patient registers with an NHS dentist, they are registered for life, unless they opt to de-register
- Dentists are paid through a 'blended' payment system involving capitation payments, personal and practice allowances and 'item of service' payment for treatments listed in the Statement of Dental Remuneration (SDR). Not all dental treatments are available on the NHS, for example, implants or purely cosmetic dentistry

Public Dental Services (PDS)

- The PDS replaced the Community Dental Service and Salaried GDS in 2013. The PDS is run by NHS boards
- PDS dentists are salaried and employed by the NHS board
- They provide a range of services, including:
  - Patients with special care needs (both adults and children)
  - Referral service for other health and social care practitioners
  - Dental care for socially excluded people who might have access difficulties
  - Specialized and specialist services, e.g. prison dentistry, sedation, and general anaesthesia
  - Access services, e.g. gaps in GDS provision, out-of-hours (OoH) services
  - Public health function—inspections, screening, health promotion, and epidemiology and teaching in undergraduate and dental core training
- The PDS may vary across NHS Boards depending on the areas served

Hospital dental services (HDS)

- The HDS configuration is similar to the rest of the UK; it treats patients as outpatients, day-case, or in-patients
- The four dental hospitals in Glasgow, Dundee, Edinburgh, and Aberdeen see outpatients with inpatient and day-case treatment available at a range of general hospitals
- It is a secondary care provider and receives referrals from doctors and dentists in primary care or consultants in other areas and specialities, including emergency dental services
- Dentists working in the HDS are salaried dentists, employed directly by NHS boards; they may be in training or career grade staff such as speciality or consultant grades

Out-of-hours services (OoH)

- Access to OoH dental care in Scotland is now mainly provided through NHS 24 who work in partnership with local NHS boards to provide a confidential telephone health information, advice, and triage service throughout the country
- NHS boards operate OoH clinical services at weekends and public holidays, and these are staffed by clinicians from the GDS, PDS, and HDS. During the week, registered patients will be referred to their own practice and unregistered to PDS access clinics for urgent care the following morning or if deemed an emergency, to an A&E service

Oral health improvement services

Within Public Health Scotland, the national Oral Health Improvement Leadership Group has oversight of the progression of the national Oral Health Improvement Programmes. This includes programmes targeted at:

- Young people (Childsmile)
- Older people living in care homes (Caring for Smiles)
- People with experience of homelessness (Smile for Life)
- People with experience of custody (Mouth Matters)
- People with additional care needs (Open Wide)

- Community-based food skills for families affected by socio-economic inequalities and/or racialized inequalities (Eat Well for Oral Health)
- People with experience of drugs (in development)

System leadership

- The CDO and the dental policy team within Scottish Government have direct lines of communication with the NHS board directors of dentistry and the wide range of key stakeholders across dentistry and oral health
- The director of dentistry in each territorial or special board works with other directors and advisers and is a conduit for strategic change, best operational practice, governance issues, and strengthening working across the interface of primary and secondary care and linking public health

Regulation

- The General Dental Council oversees professional regulation on a UK-wide basis
- System regulation is devolved with Healthcare Improvement Scotland (HIS) being the key scrutiny body for NHS hospitals and services and fully independent healthcare services (including non-NHS dental practices)
- NHS boards undertake the scrutiny of fully-NHS dental practices and mixed NHS and private practices, on a three-year rolling programme

Workforce

As of June 2023, the General Dental Council registered dental workforce in Scotland was made up of 3,993 dentists and 7,975 DCPs; the majority of whom work in primary care settings. In addition, there is a significant but unquantified number of non-GDC registrants making up the dental team, including; practice administration and management staff and healthcare support workers.

Finance

Funding for HDS and the PDS is contained within the baseline funding made by Scottish Government to NHS boards. Oral health improvement funding is made to boards by allocation from Scottish Government. Funding for GDS is retained centrally within government and, following submission of a post-treatment claim, paid directly to GDPs via the Practitioner Services Division of NHS Scotland.

An NHS dental examination in Scotland is free for all patients. For subsequent treatment, unless exempt from NHS charges, patients pay 80% of the treatment costs, up to a maximum of £384. Any costs over this maximum are fully subsidized by the NHS.

Exemption from NHS charges is available for people aged under 26, pregnant or have given birth in the last 12 months or on a low income and receiving income-related benefits. Around 40% of the Scottish population are exempt from NHS charges. Partial help with health costs is available through the NHS Low Income Scheme, for those who are not exempt, but have difficulty in paying.

Structure and commissioning of NHS dentistry in Northern Ireland

Northern Ireland is one of four devolved administrations in the United Kingdom with a population of over 1.9 million (NISRA, 2022). Political power was transferred from Westminster to the Northern Ireland Assembly in 1998. Health is included in the range of devolved powers, meaning that the Assembly has full control over this area.

Northern Ireland operates an integrated health and social care (HSC) system, which underwent significant reform in 2009 as part of the Review of Public Administration (RPA), to design a more streamlined and accountable system, putting public health and well-being at the centre of patient care. The NHS provides healthcare in England, Scotland, and Wales; the HSC system does similar in Northern Ireland. The Strategic Planning and Performance Group, in partnership with the Northern Ireland Public Health Agency (PHA) is responsible for commissioning health and social care services on behalf of the Department of Health.

Structure of HSC system

The HSC system is structured around:
- The Department of Health (DOH); responsible for policy and legislation
- The most senior dental figure within the DOH is the CDO for Northern Ireland, who provides advice to the Minister for Health on dental services and oral health
- Five HSC trusts have responsibility for the management and administration of regional HSC facilities. The sixth trust is the Northern Ireland Ambulance Service HSC Trust
- The Strategic Planning and Performance Group (SPPG), which commissions services, manages the HSC trusts, and deploys funding from the Northern Ireland Executive
- The PHA is a multiprofessional body that aims to improve and protect public health and social well-being and reduce health inequalities

Structure of dental services

A number of different models of delivery for NHS dental care exist within Northern Ireland. There are three main branches of dentistry in the region, each commissioned through the SPPG.

General dental services (GDS)
- GDS are governed by the Health and Personal Social Services GDS Regulations (Northern Ireland) 1993, with updates and amendments over the years. These regulations describe the contractual responsibilities of dentists
- The GDS is made up of GDPs who provide NHS treatment under an independent contract with the SPPG
- The majority of dentists are self-employed and the number of corporate providers has increased significantly in recent years. There are approximately 1,195 GDPs working across the country's 364 GDS practices (correct as of June 2024)

- The dental contract for dentists operates on a fee-per-item basis, based on the Statement of Dental Remuneration and administered by the HSC Business Services Organization (BSO)
- They receive approximately:
  - 60% of their gross income from item of service payments
  - 20% from capitation and continuing care payments and the remaining
  - 20% from allowances (largely paid in proportion to their NHS commitment)
- The remuneration model currently operating in Northern Ireland is largely led by demand, with expenditure mainly determined by the number of patients seeking care and the amount of treatment which the GDPs determine is required
- Commissioned high-street specialist services include orthodontics and oral surgery

Community dental services (CDS)
- The CDS is a referral-only service which provides dental care for service users whose dental care cannot be provided by a GDP
- The remit of CDS is defined by a scope of service specification document and includes those with impairments, adults in care homes, the homeless community, children, and patients who require treatment under sedation or general anaesthesia
- Dental clinicians working within the CDS are salaried

Consultant-led hospital dental services (HDS)
- Access to specialist dental care within a hospital is following referral from GDS, CDS, or other medical specialities
- Northern Ireland has one dedicated dental hospital located at the Royal Victoria Hospital in Belfast
- Dental undergraduate training in Northern Ireland is also provided on this site by Queen's University Belfast
- HDS providing oral and maxillofacial surgery and orthodontics are also located at Altnagelvin Area Hospital, Craigavon Area Hospital, Antrim Area Hospital, and the Ulster Hospital

Finance
- The Community Dental Service and Consultant-led Hospital Dental Service is delivered by various HSC trusts, each of which manages its own staff and services and controls its own budget
- NHS dental services are not provided free at the point of service for all service users. Based on individual circumstances, service users may be entitled to free treatment for assistance with the costs
- Those entitled to free treatment in primary care includes:
  - Aged under 18 years
  - Aged over 18 years but in full-time education
  - Pregnant or have had a child within 12 months before treatment commenced
  - Those entitled to some form of income support
- Individuals who are self-paying for their treatment must pay 80% of the fee, up to a maximum cost of £384
- Patients who have dental treatment provided by the CDS or HDS do not pay for treatment

Further reading

Accreditation of Performers of Level 2 Complexity Care—Application Bundle. Available at: ℘ https://www.england.nhs.uk/wp-content/uploads/2018/09/guidance-for-the-accreditation-of-performers-of-level-2-v24.pdf

General Dental Statistics for Northern Ireland. Annual Statistics 2023/24. Northern Ireland Statistics and Research Agency. Available at: ℘ https://bso.hscni.net/wp-content/uploads/2024/06/General-Dental-Statistics-Publication-2023–24.pdf

Guidance for Commissioners on the Accreditation of Performers of Level 2 Complexity Care. Available at: ℘ https://www.england.nhs.uk/publication/guidance-for-commissioners-on-the-accreditation-of-performers-of-level-2-complexity-care/

National Audit Office. Dentistry in England. Available at: ℘ https://www.nao.org.uk/wp-content/uploads/2020/03/Dentistry-in-England.pdf

NHS England's clinical and commissioning standards for dentistry. Available at: ℘ https://www.england.nhs.uk/primary-care/dentistry/dental-commissioning/dental-specialties/

Provider Assurance Framework for Commissioning of Level 2 Complexity Services—Facilities and Equipment. Available at: ℘ https://www.england.nhs.uk/wp-content/uploads/2018/09/provider-assurance-framework-for-commissioning-of-providers-of-level-2-complexity-v28.pdf

The Independent Review of NHS Dental Services 2009 (Steele Review). Available at: ℘ https://webarchive.nationalarchives.gov.uk/ukgwa/20130123200117/http://www.dh.gov.uk/en/PublicationsandstatisticsPublications/PublicationsPolicyAndGuidance/DH_101137

The dental department within the trust and health network

The hospital

A well-run dental department has an engaged consultant body that provides leadership within their regional level, anticipating and reacting effectively to local challenges. The department should work towards the strategic aims of the trust, as outlined by the board of directors, within the local area integrated care system.

Different hospitals and trusts will have varying management and departmental divisional structures. All will have a board comprising of executive directors and non-executive directors, led by a chairperson.

- Executive teams are directly involved in the day-to-day management
- Non-executive teams take a strategic role, providing independent advisory services
- The exact roles and responsibilities of each position will vary between trusts and will often be defined in a scheme of delegation, which exists at each management level. This outlines what responsibilities are assigned to named officers in the trust and is generally within a 'line management' structure (i.e. integrated governance)

Integrated governance

Integrated governance is the framework by which the trust board controls and directs the organization in order to achieve its strategic objectives. It is based on the understanding that all governance elements are important, and it is preferable to manage them together, rather than in 'silos'.

Organizational silos are discrete units in a business of experts, teams, specializations, and so forth. Each silo may have different individual goals, rather than the organization's goals. Having an embedded integrated governance structure removes these barriers and has many advantages:

- Clarity about decisions that have been made and at which level
- Provides clear escalation routes for reporting issues or concerns
- Improved accountability as everyone understands their role
- Improved communication as individuals know who to discuss issues with, thus resulting in improved clinical effectiveness
- A clear line of sight from clinical services through to the board of directors

Board of directors

The board of directors shares overall responsibility for how the organization is run, in relation to quality of services, financial performance, and the culture in which staff operate. The board:

- Provides overall strategic direction for the trust
- Ensures services provided are effective, efficient, and of a high quality
- Monitors performance
- Oversees the financial planning and control for the trust
- Is responsible for the overall culture promoted in the trust

The board comprises of the chair, the chief executive officer (CEO), executive directors, and non-executive directors:

- The chair leads the board and non-executive directors
- The CEO leads the Executive Directors and the organization
- Both the CEO and the chair appoint and review the performance of other executive and associate directors

The document 'The Healthy NHS Board 2013—Principles for Good Governance' was commissioned by the NHS Leadership Academy. It describes the role of the board:

1. Formulating strategy for the organization.
2. Ensuring accountability for the delivery of that strategy. Ensuring the organization operates effectively with openness, transparency, and candour and that systems of control are robust and reliable.
3. Shaping a healthy culture for the board and the organization.

There are three fundamental building blocks underpinning these roles:

1. The board should be informed by the external context within which it operates.
2. The board should be informed and shaped by the intelligence that provides an understanding of local people's needs, trends, and comparative information on how the organization is performing. This should be viewed together with market and stakeholder analyses.
3. The board should give priority to engagement with stakeholders and opinion formers within and beyond the organization. The focus is on building a robust, open, and healthy dialogue with patients, the public, staff, governors, commissioners, and regulators.

The chair

The chair is responsible for the overall conduct of the trust. They:

- Lead the board as it develops vision, strategies, and objectives to deliver organizational goals
- Create the conditions necessary for effective governance and overall board and director effectiveness
- Have a non-executive role—they are not involved in the day-to-day running of the trust, but instead take an overall strategic vision ensuring that the required resources are in place
- The chair appoints and reviews the performance of the CEO
- For foundation trusts, the chair oversees the council of governors

The council of governors is responsible for holding the non-executive directors to account for the performance of the board. Foundation trusts are also accountable to their members and the public, through the council of governors.

Non-executive directors

They provide independent oversight of how the trust is run, by bringing independent experience from both healthcare and other sectors (e.g. financial, legal, clinical, business skills). They may lead in making senior executive appointments and chair internal investigations or disciplinary proceedings. They are responsible for ensuring that the interests of the local community are represented. In essence, they hold the executive management team to account and offer constructive scrutiny and challenge board decisions.

The chief executive

The chief executive officer (CEO) leads the organization on a day-to-day basis in delivering the trust's strategy and they are the accountable officer to parliament. They are responsible for ensuring that the organization works effectively in accordance with national health policy, public service values, and for the maintenance of financial control. The board approves the strategy and objectives; it is the CEO's role to ensure implementation of these.

The executive management team

Led by the CEO, this team comprises the medical director, executive directors, and associate directors, who are accountable for their individual portfolios and for strategic leadership across the trust. They are responsible for the overall management of the trust, including the delivery of services, the management of staff and resources, and the development of the trust's strategic direction.

The executive directors have individual responsibilities for specific areas that include medical directors, nursing, and finance directors.

The senior leadership team

This team is responsible for overseeing the trust's operational business. Aligned with and reporting to the board of directors, they provide leadership and direction for the trust while ensuring service delivery.

The medical director

The role of the medical director (MD) varies across different organizations and trusts. They are always a member of the board of an NHS organization, with a clinical background and are almost always a hospital consultant. Formerly a strictly medical role, the position has now been expanded to include managerial duties, thus being a bridge between management and doctors. The MD's role has evolved from being merely a medical voice on the board to a fully integrated role (Good Governance Institute). Many MDs have previously held the role of clinical director of a department or directorate. The MD is a member of the executive team and they report to the CEO. The MD (along with the director of nursing) is generally one of the only clinicians on the executive board.

Their role can be divided into four main aspects:

1. Corporate responsibilities

Developing and implementing their organization's vision, values, and strategic objectives. MDs provide advice on clinical matters, including service development. They represent their organization on clinical matters to external bodies such as the media, commissioners, Care Quality Commission, patient groups, charities, academic institutions and academic health science networks.

2. Delivering high-quality care:

The MD promotes organizational efficiency and clinical productivity with a focus on cost-effectiveness. They embed a culture of high-quality, high-value care.

3. Clinical standards

The MD guides their organization in ensuring that services and policy development keep pace with statutory requirements and meets national health policy goals.

4. Medical workforce

The MD works with consultants to manage a system for job planning. They are responsible for the overall staff planning of the organization and work with the human resources director and occupational health department to ensure the trust takes steps to address any staff performance or illness issues.

Clinical directorates

Directorates are service-orientated divisions within a trust, which are focused on providing a particular clinical service. They are co-led by a clinician (the divisional or clinical director) and a non-clinician (usually the general manager). The directorate is allocated resources to provide patient care and is accountable to the board via the director of operations. Many other teams provide input and work with the directorate, such as finance, senior nursing, human resources, and general management.

The directorate is comprised of a team of healthcare professionals which may all be focused on one clinical speciality, or the directorate may oversee a number of specialities. Dental specialities in teaching hospitals may form their own directorate as the 'dental school/institute', whereas in district general hospitals, they may be linked with other outpatient services such as ear, nose, and throat (ENT), speech and language therapy, etc.

The Griffiths Report 1983 (see Chapter 1, page 3) was fundamental in strengthening the role of clinical directorates by delegating management of each clinical service to that service level. It encouraged doctors to take positions of management leadership and each speciality to self-manage their resources and funds.

Together, the clinical director and general manager are responsible for the strategic development and oversight of the operational performance of their division/directorate. This includes staffing, finance, meeting performance indicators, and business development. It is a similar but broader role than that of the clinical lead, covering a greater proportion of the hospital. Concerns that cannot be managed locally by a clinical lead are passed onto the clinical director, such as serious complaints, safety incidents, or staff management issues particularly if they involve consultants. The clinical director is responsible for the medical and dental staff, while the general manager oversees the operational managers. Staff management includes workforce planning, recruitment and interviewing, staff development, and performance management. In practice, this is carried out in collaboration with clinical leads, with the clinical director taking a lead role in the appointment of consultants.

Clinical directorates are also involved in funding support for business cases, given their responsibility for strategic planning and business development. This may include funding for new posts, capital investments, or equipment.

Clinical lead

The clinical lead is the person with overall stewardship of the department, to ensure day-to-day efficiency. They maintain clinical commitments in addition to their managerial role. They work closely with their operational manager (often called the service manager) and the lead nurse to ensure that clinical and financial targets are met. The clinical lead has a managerial role both externally and internally within the department. They provide senior managerial colleagues (such as the clinical director or executive director) with clinical analysis and opinions on implementing strategies and the daily operations of the department. More locally, as the senior clinician they have responsibilities within the department, including staffing, patient care, decision making:

- Clinical governance—ensuring that policies and procedures are adhered to, e.g. risk assessment, information governance
- Clinical performance—ensure that the department is focused on meeting clinical performance indicators
- Complaints—responding to complaints and untoward incidents
- Financial—ensuring financial viability within the department, making sure that clinical output is sufficient and costs are managed
- Business development
- Performance management of staff and job planning with consultants, in tandem with the clinical director and general manager
- Staff health and attendance issues—help is available through human resources (business partners) and occupational health departments. The latter can provide specialist support directly or through outside agencies offering confidential counselling services

Depending on the size of the dental department, there may be one clinical lead overseeing all aspects of the dental team (e.g. including all dental specialities and the oral and maxillofacial team), while larger departments or teaching hospitals may have individual clinical leads for each of the dental specialities.

Managerial nomenclature

There is no longer a standard nomenclature for managers nor a standard organizational structure, and different trusts may use different titles. The directorate may be referred to as a division, with its lead clinician being called a clinical director or divisional director. The lead manager for a division may be called a divisional manager, general manager, or speciality manager. Usually, a general manager works at the clinical level and manages operational managers (often called speciality managers), who work alongside the clinical lead of the department (see Figure 4.1).

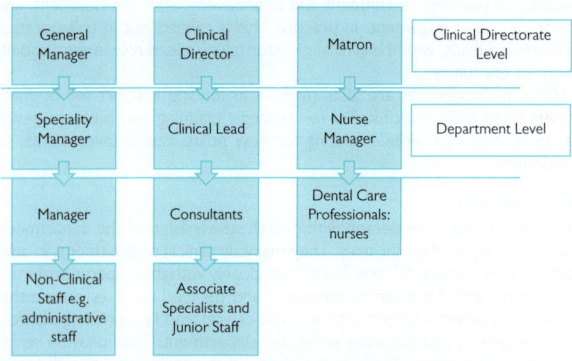

Figure 4.1 Dental department line management structure.

The wider dental health network

The government sets the overall dental healthcare policies for its country but the implementation of these is mainly carried out at a more local level. Each hospital trust must implement these policies but doing so requires the engagement of the wider dental network, outside of the hospital system. General dental practitioners (GDPs) form the main referral base for dental hospital services in addition to being the healthcare providers who carry out the majority of day-to-day dental care; thus ensuring that dental hospital facilities can focus on patients with more complex care requirements.

Local dental networks, local dental committees, and managed clinical networks all provide channels of engagement between local primary dental care providers and hospital consultants and specialists. This bidirectional engagement helps anticipate and respond to local and national concerns.

Managed clinical networks

The concept of managed clinical networks (MCNs) was initially proposed in the Scottish Acute Services Review published in 1998.

MCNs are defined as linked groups of health professionals and organizations from primary, secondary, and tertiary care, working in a coordinated manner to ensure equitable provision of high quality, clinically effective services. MCNs are not statutory bodies but instead are professionals in partnerships, often involving multiple specialities and levels of specialization.

The main benefit of an MCN is its inherent flexibility. MCNs can be disease-specific, network-specific, or in response to local healthcare circumstances. An MCN can be tailored to children's services, acute services, in response to the interests of the patient, the nature of a particular disease, etc. Clinicians may be members of multiple MCNs, which could be local, regional, national, or representative of a health board area.

MCNs are accountable to local dental networks (LDNs) via the LDN chair and in turn, to NHS England.

Membership of MCN

MCNs provide an inclusive network for stakeholders across a care pathway to meet and focus on patient services and care. Members include representatives from primary, secondary, tertiary care pathways from both the clinical and service provision aspects.

An endodontic MCN, for example, may bring together dentists with a special interest (DwSI) in endodontics working in primary care, secondary care restorative consultants, specialist endodontists, GDPs, community and special care dentists, dental public health consultants, patient representatives, practice managers, dental nurses, and more. It is a cross-representative group which facilitates discussion and resolution of issues such as access and provision of care, waiting list concerns and unsatisfactory referral pathways.

The MCN may establish a core group to lead the network which can consist of any or all the members (Box 4.1)

Establishing an MCN

NHS England's *Introductory Guide for Commissioning Dental Specialities* outlines that all dental specialist services are contractually bound to engage and

> **Box 4.1 Core group members**
> - Chair
> - Dental consultants—clinical and public dental health
> - Dental specialists
> - General dental practitioners
> - General dental practitioners with a special interest
> - Dental care professional—technicians, nurses, hygienist, practice managers
> - Patient representatives
> - Commissioning representative
> - Health Education England representative

participate within an MCN for that speciality. It outlines the core principles which MCNs must follow:
- The MCN must be managed
- There must be a defined clinical structure and strategy
- Use documented evidence base
- Must contribute to any multidental speciality, multidisciplinary, and multiprofessional MCNs
- Have a clear policy on the dissemination of information to patients
- Have a commitment from all health professionals in the MCN to practise in accordance with the network principles
- Have a quality assurance programme
- Develop its education and training potential
- All health professionals in the MCN actively participate in audits
- Have a continuous professional development (CPD) programme in place for all staff and ensure that staff are able to move within the network in ways that improve patient access and maintain professional skills
- Explore potential—allow professionals to explore better value for money, service improvement, and career opportunities

Aims and functions of MCNs

The main function of an MCN is to provide a working model where clinicians from all settings across the care pathway can liaise to focus on patient services. The type and function of the MCN will determine which stakeholders it predominantly engages with. MCNs should:
- Work with LDNs to contribute to local service planning and prioritization and to understand local health priorities
- Help meet the local dental service delivery objectives, by working with commissioners, Health Education England, and dental public health consultants
- Engage with local authorities and local health and wellbeing boards on oral health improvement plans
- Receive information on clinical needs, referral pathways, priorities, treatment outcomes, service delivery models, access to care
- Engage with stakeholders

Local dental networks

Integrated care across the community was an NHS aim as early as 2012 (Securing Excellence in Primary Care). LDNs, which are part of local professional networks, were one means of achieving this. LDNs were established to support the commissioning of local services, by facilitating the engagement of local dentists and other dental care professionals with commissioners. The rationale is that members of the LDN will have real-world information on the dental needs of their local population, and therefore a better insight into how the service should be designed.

Local dental networks are the dental local professional network (LPN). In essence, the terms LPN and LDN are used interchangeably in the context of dentistry. For reference, there are also pharmacy and optometry LPNs, which deal with primary care services only, whereas dental LPNs cover the whole dental pathway—primary, secondary, community, and out-of-hours care. This presents an opportunity for total integration of local dental commissioning and service design.

Aims and functions of LDN

- Support implementation of national dental strategy and policy at a local level
- Work with key stakeholders on the development and delivery of local priorities
- Provide local clinical leadership

The LDN liaises with:
- Primary and secondary dental care services
- Local authorities
- Public Health England
- Dental public health consultants

Composition of LDN

The LDN meets four times per year. LDN chairs attend a national assembly, also four times per year and hosted by NHS England and the office of the chief dental officer. Both of these meetings have attendees representing Public Health England and Health Education England. The LDN chair is accountable to the chief dental officer, the director of commissioning, and the local NHS England medical director.

The typical members of an LDN include:
- Clinical chair
- Manager from within the NHS England local team
- NHS England commissioners and dental leads
- Local clinicians from across the dental clinical fraternity
- Patient representatives
- Secondary care consultants
- Local dental committee (LDC) representatives
- MCN chairs
- Educational supervisors
- Others as agreed, such as dental public health consultants

Local dental committees (LDC)

LDCs are a distinct organization from LDNs but LDCs often have a role within LDNs. The LDC's role is to represent NHS dentists—those that have a performer number and work under general dental services contracts (GDS) or personal dental services agreements (PDS).

They exist in all four countries of the United Kingdom although provision in statute to be recognized and consulted exists only in England and Wales, since the NHS Act 1977. Nonetheless, local NHS representatives consult with LDCs in all countries on any matters of local dental interest.

The 110 LDCs across the United Kingdom are organized into regional groups:

- They offer advice to members, keep members up to date with new guidance, and facilitate feedback to NHS England or the BDA
- LDC members are represented on MCNs and LDNs, thus forming a cohesive link between primary and secondary dental services
- They link secondary care dental departments to their referral base in primary dental care, thus facilitating two-way communication
- Liaising with the local LDC, via an MCN can help resolve patient demand issues such as a service overburdened with referrals or a lack thereof

Further reading

British Dental Association. Local Dental Committees (LDCs). Available at: ✆ https://www.bda.org/about-us/our-structure/representative-committees/general-dental-practice/local-dental-committees/

Good Governance Institute. GGI Board Insights Paper 2: The Role of the Medical Director in the NHS. Available at: ✆ https://www.good-governance.org.uk/wp-content/uploads/2017/04/The-Role-of-the-Medical-Director-in-the-NHS.pdf

NHS England. Introductory Guide for Commissioning Dental Specialties. Available at: ✆ https://www.england.nhs.uk/commissioning/wp-content/uploads/sites/12/2015/09/intro-guide-comms-dent-specl.pdf

NHS Leadership Academy. The Healthy NHS Board 2013 Principles for Good Governance, 2013. Available at: ✆ https://www.leadershipacademy.nhs.uk/wp-content/uploads/2013/06/NHSLeadership-HealthyNHSBoard-2013.pdf

Running a department

Quality and performance management

The Next Stage Review, 2008 (The Darzi Report) emphasized quality as the organizing principle of the NHS, 'at the heart of all we do'. It insisted that quality be understood from the patient's perspective and defined it as comprising:

• Patient safety—doing no harm to patients
• Patient experience—compassion, dignity, and respect
• Effectiveness of care—measured using survival rates, complication rates, measures of clinical improvement, and patient-reported outcome measures

Performance management

Performance management is the establishment of a formal, regular and rigorous system of data collection and its use to indicate trends and measure the performance of services.

Performance indicators are commonly used across health and care systems to examine and compare performance. They either assess the efficiency of services or clinical performance and allow local (between trust departments), regional, and national comparison.

Performance management helps to:

• Identify areas of best practice
• Focus on continuous improvement and deliver improved outcomes
• Take action to improve patient care
• Ensure service aims/activity are in line with organizational strategy
• Provide an early indication of emerging issues/pressures that may require remedial action
• Identify the potential to improve the cost-effectiveness of services

Hospital performance measures

The manner in which the NHS measures the performance of a service varies over time, as it is subject to changes in policy, guidelines, or strategies.

Clinical quality and outcome measures

Clinical outcomes are broadly agreed, measurable changes in health or quality of life that result from healthcare services.

- They provide standards against which subsequent care can be compared
- They highlight areas for improvement or confirm a continued high level of care if the standards are being met
- They allow services to continually improve
- They are measured by activity data or agreed scales of measurement (see Box 5.1)
- Different hospital departments may have their own outcome measures, specific to their service and the conditions they treat
- Specific quality indicators for individual dental specialities are defined in the commissioning guidelines (see Chapter 3, page 46)
- Highly specialized services (see Chapter 3, page 54) will also define specific clinical outcome measures. Table 5.1 summarizes these for cleft services

---

Box 5.1 Examples of common clinical outcome measures

- Activity data, e.g. length of stay, readmission, or complication rates—for example, venous thromboembolism, mortality
- Adherence data e.g. guidelines, antibiotic stewardship guidance

---

Table 5.1 Clinical outcome measures used in the cleft lip/palate service

Standard	Explanation
Clinical nurse specialist visit within 24 hours of new referral	Enables the nurse to provide practical advice and reassurance, assess additional medical anomalies, coordinate onward referrals, etc.
Timely hearing assessment in children with cleft palate	Enables early intervention for hearing aids. All children to be assessed by age 1.
Further speech surgery following all palate repairs	Identifies which patients (type of cleft, severity) require further speech surgery, helping to plan services and guide families.
Five-year dental arch growth scores	Allows assessment of outcomes against the national average, demonstrate the impact of the cleft and surgery on growth.
Orthodontic Peer Assessment Rating	Degree of improvement resulting from orthodontic treatment for departmental measurements and national comparison.
CAPS-A speech outcomes	Speech assessment at age 5 using a standardized tool.

NHS Outcomes Framework (NHS OF)

This is a set of indicators developed by the Department of Health and Social Care to monitor the health outcomes of people in England.

- They provide national level accountability for NHS outcomes and are used to monitor the progress of NHS England, driving transparency and quality improvement
- They set standards that should be achieved but no prescription is given for how to do this; individual commissioners and trusts work with NHS England to determine the best way of meeting them
- All indicators are reported at a national level and the data is analysed according to characteristics such as age, gender, region, ethnicity, condition. Box 5.2 provides examples of some indicators included in the NHS OF, demonstrating that both clinical measurements and experience-related outcomes are recorded

---

Box 5.2 NHS outcome framework indicators

- Life expectancy at 75 years
- Infant mortality rate
- Employment of people with long-term conditions
- Emergency readmissions within 30 days of discharge
- Death from venous thromboembolism (VTE) related events within 90 days post-discharge from hospital
- Survival rates from all cancers (one-year, five-year)
- Incidence of healthcare-associated infection (MRSA, *C. difficile*)

Dental indicators include:

- Tooth extractions due to decay for children admitted as inpatients, aged 10 years and under
- Patient experience of NHS dental services
- Access to NHS dental services

Key performance indicators

Key performance indicators (KPIs) are a consistent way of measuring performance in the NHS. They help define and measure progress towards goals. They can also form part of the commissioning process to set targets which must be met as part of commissioning contracts. They are often the primary means of communicating performance across an NHS trust or between services. Examples of KPIs include:

- Letter turnaround time
- Length of hospital stay

Financial performance

Financial performance of a service includes the assessment of budgets or costs per episode of patient care (see section: financial management of a department, page 106).

Patient experience

There are several measures of patient experience:

PROMS/PREMS

PROMs (patient-reported outcome measures) and PREMs (patient-reported experience measures) are used to gather direct patient feedback.

- PROMs are measurable outcomes from the patient's perspective
- Data is collected through surveys and telephone calls
- While the focus is on the outcome, the questions assess the patient's health and function at certain points in time, thus giving an overall outcome of their treatment
- They evaluate the effectiveness of treatment
- PREMs assess the patient's perception of qualitative aspects of their healthcare experience
- Examples include staff introducing themselves, being seen in a timely manner, being reassured during their appointment, lay terms being used when describing investigations or surgical procedures
- They identify areas for improvement in healthcare services

The dental commissioning guidelines outline speciality-specific PROMs and PREMs allowing benchmarking and comparison between units.

NHS Friends and Family Test (FFT)

The FFT was launched in 2013 as a feedback tool to allow users to provide feedback on their experience. Revised guidance was implemented on 1 April 2020:

- The FFT must be implemented by all providers holding an NHS standard contract, a primary medical or NHS dentistry contract
- It uses a single mandatory question 'Overall, how was your experience of our service?'
- The six-point response scale is always the same, from 'very good' to 'very poor' and 'don't know'
- It includes open free-text questions, such as:
  - "Please can you tell us why you gave your answer?"
  - "Please tell us about anything that we could have done better"
- The responses to the FFT question must be submitted by the trust to NHS England each month, who measure an overall score which is published on the NHS England website
- Trusts must also publish results locally, in various manners e.g. updates on the trust's website, at patient meetings, or by displaying the 'You said—we did' posters in receptions and waiting areas

Staff satisfaction—NHS Staff Survey

- The NHS Staff Survey (NSS) is the primary method of collecting staff views about working in their organization
- It is commissioned annually by NHS England and the results are official publicly available statistics
- All NHS trusts are required to participate in the NHS Staff Survey
- The results are used to improve local working conditions and ultimately patient care
- It allows for the comparison of experiences within organizations and a comparison of organizations against the national picture
- Results are reviewed at directorate and department level

- The NSS questions are aligned with the People Promise. This is a series of aspirations that outline the actions and behaviours staff should expect from their employers and colleagues, as part of improving the experience of working in the NHS
- All staff employed by the NHS are eligible to complete the survey, including those on fixed contracts, on secondment between organizations or on leave (maternity/paternity/sickness, etc.)

Statutory and mandatory training

Appropriate completion of training requirements by staff members is important to ensure workplace safety and culture, and to avoid legal challenges for the trust:

- Statutory training is required by law. It ensures that staff have a healthy and safe working environment for themselves and their colleagues
- Mandatory training is determined by the organization based on local risk assessments and training needs analysis

NHS Performance targets/waiting times

Secondary care dental services are subject to national NHS performance targets. The most high-profile targets relate to waiting times:

- Elective treatment: 92% of patients begin treatment within 18 weeks of being referred from a GP to a specialist
- A&E: 95% of patients seen within four hours
- Cancer services: at least 85% of patients diagnosed with cancer begin treatment within 62 days of an urgent referral from their GP
- Diagnostics: less than 1% of patients should wait 6 weeks or more for a diagnostic test
- The figures above relate to NHS England. There is a target of 90% of patients to begin treatment within 18 weeks of referral in Scotland. For Wales and Northern Ireland the target is 95% to be begin treatment within 26 weeks of referral

Waiting time targets are constantly reviewed and often changed. For up-to-date information, see the www.nhs.uk website. See also chapter 5: referral management of dental patients.

Patient safety, Care Quality Commission, complaints and compliments, clinical governance

Other measures of a department or service's quality are described in detail in the following chapters/sections:

- Measuring patient safety (Chapter 6, page 170)
- The CQC—5 key lines of enquiry (Chapter 5, page 115)
- Managing complaints (Chapter 6, page 197)
- Clinical governance framework (Chapter 5, page 112) is used as a way of measuring and improving services

Referral management of dental patients

18-week referral-to-treatment standard

The NHS Constitution gives patients in England the right to access certain health services within maximum waiting times or for the NHS to take all reasonable steps to offer alternative providers. Patients have a right to start consultant-led treatment within 18 weeks of referral (or request an alternative provider). The 18 weeks referral-to-treatment standard was introduced in 2004. The 18 weeks is measured from the day the appointment is booked through the NHS e-Referral service or when the hospital receives the referral letter.

- This applies to services commissioned by NHS England only
- It does not apply to public health services commissioned by local authorities, maternity services, or non-consultant-led mental health services
- Each patient has a 'waiting time clock' (see Box 5.3)

The maximum waiting time for suspected cancer is 2 weeks from the day the appointment is booked/the hospital receives the referral letter.

Box 5.3 Waiting time clocks

Clock starts:
1. A care professional makes a referral to a consultant-led service or a referral management or assessment service, which may lead to an onward referral to a consultant-led service
2. A self-referral by a patient to these services, once the referral is sanctioned by a permitted care professional

A new waiting time clock starts:
1. If the patient becomes ready for the second stage of a consultant-led bilateral procedure
2. Following a decision to start a substantively new or different treatment that is outside the patient's treatment plan
3. If a patient is re-referred as a new referral
4. When a decision to treat is made, following a period of active monitoring
5. When a patient rebooks their appointment if they failed to attend their first appointment

Clock stops:
1. First definitive treatment starts or the patient is added to a transplant list
2. The patient is ready to return to their primary care practitioner for non-consultant-led treatment
3. A period of active monitoring is started
4. The patient declines treatment
5. A clinical decision is made not to treat
6. The patient fails to attend their initial appointment
7. The patient fails to attend any other appointment, once this appointment was clearly communicated to them and discharging them is not contrary to their best clinical interests

Since April 2015, there is no provision to pause an RTT clock.

Accountability to the standard

The National Health Service Commissioning Board and Clinical Commissioning Groups (Responsibilities and Standing Rules) Regulations 2012 (Amendment 2015) set out the standards for waiting times. NHS England collects and monitors waiting times against this by publishing monthly referral-to-treatment (RTT) data.

Breaches in 18-week RTT

The standard states that at least 92% of patients should wait less than 18 weeks. Historically, trusts were fined for failing to meet the RTT standard (up to 2.5% of income). This was stopped in 2017 due to the negative outcome of patients being prioritized based on meeting target deadlines, rather than clinical need.

Trusts that are failing to meet the target will undergo increased performance management from regulators; this could affect the trust's CQC rating. Locally agreed improvement measures would be instigated.

New approaches

In 2019/2020, the NHS National Medical Director recommended field testing new strategies to reduce waiting times, by placing greater emphasis on standards that improve clinical quality and outcomes and helping trusts modernize their care. An average wait target was proposed instead of an 18-week target. A trial period involving 12 trusts was started, measuring mean waiting times. At present however, the 18-week target is still in place.

Most waiting time clocks start with a referral from a general dental practitioner or general medical practitioner. However, referrals may also come from nurse practitioners, GP/GDPs with special interests, allied health professionals, A&E and consultants.

Referral management

Referrals to NHS hospitals for both dental and medical patients continue to increase. Management of referrals is a priority for trusts, as this controls capacity and budgets. It ensures that a service is operating at a satisfactory capacity level without excessively long waiting lists. Commissioners are responsible for ensuring that adequate clinical services are available to meet the needs of patients.

The 2010 King's Fund report 'Referral management—Lessons for success' identified ways to ensure a robust referral management system:

- 'A referral strategy built around peer review and audit, supported by consultant feedback, with clear referral criteria and evidence-based guidelines'
- Recognizing that there are risks at the point of referral, as clinical responsibility is transferred between providers
- It is not recommended for commissioners to introduce financial incentives to drive blanket reductions in referral numbers
- All referral routes need to be considered in a demand management strategy
- A total system strategy is needed, with partnership between primary, secondary, and community care
- Patient choice, quality, and efficiency must be considered

Electronic referral system (e-RS)

Referrals from primary care practitioners (GDP or GP) to secondary care providers were historically performed by the 'choose and book' service. This was a mixture of paper and electronic referrals.

As part of the NHS' 'Paperless 2020' vision, an electronic referral service (e-RS) was implemented. Over 25 million patient records were migrated to e-RS.

The NHS can securely integrate e-RS with other healthcare systems, thus providing benefits such as reducing the need to send patient referral letters and reducing demand on the NHS Telephone Appointment Line by directing patients to the 'manage your referral' website. Patients have greater flexibility to book appointments that are most convenient for them.

Due to the e-RS, secondary care services can manage referrals electronically; this reduces the processing time per referral. A standardized data set is required to submit a referral, thus reducing inadequate referrals with incomplete data.

Scenario—Dental waiting list breach

You are a restorative dental consultant and the waiting list for endodontic treatment in your department is about to breach the 18-week standard. How would you manage this?

> ### Points to consider
> - NHS maximum waiting time standards:
>   - 18-week RTT standard
>   - 52-week maximum waiting breach
> - Potential for harm to patients with excessively long waits
> - Reputation of the department/hospital trust
> - Current staffing levels
> - Need to deliver timely care without compromising treatment quality

Immediate term management
- Arrange urgent team meeting, with input from relevant clinical, management, and admin staff
- Validate the waiting list—by phone, letter, or validation clinics
  - Check that patients still live locally and want/need treatment
  - Some patients may have relocated or sourced treatment elsewhere
  - Check referrals are appropriate for services offered
  - Check all relevant information has been included within the referral, e.g. radiographs, general dental status, medical history
- Check existing clinic capacity is being fully used
- Consider letter of explanation to patients/referrers

Intermediate management
- Review (audit/service evaluation) of clinical activity to assess maximum capacity and current level of efficiency:
  - Number of clinicians and nurses
  - Number of clinical rooms/equipment
  - Number of clinical sessions available
  - Skill mix available—ratio of junior doctors/dentists, fellows, specialists, consultants

- Review timing of appointments within the clinics
- Change the clinical profile
  - Balance of 'new patient' clinics and treatment clinics
  - Adjust acceptance criteria to limit the number of new patients, e.g. only complex cases
  - Discharge those patients in 'active monitoring' to general dental practitioner, to be re-referred as needed
- Implement waiting list initiatives—schedule additional clinics to reduce the backlog. This can be done in the department with staff working overtime or in other trusts
- Close the waiting list—this should be a last resort and is generally not recommended, but if the service is severely restricted, it may be necessary to close the waiting list. Referrers should be informed and communications updated to reflect this, e.g. the website

Long-term management
- Formally change the referral criteria to reduce the number of referrals:
  - Liaise via the Managed Clinical Network
  - Educate referrers through training courses
  - Use an electronic referral proforma requiring specific data input to enable referral submission, thereby reducing incomplete or inappropriate referrals
- Increase clinical capacity and clinical efficiency to meet higher demand
  - Redistribute clinicians—for example, establish resident dentist clinics with a circulating supervising consultant (change in skill mix of clinicians)
  - Formulate a business case for increasing capacity with additional staff, facilities, and equipment
  - Standardise clinical protocols—clear, evidence-based guidelines for treatments and referrals can reduce unwarranted variation and improve efficiency
  - Extend appointment slots for complex cases—this can prevent repeat visits due to incomplete assessments or treatment delays
  - Use new technology—e.g. chairside digital scanning may reduce time spent on impressions or enable nurse-led records clinics
- Ensure that regular meetings are scheduled with management so that waiting list times can be reviewed. If there are any potential issues these can be managed proactively preventing waiting list breaches and using demand/capacity models
- Ensure that treatment is started (and completed) in a timely fashion once patients have been assessed. This could be internally audited

Scenario—Insufficient referrals

Scenario: You are a dental consultant working within the NHS. How would you manage a situation where there are insufficient referrals to your department and underutilized clinical capacity?

Patient referrals may sometimes undergo variation which is within a normal range. However, if through auditing patient referrals and the number of patients in active treatment, it becomes apparent that the department is functioning at a level below its operational capacity, it may be necessary to intervene.

Immediate actions
- Recognize that there are two issues—insufficient referrals and under-used clinics
- Check with the administrative team that referrals are being uploaded and directed to the appropriate consultant for triage in a timely manner
- Check if any contact details for the department have changed and ensure that referral information on the website is accurate
- Request that management gather information on previous referrals over a 5-year period, to examine patterns, and compare with current referral rates. Assess whether referrals were internal (from other departments within the hospital) or external. Look at referral patterns at different times of the year
- Assess which clinics are being underutilised and if it affects one clinician or multiple clinicians and what level are they e.g. consultant/trainee
- Check that all activity is correctly recorded to determine if the clinics are truly being underused. For example the patients being seen may be complex, requiring multidisciplinary care team (MDT) input but this is not being reflected on the appointment booking system or clinical coding. Ensure that all clinical activity and clinicians who see patients are accurately recorded e.g. ad hoc appointments
- Ensure that appointment letters are sent out in a timely manner, along with text message reminders. Review the departmental DNA (did not attend) rate
- Arrange a departmental meeting with all relevant consultants, treating clinicians, and the lead dental nurse to discuss the situation and identify contributing factors, e.g., changes in clinical practice, lack of equipment preventing treatment, or insufficient administrative staff for booking appointments

Determine whether there is a genuine reduction in referrals by assessing the local population and estimating the proportion expected to require your department's services. Review the original documents related to the commissioning of your service. Assess whether the assumptions on which they were based remain relevant to the current situation.
- Any local contributing factors (e.g. a local industry shutting down resulting in residents leaving an area, a lack of NHS dentists seeing patients and thus onward referrals)
- Changes in supply: has a new hospital or specialist clinic opened which may be treating some of the population, is there another department within your trust seeing some of the patients, has another nearby hospital changed their acceptance criteria/catchment area
- Consider a change in patient choice not to attend the department e.g. due to a previous long waiting list or departmental reputation. If so, engage with patient groups/patient representative on the trust board. Check if any issues were raised through the patient advice and liaison service (PALS)

Increase awareness of your department's services
- Liaise with the managed clinical network (MCN) or integrated care board (ICB) to ensure that local referring doctors and dentists are aware of the service

- Communicate with newly graduating clinicians through clinician forums/training programmes
- Establish a strong online presence with clear information about the services provided, the clinical team, expertise, and the referral pathway
- Ensure there is a well-functioning e-RS to streamline referrals
- Hold a department open day for patients and clinicians to visit the service and meet the team

Other things to consider:

- If you have trainees within your department, consider if they are getting sufficient clinical exposure and experience for their training. You may need to inform their education supervisor and training programme director. Trainees may need to attend another unit for sufficient patient exposure for training

Setting up a dental service

The aim of setting up a new service or modifying an existing one is to achieve a fundamental improvement in patient care, as well as the quality and sustainability of the service. Substantial service change generally refers to a 'substantial shift or variation in the way frontline health services are delivered, usually involving a change to the geographical location where services are delivered' (from: Support and Guidance Toolkit). Proposals for a new service or changes to an existing service require commissioner ownership, support, and leadership, even if the individual provider is the proposer and intends to facilitate the daily operations. This ensures that proposals are aligned with commissioning intentions.

From inception to implementation, a clear pathway is required (see Figure 5.1), this is applicable when:

- Setting up a service
- Service reconfiguration/substantial change
- Service decommissioning

Discussion and proposal

Assess clinical patient need

Clinical patient need may be assessed through:

- Audit referrals
- Joint Strategic Needs Assessment (JSNA)—local assessments of current and future health and social care needs, produced by integrated care boards (ICBs) and local authorities
- Survey referring practitioners, local GDPs, and GPs
- Review NHS policy documents and national surveys, such as the Adult Oral Health Survey
- Consider training and development needs, for example, the training of future dental specialists

Review the existing service provision

- What services are currently provided?
- What additional services are required?

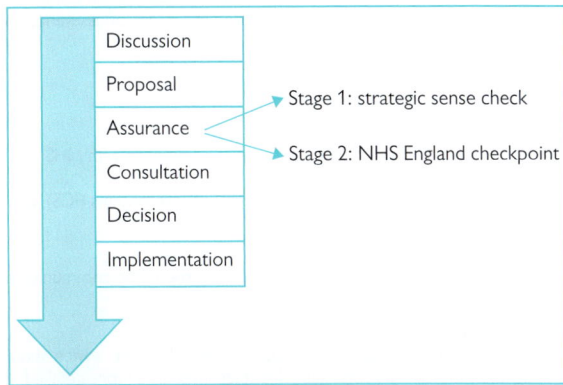

Figure 5.1 Phases of service change.

- What infrastructure is required to establish this additional service?
- Which other providers currently offer this service, and how is it delivered?

Decide what the priorities are for the new service
- Liaise with NHS England and local integrated care board (ICB) to help determine commissioning healthcare priorities
- Review Joint Health and Wellbeing Strategies (JHWS)—these are the strategies and priorities for addressing needs identified in JSNAs

Design the service
- A clinically led group should oversee the service design and development of proposals
- Engage internal stakeholders, both within the department/trust and with ICB
- Develop a business proposal/case that outlines a detailed case for change, supported by evidence and specific service configuration options
- Devise the financial proposals, outlining capital, revenue, sustainability, and financial targets. Capital financing proposals require NHS England approval

Assurance

NHS England assures service change proposals prior to public consultation. The assurance process is an objective assessment of the evidence for the proposal with considerations of cost, benefit, risk, etc. An effective assurance process gives confidence to staff, patients, and the public that the proposals are well-evaluated, will deliver real benefits and that all views have been considered.

Most proposal assurances take place at a regional level. However, some service changes require a more detailed level of assurance, including national decision-making and advice from Clinical Senates. Examples include large-scale proposals with significant financial implications or those involving multiple organizations and a broad geographical scope. These proposals require assurance from the Investment Committee or the Chief Financial Officer of NHS England. NHS England has a two stage assurance process.

Assurance stage 1: strategic sense check
This is a formal discussion between commissioners leading the change and NHS England. It determines the level for the next stages of assurance and decision-making. Areas of focus include:
- Alignment with the government's four tests (see Box 5.4)
- Proposal for change and options appraisal
- Potential risks, mitigating factors, and impact assessment
- Level of stakeholder engagement
- Required resources and capital. Discussions commence with NHS England finance teams at this stage
- Alignment between commissioners, integrated care systems (ICS) and other partners
- Development of a business case

The decisions made at the strategic sense check should be communicated formally to the commissioners in writing.

Assurance stage 2: NHS England checkpoint
This occurs before any public consultation. Clinical Senate advice should be sought for substantial proposals. This stage involves a more detailed assurance of the proposal. An assurance panel may be established by NHS

England. The financial viability, deliverability, and strategic alignment of the proposal, as well as its impact on other commissioners, will all be considered in relation to national priorities. The panel will deliver a report to NHS England with outcomes:

- Assurance received: NHS England advises commissioners can proceed
- Partial assurance received: commissioners can proceed but additional work is required on the proposal
- Assurance not received: NHS England advises not to proceed with the proposal

Financial proposal

Financial evidence must be considered at stage 2. If capital funding is required, NHS England will assess the proposal to ensure that the level of capital expenditure is affordable in revenue terms and will be sustainable. Service proposals must be assessed to be financially viable by NHS England prior to public engagement and consultation. Support for funding must be obtained in writing from NHS England.

A pre-consultation business case is devised and the proposal evaluated against the government's four tests of service change (see Box 5.4)

Box 5.4 All service change should be assured against the government's four tests:

1. Strong public and patient engagement
2. Consistency with current and prospective need for patient choice
3. Based on clear clinical evidence base
4. Support for proposals from clinical commissioners

Consultation

Following decision-making, the proposing organization announces the decision to the public for public consultation:

- Patients and the public
- Staff
- Media
- Health and well-being boards
- Local authorities
- Local Healthwatch and other relevant bodies

Decision

A Decision-Making Business Case (DMBC) is devised following the consultation and assurance process. This shows how all the views obtained have informed the final proposal and that the proposal is sustainable in service, economic, and financial terms.

A Strategic Outline Case for capital funding is then submitted to NHS England, once successful public and local authority consultation has occurred.

Implementation

An implementation plan is devised to outline the changes, responsible parties, and timeline. NHS England's local team will support commissioners during this stage.

Business plan and business cases

A business plan is a summary proposal for the overall development of a service or organization, while a business case is a structured plan or proposal for a specific aspect of the service.

The business planning process

Business planning is a process which integrates:
- Forecasting the types of service to be supplied
- The volume of demand for those services
- Assessing any internal demands on the service, considering available resources—including money, premises, equipment, staff and their specific skills
- The aim is to ensure maximum output, quality, and safety of patient care and customer satisfaction, within the boundaries of financial viability

The business planning process (see Figure 5.2) follows a logical system and may involve staff from clinical and support departments. This allows a thorough analysis, choice, and implementation of the chosen schemes. The aim is to answer three questions:
- Where are we now?
- Where do we want to be?
- How do we get there?

Within the business plan there may be several separately identifiable, fundable, and implementable schemes. Each of these will have a business case.

Mission statement

Every department, service, or trust needs a mission statement to plan successfully. This is informed by its values and the context within which it works. It should define the organization's purpose, provide an outline of its strategy, outline its policies and standards of behaviour and define its values. The mission statement is followed by the more detailed aims and objectives of the service.

External analysis

The STEEPLE acronym is used to identify specific outside influences on the service's ability to provide safe and effective services. The categories of external influences used are: social, technological, economic, educational, political, legal, and environmental. They can be used in the next stage, which asks, 'What is its impact on us?' and 'What are the options for dealing with that impact?'

Porter's Five Forces is a technique used to identify external competitive forces, including the threat of new entrants, substitute services, existing rivalry, supplier power, and customer power. It aims to answer the question: 'What are the external threats to our ability to carry on providing safe and effective services?' These are an essential part of answering the question 'Where are we now?'

Internal analysis

Internal analysis consists of a position audit or capability profile. This is a profile of the current service and provides a baseline against which the changes proposed will be measured. It covers:
- Resources: the finances and the staff

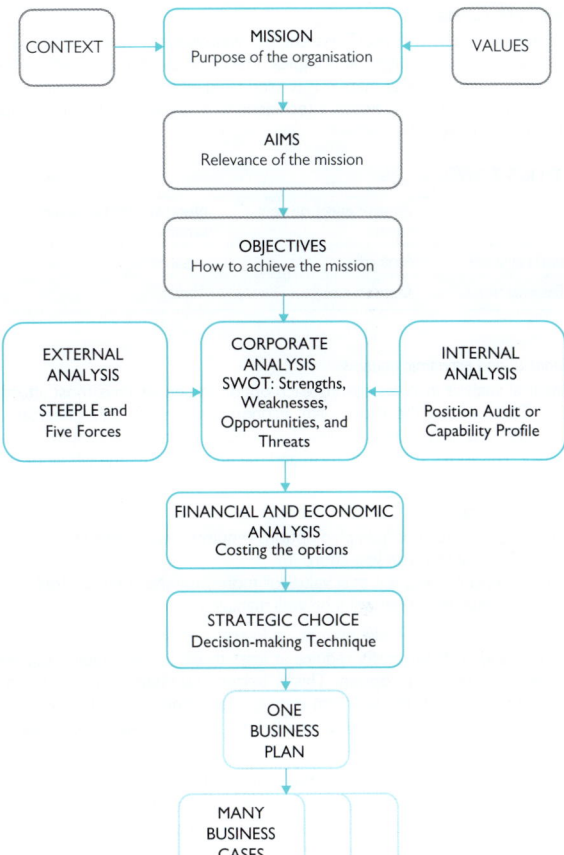

Figure 5.2 The business planning process.

- Services: how much work the service undertakes and what type
- Systems: the process by which patients are treated, often expressed as a care pathway
- Organization: the organizational structure of the service
- Results: the achievement of quality standards
- Returns: the financial over/underspend on the current service

Corporate analysis

Techniques such as SWOT (strengths, weaknesses, opportunities and threats) are used to organize complex internal and external influences on the service into a useful matrix. It is used to identify factors impacting the service as it currently is, not as a technique to analyse or justify any choice of scheme (Table 5.2).

Table 5.2 SWOT analysis

	Positive effect on your service	Negative effect on your service
Internal factor	Strength	Weakness
External factor	Opportunity	Threat

Financial and economic analysis

Financial analysis involves costing each option to see which is most affordable. This looks at the short term. Economic analysis is only undertaken for larger business plans and identifies which option is the best value for money. This looks at the long term and the effects across the whole of the public sector.

Strategic choice

Choosing between business plan options requires passing three tests:
- The financial test: can you afford it?
- The economic test: is it best value for money for the public sector?
- The management test: will it be well managed?

Where there are multiple options, a formal decision-making method is recommended. Most trusts require at least three options. Doing nothing should be listed as an option. This is better described as 'do minimum' as it involves doing the minimum required to maintain high-quality health services. Counterintuitively, this can often be the most expensive option.

Stakeholder involvement

If the business plan affects others, their input and advice should be obtained. This may be through discussion at a staff/consultant clinical governance meeting. Support teams which could be approached include finance, human resources (HR), IT, security, estates, the transformation team and information governance. A supportive letter from others may contribute to the business plan being successful.

Business case

A business case is a structured plan for development of a specific aspect of a service. It is a requirement in the NHS as part of the procurement process to support decision-making. A business case is required when requesting funding larger than a specified amount. This varies between trusts (usually £5,000–10,000). Below this, approval can be obtained within the department, usually by the service manager and speciality lead, as long as it is within the departmental budget.

Many NHS trusts have business case templates available on the trust intranet or from the service manager. This should be reviewed prior to

starting a business case to understand the information required. The template and process for approval may vary based on:
- Whether new funds are required or the existing budget can be used
- The value of the investment
- Whether it involves capital or revenue expenditure
- Whether it is an emergency business case

Higher value business cases have ten central aspects:
1. Executive summary: overview of the ultimate goal and the preferred option to achieve it. Provides a summary of the proposed option, financial, and non-financial benefits, KPIs (both financial and non-financial), quality/safety and productivity implications, management, project plan and the risks of not implementing the proposal. Details of meetings and the involvement of other staff are required to show support for the business case.
2. Profile/background: a summary of the service and how it currently operates. It includes the capability profile or position audit.
3. Strategy and goals: the organization's vision and future plans, the rationale behind them, and an indication of what success would look like. This includes the mission statement, vision statement, or statement of values. Each business case should show how it supports the department's or organization's business plan.
4. Market assessment: a high-level analysis of the current health economy including private providers, includes STEEPLE and Porter's Five Forces.
5. Service development plans: outlines how services will change and how this is aligned to the SWOT analysis.
6. Finance: evidence of how the levels of income and expenditure make the case affordable, including financial analysis. Funding may be available within the trust from existing revenue budgets, from savings or additional funds from commissioners or charitable sources.
7. Economics: how the long-term economic consequences mean the proposal is in the best interests of the public sector.
8. Risk: what could go wrong and how to mitigate against this. Includes the risk register.
9. Leadership & workforce: how your organization's management operates and the attitude surrounding the workforce.
10. Governance: the project plan for implementation together with details of how implementation will be organized and managed. Details of meetings and involvement of other staff are required to show support for the business case.

Trust templates may also require:
- An options appraisal—including impact on activity, research, space
- Proposed recommendation in further detail
- Equality impact assessment and/or health inequalities assessment
- Review of patient user experience
- Benefits realization and benefit owner assessment—detailing patient safety, quality, and experience
- Sustainable development considerations

Common components of lower value business cases include:
- Executive Summary
- Background and rationale for change

- Potential benefits
- Financial implications
- How it aligns with the department and trust strategy and targets
- Options appraisal, including the impact of doing nothing
- Impact on other areas of the trust: demand, capacity, resource
- Suggested implementation plan and timeframe

Most templates require designated staff for the project, including a responsible officer (usually the service or general manager), executive sponsor (if any), clinical lead, divisional lead, finance lead, and human resources lead. The acronym ROBRICES (reasons, options, benefits, risks, income, cost, evaluation, and stakeholders) (see Tables 5.3a and 5.3b) can be used to inform the contents of a business case.

Approval process

Prior to submission, sign-off may be required from the executive sponsor, divisional director of operations, divisional medical director, HR business partner, senior finance partner, head of contracts, commercial finance, procurement, and strategy. Additional supporting signatories may be required if other departments are affected.

Reasons for failure

Common reasons (and mitigations) for business case failure include:

- Failure to outline the mission statement—have a shared understanding of the purpose of the service among key stakeholders
- Failure to set the scene—identify the major drivers for change and present them in the most compelling way
- Failure to involve the team—include key decision-makers and stakeholders in evidence-gathering, analysis, and decision-making
- Failure to generate innovative options—create a long-list and narrow it down to an appropriate short-list
- Failure to appraise options—undertake an options appraisal of multiple competing options with many different features
- Failure to undertake a full financial and economic analysis
- Failure to make a decision
- Failure to undertake a sensitivity analysis—identify the robustness of the decision-making when subjected to changes in input assumptions
- Failure to assess risk and plan the project management—identify and measure risks inherent in the development proposed and appropriate strategies to manage them

External approval

For high-value business cases, external review is required by the NHS England Project Appraisal Unit. This is a team of experienced capital investment and estates professionals.

The approval authority varies by the financial value of the investment or transaction. Examples include the NHS England Director of Finance for the relevant region (£1 million) or NHS England Investment Committee (£20 million). Details may be found in the 'NHS England Business Case Approvals Process Guidance'.

Table 5.3a ROBRICES (reasons, options, benefits, risks, income, cost, evaluation, and stakeholder) assessment for common dental business cases

	New consultant	Cone-beam computed tomography (CBCT)	MDT clinic, e.g. hypodontia
R	Waiting list Provide training Safe service provision	Best practice Clinical need Increase income	Clinical need Develop/defend service
O	No change Waiting list initiative Locum Therapist/Hygienist New trainee Staff grade	Outsource	No change Outsource referrals
B	Reduce waiting list Increase activity/income Increase training provision Increase skills	Meet clinical need SEDENTEXCT guidelines Income generation Reduce review appointments	Multidisciplinary care Improve training Reduce patient delay
R	Lack of resources (dental chair, nurse) Increase cost	Training/installation Increase waiting time in clinic	Under-used Stretch current resources
I	Payment by results Private income Reduce RTT fines	Reduce outsourcing Private Income	MDT in PbR models Increase trainees
C	Salary Support Consumables	Installation Software Updates Training	Staff costs Reduction in other activity
E	Income Waiting List Reduced fines Appraisal	Utilization Income	Utilization Income Patient satisfaction Treatment time
S	MCN Deanery RCS	Radiology Primary care services/MCN Information governance team Immediate care team (ICT) team	Trust Patients MCN Deanery Restorative Department

Table 5.3b ROBRICES for common dental business cases

	Intraoral scanner	Surgical equipment, e.g. TAD kit, WAND
R	Increase efficiency Patient data protection	Improve patient care, safety, experience, outcomes Reduce treatment time
O	No change	No change Alternative equipment types if relevant
B	Patient comfort Facilitate virtual clinics Improve patient communication Clinical efficiency Reduce models storage requirements	Treat patients with greater complexity Increase quality Improve trainee experience
R	Information governance risk Training/installation	Training External validity of proposed benefit
I	Improve clinical efficiency and virtual clinic utilization	Trainee Improved clinical efficiency (more patients seen)
C	Capital cost Scanner tips cost Licensing cost	Equipment, training Infection control Sterilisation Consumable costs
E	Utilization Patient satisfaction	Audit patient satisfaction
S	Caldicott Guardian Information governance ICT/ICT security Records management Medical equipment safety team Sterilization team Patients Space management team Dental laboratory	Sterilisation Theatre staff Medical equipment safety team Dental nursing team

Business cases will be assessed, scored and prioritized against a standard scoring system based on the trust objectives with reference to the risk register. Final approval depends on the value of the investment (see Table 5.4).

Table 5.4 Examples of the boards that may give final business case approval

Board	Value
Executive directors	Up to £50,000
Capital control group	Up to £100,000
Management board	Up to £1 million
Trust board including CEO and CFO	£1 million +

Outcome

The following are possible outcomes of a business case:
- Approved
- Approved subject to timing of funding or partially funded
- Denied, subject to changes
- Denied

Implementation

Once approved, the business plan or case must be implemented according to the project plan submitted. The investment team will contact the responsible officer to complete a benefits realization, which includes confirmation that implementation of the project for which the business case was submitted is proceeding as planned. If there is any deviation, an explanation will be required.

Scenario—Introduction of new technology

You start work as a new consultant and would like to introduce intraoral scanners in the department to replace traditional alginate impressions. How would you go about doing this?

This is the 'shopping list' approach to planning which wrongly inverts the entire business planning/business case process. Instead, you need to demonstrate the process that led to the identification of intraoral scanners as the best solution, rather than deciding on a preferred option first and then seeking justification for it. The danger of inverted planning (justifying your choice after the fact) is that public money is spent on personal preferences, rather than on solutions that most improve patient care or efficiency.

Once this has been established:
- Check the trust budget/policy
- Research on intraoral scanners—are they currently being used in the department/dental hospital/lab, other departments in the same hospital, other departments in different hospitals? If so, which ones?
- Undertake a literature review, which scanner make/model is more efficient for your speciality, if the hospital is already using a specific scanner, is this manufacturer good enough for you? Will the trust allow the use of different makes of scanners in the same hospital?
- Discuss with colleagues within and outside the trust who may have experience or invested in this technology
- Discuss at a local consultant meeting to gauge views and experience
- If there is interest in proceeding, conduct further research into costs and support, involve the service manager, directorate finance team, information governance (IG), ICT, dental laboratory, and transformation team for advice

What financial aspects may you consider?
- Review your trust and service's current financial position. Are there currently any emergency measures for funding new equipment
- Financial information:
  - Initial outlay—cost of buying and installing the intraoral scanner
  - Running costs—data storage, manual storage of models, staff time/appointments, resources to set up and maintain. This may be presented as costs in year 1, 2, etc. following implementation

- Cost savings—this may be detailed in the 'do nothing/minimum option'—current and projected cost of impression materials, tray, fixative, disinfectant, nurse time, clinician time, transport to lab, lab technicians to pour, base, label, and store
- The cost of storage should be considered—saving on storage space internally and externally vs. paying for yearly subscription of software, data storage

What clinical governance aspects would you consider?

- Clinical effectiveness and research—conduct a literature review to assess potential benefits and risks. Discuss with colleagues in other units or seek advice from a professional society
- Information governance (IG)—seek advice from the IG team. As there is a change to patient data processing, a data protection impact assessment (DPIA) may be required. Establish how information will be stored, accessed, and retained within data retention guidelines. If data is being sent externally (laboratories), data protection agreements (DPA) may be required
- Risk management
  - Risk of no change—falling behind technologically, inability to use new technologies and treatment modalities
  - Risk of failure of the intraoral scanning system—a backup plan should be in place. Materials and skills for taking physical impressions should be retained
  - Establish how ICT support will be provided, internally or externally?
  - Update the business continuity plan (BCP)—this document contains critical information required for the service to continue operating during an unplanned event (e.g., loss of power)
  - The scanners should be placed on the information asset register (see Chapter 8)
- Clinical audit/service evaluation—this may help assess the effectiveness of current processes in regards to quality, efficiency and cost. Digital scanning may reduce issues related to distortion of impressions or delays in appliance manufacture. Prescriptions and scans can be sent to external labs within seconds, compared to the process of disinfecting, logging, and transporting physical impressions
- Education and training—consider the time required to train staff and the need to cancel clinics
- Patient involvement/benefits—digital scanning may improve patient satisfaction, comfort, and time efficiency, particularly for individuals with additional needs, a gag reflex, or trauma history. How will these benefits be measured—PROMS/PREMS? Is there supporting research available?
- Staff involvement/communication with the team—all stakeholders should be involved, this includes nurses, laboratory staff, clinicians, and administrative staff

What might you consider when deciding the make, model, and supplier of the intraoral scanner?

- The start-up and running costs
- Medium and long-term serving agreements/costs
- Licensing restrictions (number of scans)
- Ability to integrate clinical and laboratory processes
- Ability to integrate with the current 3D team—if present in the trust

- Ability to integrate with current electronic patient record system
- Associated software packages
- Acceptability to all clinical specialities and the dental laboratory
- Compliance with IG and GDPR
- The experience of the supplier in facilitating adoption of this technology in an NHS trust environment (particularly regarding IG)
- Whether suppliers are on the NHS suppliers list

Scenario—Increasing clinical capacity

You are the clinical lead of your department and realize that the pressure on the waiting list is becoming unmanageable, and your department is consistently falling short of trust targets. What actions should you take?

Immediate:
- Establish the trust targets, e.g. 18-week RTT
- Review the number of patients on the waiting list. Are they waiting for an initial consultation or to start treatment?
- Validate the waiting list (see scenario: dental waiting list breach)
- Establish why the waiting list has increased. Is it due to an increase in referrals or due to reduced clinical capacity?
- If clinical activity has reduced, establish the reason—will this be temporary or permanent?
- If there has been an increase in referrals—establish why e.g. changes to other local services, increased prevalence of a condition?
- If patients are waiting to start treatment, are we coding correctly?
- Can we stop the clock for some, e.g. start interceptive treatment
- Look at clinic utilization
- Review capacity of all consultants and clinicians, e.g. associate specialist, new patients vs. treatment sessions and review appointments
- Review capacity of trainees and therapists under supervision
- Where there is a risk to patient safety, take immediate steps—such as vetting and prioritising referrals
- Is there capacity and scope for nurse led clinics?

Short term:
- Review clinic capacity
- Gather further information to establish why the waiting list has increased. This may include an audit, service evaluation, discussion with colleagues and the wider team
- Can the team accommodate additional patients, e.g. 1–2 additional new patients per clinic. Consider adjunctive services e.g. radiology, dental lab, medical photography
- Is there a possibility to convert treatment sessions to new patient clinics?
- Backfill empty slots with new patients
- Consider nurse led clinics
- Audit and review attendance rates. Identify patterns and introduce strategies such as text reminders or telephone follow-ups
- Introduce virtual or telephone consultations to reduce pressure on in-person appointments

Medium term:
- If staff members are on long-term absence, a locum may be justified
- Consider if there are available clinical sessions which may be used

- Review team job plans to ensure that clinics have an appropriate balance of direct clinical care (DCC) activity
- Consider adding the issue to the risk register, depending on the impact on patient care. If there is a patient safety concern, this may need to be addressed as an immediate or short-term action
- Engage with local MCN/ICB to ensure referrals are appropriate and alternative pathways such as community care are being fully utilised

Long term:

- Business case for a new consultant/associate specialist colleague or if there is scope for supervision, a new therapist/trainee

How would you determine which type of staff member is required?

- An options appraisal would highlight the best option (see Table 5.5)
- Where the treatment waiting list is the concern, a therapist or associate specialist may be the most cost-effective measure
- A consultant would be required where new patient clinic/joint clinics are the concern

Table 5.5 Staff options appraisal

	Consultant	Associate Specialist	Hygienist, therapist, orthodontic therapist	Trainee
'Supervision	None. Increases supervision	Some supervision may be required	Supervision required, initial training time may be required	Supervision and additional time for training
Cost	Most expensive	Less expense than consultant	Less expense than associate specialist	No cost associated
Service development/ (SD), direct clinical activity (DCC)	Significant involvement in SD. 75% of activity DCC	Some involvement, 90% DCC	Limited involvement, all sessions are DCC	Some involvement (greater for post-CCST trainees) in SD. DCC variable as training time is required
Clinical efficiency/ flexibility	Greatest clinical flexibility	Treatment only	Treatment only	Treatment and new/joint clinic capacity. Variable increase in capacity—risk of inconsistent appointment or trainee experience/skill

References

NHS England Business Case Approvals Process Guidance. Available at: https://www.england.nhs.uk/bus-case/

NHS Standards of Procurement (2016). Available at: https://assets.publishing.service.gov.uk/media/5a8071c2e5274a2e87db9d90/Standards_of_Procurement.pdf

Procurement

NHS procurement

The NHS purchases large quantities of goods and services to enable it to run its day-to-day services. This process is called procurement.

NHS procurement is a complex area involving legislation, guidance, and policy. Advice should be taken from procurement professionals to avoid unnecessary costs and delays. NHS procurement is governed by both World Trade Organization (WTO), Government Procurement Agreement (GPA) and UK principles. These include:

- Transparency and fairness—procurement must be advertised appropriately, with clear information about the process, requirements, and evaluation method
- Proportionality—the procurement approach must be proportional to the risk and value, so it does not discourage bidders
- Non-discrimination—consistency of procurement rules
- Equity and equality—giving all providers equal opportunity

There are NHS Standards of Procurement, issued by the Department of Health in 2012 and since updated that define good procurement practice through 18 standards arranged under four domains: leadership, process, partnerships, and people.

Non-pay expenditure in the NHS covers all third-party expenditure. This includes all clinical and non-clinical supplies and services, pharmaceuticals, capital expenditure, infrastructure works, maintenance, utilities, rent and rates, healthcare purchased from independent sector providers, as well as professional services.

The NHS must be transparent about how it spends public money and awards contracts. This is so that it:

- Stays within the law
- Is fair to business
- Secures the best outcomes for patients and service users
- Assures taxpayers they are getting good value for money

The NHS in England must publish all procurement opportunities and the awarding of contracts above £25,000 on 'Contracts Finder'. Suppliers may search for contracts over £12,000 (including VAT) advertised by the government and its agencies. Scotland, Wales, and Northern Ireland have their own dedicated public sector procurement websites. This transparency facilitates easier access for small businesses and voluntary sector organizations to engage in NHS procurement, promoting fair and open competition.

A common method of buying products and services in the NHS is through framework agreements. Suppliers undergo a tendering process and meet the specified requirements to be accepted on a procurement framework. NHS buyers can subsequently place orders without the need for a lengthy full tendering exercise and they can select from the list of accredited vendors.

A trust is likely to have several procurement policies:

- Purchasing of capital policy—for expensive items due to last more than one year
- Purchasing of medical equipment policy
- Purchasing of supplies policy—for consumable items

In the NHS, organizations supplying any equipment or services must be part of the supply chain. This registration is required to ensure it is a legitimate entity to reduce the risk of fraud. It is important to avoid any conflict of interest between the applicant and the organization that is supplying the equipment/service.

Medical equipment

Aspects of medical equipment policy relevant to dentistry include:
- All medical equipment must be properly procured, maintained, and disposed of at the end of its life
- All medical equipment procured must be CE marked, meet relevant guidelines, and be suitable for its intended purpose
- All staff should be aware of the procedures to follow relating to procurement, repair, maintenance, and disposal of equipment
- All staff should be aware of the procedure for reporting medical equipment incidents, training for users and parents, requesting equipment repairs, and decontamination procedures

Purchase order process

Goods and services are procured in the NHS through a standardized purchase order process which works in multiple settings across the NHS. The names of the stages may differ, but the principles or purchasing remain the same. This applies for all goods and services and for all agency staff:
- Idea –what you wish to buy
- Specification—details of the product
- Quotes –a minimum of three competitive quotes from different suppliers based upon the same specification
- Check affordability—ensure adequate funds are available
- Purchase requisition –place an internal requisition to the supplies department requesting that they order it on your behalf
- Purchase order (PO)—the supplies department place an external order. This is the official, external, sequentially pre-numbered order
- Delivery—the goods or service are delivered. This may involve other services such as equipment setup, portable appliance testing (PAT), calibration, and staff training
- Delivery note—the goods or service may come with a delivery note from the supplier
- Goods received note—fulfil internal requirements to check that the goods are undamaged, of acceptable quality and follow local systems to acknowledge receipt
- Invoice—if an invoice is received, follow local procedures and, if necessary, authorize and financially code it and then send to the payments department
- Invoice matching—finance will carry out financial safeguarding checks, including checking that the goods or service were officially ordered. They may use a 'No PO no pay' system. Further checks will include that the goods have physically arrived, been checked and are of acceptable quality and quantity, and that the price is within tolerable limits of the original quotation

- Wait—finance will usually wait until the end of the 30-day credit period before making payment to a supplier
- Payment—transfer of funds from the organization's bank account to the supplier

Fraud

The scale of procurement means the NHS is vulnerable to fraud (see Chapter 7, section 'Fraud and bribery')

To reduce the likelihood of fraud, a standard control is separation of duties. This divides the process between two or more people so that no one person handles the entire procurement process. The most common separation is into:

- The person holding the budget
- The person getting quotations and placing orders
- The person paying invoices

Financial management of a department

The method by which NHS organizations are funded by commissioners for the work their services provide is often different from the way in which the services themselves are funded. There are a variety of payment mechanisms through which payments are made to organizations.

Payment mechanisms

Block contracts have been widely used throughout the UK and continue to be the main payment system for hospitals in Scotland, Wales, and Northern Ireland. In England, the national tariff (payment by results) dominated payments until the 2020 coronavirus pandemic. New, integrated models of care mean that other ways to pay providers may become more dominant.

Block contracts

A block contract is an agreement made between a commissioner and a provider to enable payment to be made in exchange for providing access to a defined service. This service is usually broadly defined. The block contract might include details of the volume of activity expected.

The value of a block contract may be determined based upon the historic cost of providing the service or through a zero-based approach, using evidence of patient need.

Advantages:
- The amount is fixed and predictable. The total financial value is known and services/trusts can plan with certainty
- The process is less time-consuming and more efficient to agree and implement. No time-consuming calculations are required
- Useful to maintain control of activity volumes

Disadvantages:
- The service may not be provided to the activity levels anticipated
- Does not take into account changes during the year such as increased patient demand or changes in the cost of providing the service
- Lacks financial incentives to improve efficiency or increase service volumes

Payment by results (PbR)

Payment by Results (PbR) is a system of paying NHS healthcare providers a standard national price or tariff for each patient seen or treated. A tariff is a standardized price list for payment to providers for completing procedures, interventions, and delivering services. A national tariff is used for much of acute care in England.

The national tariff comprises a list of Healthcare Resource Groups (HRGs), which categorise procedures and services into clinically meaningful groups, each with an associated price (See Box 5.5).

Advantages:
- The more work providers do, the more they are paid. This encourages providers to provide more activity and treat more patients. This can lead to reduced waiting times
- Payment at an average cost rewards lower-cost providers and penalizes higher cost providers. This can encourage higher cost providers to become more efficient

> **Box 5.5 The national tariff**
> - The national tariff is based on three aspects: classification, currencies, and cost and activity
> - Classification—Following discharge, a clinical coder uses the patient notes to classify treatment received into a standard format called codes. Two standard clinical classifications are used to cover diagnoses (ICD-10) and interventions (OPCS-4)
> - Currencies—A currency is a unit of healthcare for which a payment is made. The tariff currently uses HRGs as the currency for admitted patient care and outpatient procedures. Whilst treatment function codes (TFCs) are used to set prices for outpatient attendances
> - The price of each TFC varies based on attendance, clinic type or consultant speciality
> - The price of each HRG varies based on the diagnosis, intervention and complexity
> - Complexity may be based on age, complications, comorbidities or length of stay
> - Cost and activity data—Providers collect and record the cost they incurred by providing services. The national price (or reference cost) is based on either the average cost of providing services from a previous year, including inflation, and reduced by an efficiency target, or on a best-practice calculation

Disadvantages:
- Incentivizes activity rather than quality. Quality may be sacrificed in pursuit of volume of activity. Contracts pay for what is measured rather than what truly matters
- Organizations are incentivized to focus on delivering the contracted work, rather than prioritizing clinically necessary interventions or coordinating effectively with other providers
- Complexity may not be recognized and appropriately funded

Capitation

Capitation-based payment systems operate on a per-head basis. Commissioners agree fixed financial amounts within a contract to pay providers based on the number of patients who will have access to the service. The service provided is specified and the payment linked to the population covered by the service.

In England, most sustainability and transformation plans (STPs) aim to move towards an outcome-based capitation-based contracting system.

Advantages:
- Service providers have the flexibility to deliver care in a way that best meets patient needs and achieves optimal outcomes
- Joined-up working between and within organizations leading to more integrated care
- Low transaction costs, making it more efficient than other payment systems

Disadvantages:
- Providers are paid regardless of what they deliver—enabling them to provide as little care as possible to minimize costs

- Payment is based on the population and not the level of demand within that population. Changes in demand can cause challenges

Payment for performance

Commissioners reward providers financially for stretching performance or quality targets. Payment for performance schemes pay providers based upon an array of quality or performance metrics.

There are three categories of quality metrics or indicators used in payment for performance schemes:
- Patient outcomes, including those reported by patients
- Process measures, including measures such as waiting times and screening rates
- Clinical process measures

Advantages:
- Focuses relationship between commissioners and providers on improvements to the quality of service, both in inputs, processes, and outcomes

Disadvantages:
- Financial incentives are used to manage only those narrow measures which are measured, and quality of care overall may worsen due to perverse incentives

Understanding budgets and spreadsheets

Budgets are plans based upon estimates for the future. They include financial budgets, staffing budgets and activity budgets:
- Financial budgets—the financial plan expressed in £ and listed in detailed categories under pay, non-pay, and income budget subheadings
- Staffing budgets—the staffing plan expressed in whole time equivalents (WTEs)
- Activity budgets—the activity plan expressed in the activity measures relevant to the service

All three aspects of a budget must be negotiated and agreed on and in balance with one another. There should be enough money to employ the staff to do the work expected, safely and effectively. Budgets are often confused with allocations. Allocations are fixed, arbitrary, and imposed, while budgets are negotiated and agreed. Dental consultants should be able to interpret budget sheets to ensure the financial health of their departments.

Methods of setting budgets

Budgets can be set in different ways, usually one of:
- Historic based budgets—current budget is based upon last year's budget plus pay awards, inflation, agreed funded developments, less any cost saving targets
- Zero-based budgets—this year's budget is set based upon evidence, using best practice, forecasting activity
- Activity based budgets—rather than setting a fixed budget for the year, there is a standard cost for each unit of activity undertaken. At the end of each month the activity undertaken is counted, multiplied by the standard cost and that amount is the budget for the previous month

The meaning of income and expenditure

Income refers to the amount earned by the service, while expenditure represents the costs incurred. This is not the same as the amount of cash which has been received and paid, as there is often a timing difference between earning income and receiving payment and incurring the cost and payment. The budget/expenditure reports sent to departmental managers are created on an income/expenditure basis and not on a cash basis. They are not bank statements and do not show the timing of cash receipts and payments.

Plus or minus?

Accountancy uses debits and credits and not pluses and minuses. When reporting financial results accountants are faced with a choice: do they show the expenditure spent as a plus or a minus? Do they show income earned as a plus or a minus? Practice within the NHS varies, expenditure may be shown as a positive figure or blue/black/red. Negative figures may be in brackets or with a minus sign; before the figure (a leading minus) and sometimes after the figure (a trailing minus).

Financial year

The calendar year, tax year, and NHS financial year are all different. The calendar year runs from 1 January to 31 December. The UK tax year runs from 6 April to the following 5 April. The NHS financial year follows that of the UK Government and runs from 1 April to the following 31 March.

Income and expenditure

Budget statements are created on the accruals basis of accounting. This is not the same as the cash basis. The accruals basis of accounting counts each transaction at the point at which the value of the goods or service are transferred, not at the point at which the cash is transferred.

Explanation of columns on the Budget Statement

- Monthly Budget £—the total amount of money planned to be spent (expenditure) or earned (income) in the last financial month. It is not necessarily a twelfth of the annual budget, as the amount planned can vary over the financial year, such as summer or winter peaks or differences in income or expenditure due to the length of the month or number of bank holidays. This heading may also appear as 'Current Month Budget £'
- Monthly Actual £—the total amount of money that was spent in expenditure or earned in income in the last financial month. The calculation is based on the accruals method of accounting, recognizing the amount on the day that it is spent or earned and not the day on which the cash changes hands. This heading may also appear as 'Current Month Actual £'
- Monthly Variance £—the difference between the plan and the actual for the previous month. A positive variance is an underspend on the expenditure budget or an under-achievement on the income budget, or vice versa Budget − Actual = Variance. Sometimes this heading appears as 'Current Month Variance £'
- Monthly Budget WTE—staffing levels are measured in whole time equivalents (WTEs). One nurse working 37 ½ hours per week is one whole time equivalent, while two nurses working 18 ¾ hours per week are one whole time equivalent. The monthly budget WTE is

the planned number of hours in the month expressed in whole time working. This heading may appear as 'Current Month Budget WTE'

- Monthly Actual WTE—the actual number of hours worked expressed in WTEs. This heading may also appear as 'Current Month Actual WTE'. There are three possible actual WTEs, those of contracted, worked, or paid WTEs. Which WTE is used can vary by trust and would be confirmed by the finance team. Sometimes this heading appears as 'Current Month Actual WTE'. However, there are timing differences which may complicate this, such as additional hours one month may not be counted until they are paid in the next month. Staff on maternity leave or long-term sick leave may appear as 'worked WTE' when they have not been in the department for months
- Monthly variance WTE—the difference between the planned staffing levels and the actual staffing levels expressed in WTEs. This heading may also appear as 'Current Month Variance WTE'
- Account code—the part of the financial code which stands for the type of expenditure. Sometimes this heading appears as the line number or subjective code (as it is the subject of the income or expenditure)
- Account description—a description of the type of expenditure or income. This is often truncated due to a limit in the characters available. The finance team can list the items charged to each account
- Annual budget £—the total amount of money planned for the year, either income or expenditure. This is the total amount each budget holder is held responsible for. This heading may also appear as 'Cumulative Year Budget'
- YTD (year to date) budget £—the cumulative amount of budget which was planned to be appropriate for the financial months of the financial Year to Date. This heading may also appear as 'Cumulative Budget £'
- YTD actuals £—the cumulative amount of income or expenditure for the financial year to date. This heading may also appear as 'Cumulative Actual £'
- YTD variance £—the difference between the cumulative amount of budget and the cumulative amount of income or expenditure for the financial year to date. This heading may also appear as 'Cumulative Variance £'

Cost saving in a department

Making savings is often referred to as efficiency savings, value for money targets or cash releasing efficiency savings (CRES). Effective financial management involves managing patients, staff, equipment and materials efficiently.

Dental consultants may be required to make efficiency savings within their service. This can be a sensitive issue, short-term savings may lead to long-term costs, ultimately proving to be a false economy. Measures should ensure patient safety, quality, access to care, and staff morale. Examples of measures that may be taken include:

Review the current budget.

- All aspects of the budget should be reviewed and validated. Ensure that all expenses (staffing, consumables) or charges from other services (ICT, estates) are correctly allocated to the service

- Confirm if the budget is specific to your department and not shared
- Establish the payment mechanism—a block contract requires efficiency, whereas PbR may allow an increase in clinical activity
- In block or capitation funding, it may be possible to negotiate better funding for under-compensated services. Engage with commissioners to ensure funding reflects the true cost of services provided

Consumables:
- Review current stock levels—identify any unused or near-expiry items and adjust ordering practices accordingly
- Return unwanted or excess stock
- Review suppliers and negotiate better rates where possible. Consider re-tendering or bulk purchasing for cost savings

Fixed/building costs:
- Confirm the department/service is being charged correctly for any premises that it rents
- Consider relocating clinics—either physically or establish virtual consultations to reduce costs

Clinical/Staff efficiency:
- Review whether staff are being used efficiently, a service evaluation or audit may identify areas for improvement
- Provide training and support for underperforming staff
- If there is excess capacity, consider whether any staff would like to reduce hours, take unpaid annual leave or are approaching retirement. Such conversations should be undertaken sensitively, advice and support from HR should be sought
- Change timetabling to use staff and clinic capacity more efficiently
- Outsource services—e.g. dental laboratory or medical photography
- Repatriate outsourced services where cost-effective
- Convert locum staff posts into substantive roles, as this may reduce costs
- Adjust the workforce skill mix—employment of hygienist/therapist/orthodontic therapist or trainee
- Provide training to increase the skillset of nurses and other DCPs

Income generation:
- Ensure activity is coded and coded correctly to ensure payment
- Increase the services provided—establish MDT services such as hypodontia, orthognathic surgery
- Where clinic rooms are under-used, can these be given or 'rented' to other services
- Many aspects of clinical efficiency are common with referral and patient management—such as reducing DNA/short notice cancellations, appropriate clinic utilization, the number of review/follow-up patients, discharging where appropriate (see pages 85–86)

Increase private income generation:
- Explore dental research funding—apply for grants or funding for research projects
- Develop educational partnerships—CPD courses for professionals, a funded resident may bring additional income to the service or department

Clinical governance

Clinical governance is a framework through which the NHS continuously improves the quality of patient care. Clinical governance is considered to have seven pillars:

- Clinical effectiveness and research
- Clinical audit
- Risk management and patient safety (see Chapter 6)
- Training and education
- Patient experience and public involvement
- Information governance and management (see Chapter 8)
- Staffing and staff management (see Chapter 7)

There is some variation in these pillars and the following may also be cited: communication, resource effectiveness, strategic effectiveness, governance, and leadership and learning effectiveness.

Clinical effectiveness and guidelines and quality standards

Clinical effectiveness is defined as 'doing the right thing at the right time for the right patient'. It involves:

- Adopting an evidence-based approach
- Implementing guidelines and standards to ensure optimal care
- Changing practice, developing new protocols based on experience and evidence, if current practice is shown to be inadequate
- Conducting research to develop the body of evidence available

Clinical guidelines and quality standards

Guidelines are evidence-based recommendations on how clinicians should care for people with specific conditions. They may relate to providing information and advice, prevention, diagnosis, treatment, and longer-term management. Guidelines are not always appropriate for all patients and clinicians should use their judgement.

Quality standards describe priority areas for quality improvement in a defined area of health or social care and include:

- Quality statements—that are aspirational but achievable
- Quality measures—that can be used to assess the quality of care or service provision specified in the statement

Quality standards aim to:

- Enable clinicians to make decisions based on the latest evidence and best practice
- Allow commissioners to be confident that they are purchasing high-quality and cost-effective services
- Inform service providers and users the quality of service they should expect to provide or receive
- Allow benchmarking against other services

Clinical audit

Clinical audit aims to improve patient care and outcomes by reviewing current practice against a recognized 'standard'. Examples of standards include clinical guidelines, local policy, or advice issued by a professional body. It is often termed an audit cycle as further monitoring is used to confirm improvement once changes are implemented. The clinical audit process involves:

- Selecting a topic
- Establish a standard
- Data collection
- Analysing data against standards
- Implementing changes
- Re-audit

Quality improvement programmes

Quality improvement programmes (QIPs) aim to improve the patient experience. They involve reviewing current practices and designing ways to improve. Unlike clinical audits, QIPs allow creativity by enabling improvements in areas that might not have easily identifiable 'standards'. They involve incremental changes and measurements to test the impact of changes and are conducted over a longer time period.

They can be undertaken using the plan, do, study, act (PDSA) framework.

Service evaluation

A service evaluation assesses or measures current practice within a service. It helps to produce internal recommendations for improvements such as informing a business case. It is not intended to be generalized beyond the service area.

The differences between research, clinical audits, and service evaluations are summarized in Table 5.6.

Training and education

All staff should be supported to maintain competency and develop their skills. Professional development is lifelong and involves:
- Continuing Professional Development (see Chapter 7, page 285)
- Appraisal and Revalidation (see Chapter 7, page 244)
- Taking relevant exams
- Trainee management (see Chapter 9)

Patient experience and public involvement

Patient and public involvement (PPI) ensures that patients are involved in decision-making processes so that services suit them and it allows for feedback to improve quality and suitability.

This may be implemented through:
- Patient feedback surveys (see 'Patient experience', page 81)
- Involvement of PALS in handling issues with patients
- Local Involvement Networks (LINks) which enable communities to influence local services (previously known as 'patient forums')
- Foundation Trust Board of Governors who are elected by members of the local community
- NHS trusts will have patient groups who may be consulted
- National patient support groups, e.g. cleft patient groups

Staffing and staff management

This encompasses recruitment, performance management, encouraging staff retention by motivating and developing staff, and providing good working conditions. See staff satisfaction (page 81), and Chapters 7 and 9.

Table 5.6 The difference between research, service evaluation/improvement and clinical audit. Adapted from 'Defining Research' National Research Ethics Service

	Research	Service evaluation/ improvement	Clinical audit
Purpose	Conducted to generate new knowledge. Documented methodology which allows results to be extrapolated or applied from the study sample to a larger population	Define or judge current service, or deliver and measure improvements in quality of current service	Establish whether the quality of a service meets a defined standard Produce information to inform delivery of best care
Question/ hypothesis	Generate a new hypothesis or test a hypothesis	'What standard does this service achieve?' Seeks to improve within that service only	'Does this service reach a pre-established standard?'
Aim	Clearly defined aims and objectives to answer a specific research question(s)	Measures current service without reference to a standard	Measures against a standard
Interventions	Involves evaluating or comparing interventions. Not all research involves interventions	Intervention already in use or new in that context only. Treatment choice based on guidance, professional standards, and/or patient	Intervention already in use only. Treatment choice based on guidance, professional standards, and/or patient
Data	Usually involves collecting data that are additional to those for routine care or service	Usually involves analysis of existing data but may also include administration of interview/ questionnaire	Usually involves analysis of existing data but may include administration of interview/ questionnaire
Participant allocation	May involve allocation to an intervention	No allocation. Intervention chosen independent of the service evaluation	No allocation. Intervention chosen before audit
Randomization	May involve randomization	May involve randomization for sampling, but not for treatment	May involve randomization for sampling, but not for treatment

CQC and dentistry

The Care Quality Commission (CQC) is the independent healthcare regulator in England (see also: Chapter 2; NHS Regulators; CQC). It has been a legal requirement for primary care dental services to register with the CQC since April 2011. The CQC shares information with other organizations and has a Memorandum of Understanding with the General Dental Council (GDC) and the Parliamentary and Health Service Ombudsman. When inspecting dental practices, inspectors are accompanied by dental advisors.

CQC inspection

The CQC carries out inspections that focus on assessing whether the care is safe, effective, caring, responsive, and well-led. These five domains/standards are further divided into questions called 'key lines of enquiry' (see Box 5.6). These each have prompts, questions, and potential sources of evidence to direct the CQC inspection.

Box 5.6 Sample of some key line of enquiry questions

Safe

- Safeguarding and protection from abuse in all systems, processes, and practices
- Managing risks—how are they assessed, mitigated, and monitored
- Safe care and treatment
- Medicines management
- Cleanliness and infection control
- Safe equipment
- Learning when things go wrong

Effective

- Assessing needs and delivering evidence-based treatment
- Monitoring outcomes
- Ensuring and updating staff skills and knowledge
- All staff and teams working together
- Health promotion and prevention

Caring

- Patients treated with kindness, respect, compassion
- Patients actively involved in making decisions about their care
- Patients' dignity, independence, and privacy respected

Responsive

- Do patients receive personalized care that is responsive to their needs?
- Are complaints and concerns listened to?
- Timely access to care and treatment

Well-led

- Clear vision to deliver high-quality care
- Governance framework suitable, clear responsibilities, risks and regulatory requirements understood
- Service users engaged
- Does the service strive to continually improve?
- Culture of the organization

The principles of CQC visits:
- Visits are unannounced unless there is a significant reason to inform the hospital/clinic in advance. This ensures that CQC can see a true representation of normal daily activities
- Most clinics, hospitals, and social care services are visited once per year
- There are three possible types of visits:
  - Themed: these look at a specific theme in response to current issues
  - Responsive: a visit at any time in response to an identified outcome or if serious concerns
  - Scheduled: the visit is planned in advance but is carried out at any time
- The CQC continually review the information which they hold about a service from sources such as inspection reports, contract monitoring reports, information from the public and from reports which the service themselves submits to CQC (such as complaints, safeguarding issues, etc.). This information is used to determine which type of inspection the CQC will plan
- The inspector will decide which key line of enquiry their visit is focused on

A four-point rating scale is used to issue an outcome: outstanding, good, requires improvement, and inadequate.

Outcomes from CQC inspection if concerns are identified
- Issuing warning notices—notifying a provider that they are not complying with a standard/legal requirement
- Civil law enforcement action—by imposing or changing a condition of registration, suspending or cancelling a provider's registration
- Criminal law proceedings—if harm has been caused to patients or statutory obligations were not met. This may lead to a fixed penalty notice, caution, prosecution, court conviction, or imprisonment

Updates to the CQC inspection process

The CQC has been developing a new inspection framework (CQC pyramid, see Figure 5.3), with pilots started in August 2022. It moves away from routine inspections and towards people's experience of the service. The rating scale (outstanding, good, requires improvement, inadequate) remains the same along with the five questions of: safe, effective, caring, responsive, well-led. However, the assessment process is changing.

CQC single assessment framework
The CQC is changing from three assessment frameworks (for hospitals, adult social care and primary medical services) to a single framework. This will establish one assessment process, set of expectations, and definition of good-quality care. The 'specific evidence and quality indicators' pyramid layer (see Figure 5.3) will gather and assess data specific to the individual service.

Topic areas for assessment
There are currently around 335 key lines of enquiry and prompts. These will be streamlined into six core elements, which represent the 'evidence' section in the CQC pyramid (see Figure 5.3).
1. People's expectations
2. Feedback from staff and leaders

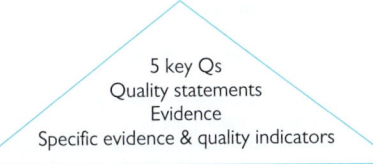

5 key Qs
Quality statements
Evidence
Specific evidence & quality indicators

Figure 5.3 CQC pyramid.

3. Feedback from partners
4. Observation
5. Processes
6. Outcomes

Quality statements are being introduced, using 'I' and 'we' statements. This is to focus on person-centred care, for example 'I have a care plan that is seamlessly transferred between different services' and 'we as a hospital work in partnership with other care services'.

Nature and timing of inspection
The physical inspection of a premises will be one component of a broader assessment process. A rolling assessment of quality and risk will occur. Other assessment methods will be used such as surveys, focus groups, feedback from staff and submitted evidence.

Preparing the department for a CQC visit

A hospital and department that fosters a culture of openness, transparency, and honesty and which has robust reporting systems in place should not need to do any additional preparation for an inspection. Staff should be up-to-date with required training and the hospital should be operating safely and efficiently.

Throughout the year
- Ensure that reporting of notifications is continuous, so the CQC have a clear picture of the service
- Ensure that there is a clear framework in place for learning from any incidents and action taken to further minimize risks
- Ensure that regular patient feedback is invited
- Ensure that any patient information documents, posters, guidelines are contemporaneous
- Ensure that key documents are prepared, for example, significant event forms, audits, outcomes, risk assessments, health and safety documents, staff training logs, policies and procedures, action plans from previous surveys, learning from complaints, minutes of clinical governance minutes

General preparation suggestions
- Staff are dressed in appropriate clinical uniform and wearing name badges
- Notice boards are up-to-date
- Alcohol gel is available in appropriate locations and immediately upon entry

- Offices are neat, tidy, and secure
- Staff are confident in how to raise concerns and how to locate hospital policies. They are familiar with their line manager and how to reach them
- Staff are familiar with the incident reporting system
- Appraisals and mandatory training are up-to-date
- Staff are aware of hospital and departmental activity, for example, concerns that have been raised, patient safety initiatives, lessons being shared, etc. Staff are not required to have an in-depth knowledge of the hospital service but to understand their own area and where to access further information and how to escalate concerns

During a CQC visit
- The members from the CQC team will introduce themselves, provide identification and ask to speak to the nominated/senior individual in charge
- They will confirm if the visit is scheduled, themed or responsive and which standards they are inspecting
- A room will be required to host them for their visit
- Patient care and clinical activity should not be interrupted but continue as usual
- The CQC visitors may wish to undertake 'process tracking' and process map the service by following a patient's route through the service or focus on one specific area of it
- They will have both formal and informal discussions with staff, service users, etc.

At the end of an inspection
- Feedback will be provided and the inspectors will use a 'judgement framework' to decide if a service is meeting each regulation
- Findings from the inspection will be shared. If regulations are not being adequately met, the level of discrepancy will be outlined (mild/moderate/major) and an action plan devised
- A formal report will be sent in due course
- The CQC website will display the findings from the inspection and give the hospital/service an overall rating
- Compliance or enforcement action may be taken if there are serious breaches of regulations. If deemed to be high risk and unsafe, the service could be shut down or prevented from seeing patients

Leadership and management

There have been a number of high-profile cases in healthcare where patient safety/care have been compromised, often over many years. These have been attributed, at least in part, to failures in leadership which is why aspects of leadership feature on the healthcare landscape. Management and leadership is one of the learning domains in the General Dental Council's framework. Leadership in the dental setting is a unique combination of needing the skills to deliver effective patient care while also running a successful department.

There is a difference between management and leadership:
Management involves:
- Implementing policies, procedures, and systems to optimize processes and achieve desired outcomes
- Focusing on planning, organizing and coordinating activities
- Aiming to achieve specific goals and objectives
- Managers typically oversee day-to-day operations

Leadership involves:
- Inspiring, influencing and motivating individuals/groups to work towards a shared vision or common goals
- Leaders set overall direction, vision and drive organizational change
- Approach challenges and problems with a focus on innovation, adaptation, creativity, and long-term vision
- Leaders are comfortable navigating uncertainty and ambiguity

Levels of leadership

Levels of leadership (see Figure 5.4) have been outlined, each representing a progression in leadership development, and deeper engagement at each stage (Maxwell 2013).
1. Positional—leadership derives from job title or position. Compliance is often driven by authority rather than genuine commitment.
2. Permission—leaders establish rapport and trust based on relationships rather than mandates. People give the leader permission to lead them.
3. Production—leaders showcase results and efficacy, earning respect through demonstrated competence and achievement. People follow level 3 leaders because of their track record.
4. People development—leaders prioritize nurturing and empowering team members, fostering growth and a culture of mentorship and development.
5. Pinnacle—pinnacle leaders are the highest level of leadership, leaving a lasting impact and creating a legacy of positive change and empowerment. This is the hardest level to attain. Followers are inspired by the leader's character and vision.

Leadership styles

These are approaches that reflect the leader's behaviour, attitudes, and interactions with the wider team (see Box 5.7).

Managing change

Embracing change in everyday clinical practice is essential to ensure that patients receive the best possible care. It means adopting new treatment modalities, understanding, and applying innovative technologies, and

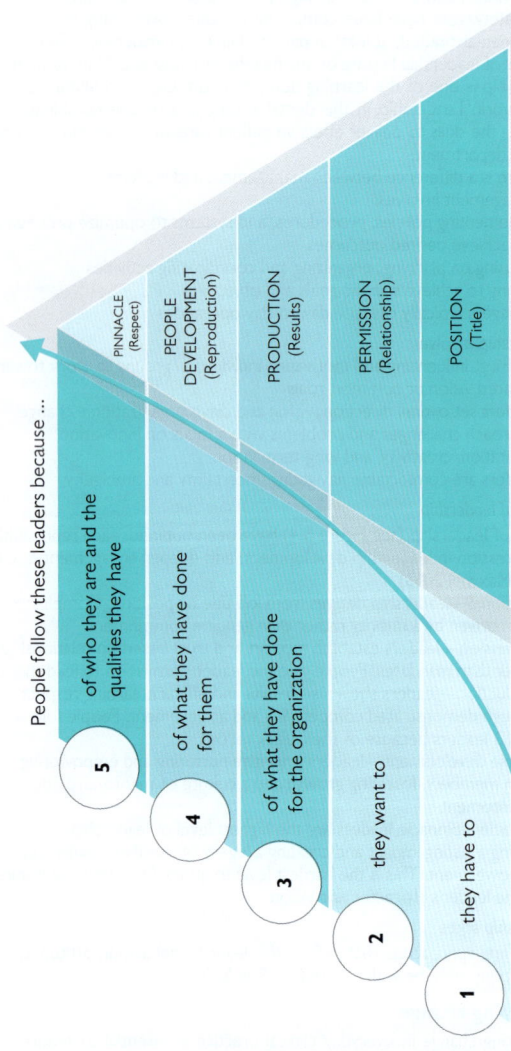

Figure 5.4 Maxwell's 5 levels of leadership.

> **Box 5.7 Styles of leadership**
>
> **Autocratic** (authoritarian): centralized decision-making and minimal input from team. Relies heavily on the leader's directives.
>
> **Democratic**: encourages participation and collaboration, fostering a sense of ownership and engagement. The leader makes the final decision, having taken soundings from others in the team.
>
> **Laissez-faire/delegative**: delegates authority to team members, allowing them significant freedom to make decisions.
>
> **Transformational**: inspire and motivate their teams through a compelling vision, encouraging innovation and collective achievement.
>
> **Transactional**: focus on setting clear expectations and providing rewards or consequences based on performance. It is a results-driven approach. It is particularly effective in situations where tasks are routine or require strict adherence to procedures.
>
> **Servant**: prioritize serving the needs of their team members and patients and facilitating their development by providing guidance and emotional support to help them succeed. A servant leadership style is seen as advantageous in dentistry (Certosimo 2009).
>
> **Situational**: adapt to the often-changing needs of their teams. The leader is flexible and understands that different situations demand a different type of leadership.

understanding updated clinical guidelines and protocols. Outside the clinical sphere, organizations are also changing, often as part of a wider improvement and efficiency plan.

Change management models

Change management requires a structured approach to guiding individuals, teams, and organizations through transitions from the present to future state to achieve successful outcomes. There are many change management models. Examples include:

- Kotter's 8-Step Change Model: Developed by Dr John Kotter, this model provides a step-by-step approach to leading change
- ADKAR Model: ADKAR stands for awareness, desire, knowledge, ability, and reinforcement. These highlight the five key elements required to implement change
- Lewin's Change Management Model: This model highlights three stages: unfreezing, changing, and refreezing to capture the future state
- PDSA (plan—do—study—act) cycle: this is a dynamic framework which enables testing of change initiatives which can identify problems. It focuses on the translation of ideas into measurable actions (see Figure 5.4)
  - Plan: identify objectives and potential solutions
  - Do: the plan is implemented on a small scale. This allows for testing without widespread impact, reducing potential risks
  - Study: analysing the results and outcomes, assessing whether the interventions achieved the desired improvements and identify any unexpected consequences or barriers
  - Act: integrating the lessons learned and making adaptations as needed

Regardless of the model chosen, there are key features which any change management process should have (see Box 5.8).

> **Box 5.8 Important considerations when managing change**
> - Clear vision and objectives—Define the objectives and ensure that everyone understands the purpose, vision, and direction
> - Clear communication—Communicate openly and transparently throughout the change process. Address concerns, share relevant information, and provide regular updates. This helps to build trust and alleviate uncertainty
> - Involvement and participation—Involve the team in the change process. This helps to instil a sense of ownership and commitment
> - Skill Development—Identify the skills and competencies required for the change. Provide training and support to help individuals acquire these necessary skills
> - Monitoring—Establish mechanisms for monitoring progress and assessing the impact of the change

Motivators and resistance to change

Change management is a continuous process, recognizing that change is inevitable and requires ongoing evaluation and adjustment. It relies on external and internal motivators:
- External motivators such as pay, reward, and recognition
- Internal motivators are linked to values and personal satisfaction in completing meaningful tasks
- Change management works when both co-exist

Without a clear vision for change and effective communication, the pace of change can falter. It is important that everyone understands the purpose and benefits of the proposed changes. Without this, there is likely to be resistance to change. Human beings are naturally resistant to change, especially when it disrupts established routines or threatens perceived stability. Resistance can also stem from fear of the unknown, loss of control, or scepticism about the benefits of the change.

References

Certosimo F (2009). The servant leader: a higher calling for dental professionals. *J Dent Educ*, 73:1065–8.

Maxwell JC (2013). *The 5 Levels of Leadership: Proven Steps to Maximize Your Potential*. New York: Center Street.

Artificial intelligence and dentistry

AI refers to computer systems being able to think like and perform tasks in an intelligent manner, similar to humans. Machine learning (ML) is a method by which computer systems can learn autonomously and not rely on explicit instructions provided by humans. Deep learning is a subset of ML, and uses multilayered neural networks to simulate the complex decision-making power of the human brain.

Generative AI is a subset of AI whereby computer systems can create new data and content including text, images, and videos. One of the earlier applications of Generative AI was DALL-E, released in January 2021, which could create images based on descriptions provided as text. The technology really came into the public spotlight when OpenAI released a chatbot, called ChatGPT in November 2022. Touted as something that can pass medical and law exams, help write a presentation or essay, and transform many jobs, it reached a million users in less than one week after launch (Statista, 23 January 2023).

How can AI help hospitals and dentistry?

While AI and related technologies holds much promise, it is not a silver bullet that will magically transform a dental department in a hospital. AI can help, and by considering two dimensions which come together, it creates a framework to help identify use cases (see Figure 5.6 and Box 5.9).

The first dimension is the 'areas' non-clinical or back-office, increasing productivity and enhancing the delivery of care. The second is the 'stages' of the patient's journey when receiving care—plan, prevent, deliver, and manage (see Figure 5.5 and Box 5.9).

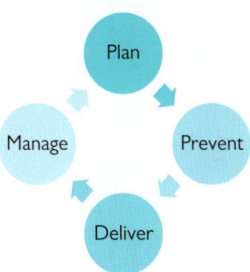

Figure 5.5 The stages of the patient's journey.

What are the challenges and considerations?

Healthcare settings are complex and sensitive, and the successful adoption and scaling of AI has challenges that can be identified across three categories—people, systems, and technology.

1. People (clinicians, operational admin staff, patients and families)
- Users need to be able to understand, trust and have confidence in the output of the solutions

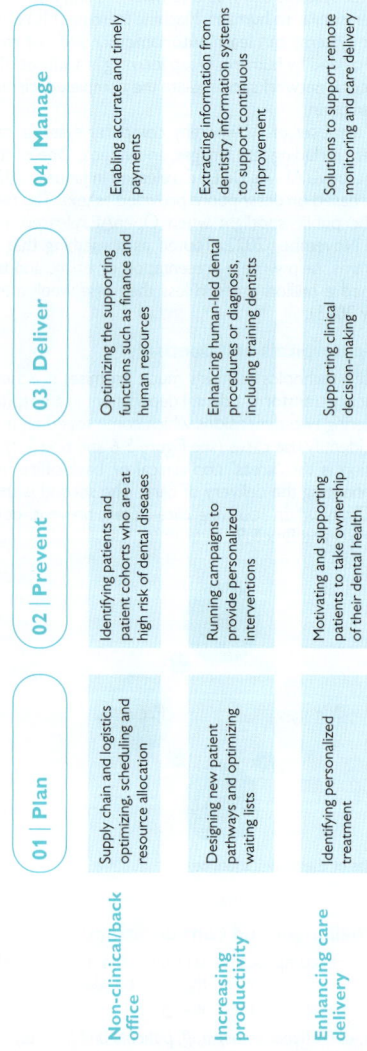

Figure 5.6 Framework for uses of AI.

Reproduced from Gunatilleke, J., 2023. AI in dentistry: understanding and realising its full potential. *Faculty Dental Journal*, 14(3), pp. 108–11.

> ## Box 5.9 Examples of AI use cases within dentistry
>
> ### Waiting list optimization
> There are several challenges with long waiting times: the patient's condition can deteriorate, the optimal timing for treatment such as orthodontics may be missed, GDPs may send referrals earlier than needed to compensate for a long wait time which further increases the list length and number of rejections.
>
> AI can help 'order' waiting lists based on risk and clinical need, rather than when a patient was referred. It can also help predict patients that are likely to not attend for appointments and allow proactive communication to reduce the likelihood.
>
> ### Motivating and supporting patients take ownership of their dental health
> Suboptimal basic oral health and diets high in sugar are still prevalent issues in dentistry. Dentists may not have the time or adequate incentives to support behavioural change.
>
> AI powered chatbots that interreact with patients and prompt, remind and coach patients in an individualized way (adapting based on responses) could help.
>
> ### Identifying patients and patient cohorts who are at high risk of dental diseases
> With increasing demand and long waiting lists, acceptance criteria for treatment in dental departments are skewed towards complex cases.
>
> AI can support more sophisticated risk stratification of patients to identify patients that should be treated within a hospital dental department, when they should be treated and help identify patients that don't meet the criteria immediately but are likely to need treatment in the future (see Box 5.10).
>
> ### Enhancing human-led dental procedures or diagnosis, including training dentists
> AI could support dentists identify pathology in diagnostic images or plan orthodontic procedures based on outcome prediction or implant planning based on optimal placement.

- The relevant individuals need to have the knowledge and confidence to make informed decisions on what solutions to buy and use
- Stretched frontline staff need headspace and protected time to engage with the development and to support implementation of AI solutions

2. *Systems (deployment ecosystem e.g. NHS hospital, dental department)*

- AI solutions need to integrate into established dental pathways and with the wider healthcare processes within a hospital, and to not cause extra burden or demand
- AI solutions need to comply with legislation and regulations including data privacy, patient safety, and medical devices
- Compliance with public procurement rules and alignment with funding flows and mechanisms

3. Technology (the solution itself, the data input it requires and other systems that it needs to 'talk to')

- AI solutions require access to high-quality input data, which must be available as regularly as required
- To prevent manual work and errors, the solution needs to be connected with other relevant systems to access input data and share results
- The data feeding the systems needs to consider and overcome potential biases. The solution also needs to account for local demographics and different patient cohorts

How can we increase the likelihood of success with AI?

Following the subsequent three steps when designing, deploying, and operating AI will help to increase the likelihood of successful adoption and incorporation into the workplace.

1. Solve a real problem (the importance of the use case)

- Always start with the problem you are trying to solve and don't get carried away with technology or the solution, no matter how exciting it might be (success is unlikely if trying to shoehorn a solution into a problem)
- In an environment where there are lots of challenges, pick a problem that is important enough to get the resources it needs and where the impact makes the most difference
- Think strategically and develop a 'roadmap', start with quick(er) wins that will have an impact and help get buy in for more complex and ambitious initiatives later

2. Consider the lifecycle of AI solution development

- The lifecycle has several stages and five groups of stakeholders that need to work together (see Figure 5.7)
- At each intersection in the grid, there are key activities that need to be completed
- It is important to consider a pilot phase before full implementation
- Dentistry operators and systems (i.e. department managers, clinical leaders) have responsibilities to help develop the business case, make sure the solution meets requirements, and allocate resources needed to deploy, evaluate, monitor, and improve the solution

3. Strengthening the enablers (organizational, regional, or national level)

- The enablers include access to good data, compliance with regulation, collaboration, integration with existing workflows, and robust underlying infrastructure. Staff need to have the skills to support implementation and use
- Some of the required enablers can be provided by an individual hospital organization; some requires national level policy making, decisions, and funding
- Linking up with other hospital departments and supporting functions (e.g. IT, finance, procurement) within a hospital will help share solutions and underlying infrastructure investments, develop strategic partnerships with suppliers and provide opportunities to share best practice and avoid common mistakes

	01 Identify Solve the right problem	02 Design Do it with the right people	03 Develop Safe, effective, and scalable	04 Implement Pilot, evaluate, refine, and scale	05 Monitor and improve Realise benefits and compliance
Innovators	Develop problem statement and use case	Work together to develop value proposition	Embed enterprise standards, and evidence model	Change management, and clinical safety	Continuous improvement and regulatory duties
Dentistry operators and systems	Support idea validation and refinement	Provide insights on workflows and value proposition	Provide feedback on solution and outputs	Allocate resources and support validation	Provide feedback and support regulatory monitoring
Funders	Clear info on funding process and criteria	Provide insights on value proposition and payment flows	Provide insights on value proposition and payment flows	Assess initial benefits against criteria	Assess longer-term and ongoing benefits realization
End users	Support idea validation and refinement	Provide insights on workflows and value proposition	Provide feedback on solution and outputs	Provide feedback on solution and outputs	Provide feedback and support regulatory monitoring
Regulators	Understand use cases to ensure regulation fits	Support early embedding of compliance activities	Support early embedding and compliance activities	Support evaluations and corrective actions	Support ongoing compliance

Figure 5.7 Stakeholder and activities in AI solution development.
Reproduced from Gunatilleke, J., 2022. Artificial Intelligence in Healthcare: Unlocking Its Potential. N.

> **Box 5.10 Existing dental AI technologies in use or development**
>
> **Diagnosis**
> - Second Opinion® by Pearl is an AI platform that detects pathology from dental radiographs, with the ability to detect incipient caries and signs of periapical pathology
> - CariesNet is a proposed system to enhance the diagnosis of dental caries from radiographs
> - Diagnocat uses AI to provide radiological reports for CBCT as well as well as plain film radiographs
>
> **Monitoring**
> - Dental Monitoring® offers a software-as-a-service (SaaS) AI platform for dental care. Its main product uses AI to review intraoral photographs which the patients themselves submit. They use their image database to help detect oral hygiene, periodontal disease, tooth movement and progress of orthodontic treatment, including when archwires become passive
>
> **Record-keeping and administration**
> - DentAI® uses speech recognition technology to automatically input any clinical findings during a dental exam into the patient's electronic record, obviating the need for the dentist or assistant to input clinical findings manually
> - Overjet dental AI automates administrative tasks, detects coding and billing errors, identifies potential treatment opportunities with real-time data analysis

Further reading

Gunatilleke J (2022). Artificial Intelligence in Healthcare: Unlocking Its Potential. *N. Janak Gunatilleke*.

Gunatilleke J (2023). AI in dentistry: understanding and realising its full potential. *Faculty Dent J* 14(3):108–11.

Statista. Available at: ✋ https://www.statista.com/statistics/1360613/adoption-rate-of-major-iot-tech/

Sustainability in dentistry

Dentists can help support sustainable healthcare systems by incorporating sustainability principles into daily practice, emphasizing waste reduction, efficient energy use, and responsible procurement of materials. Active participation in education that integrates sustainability concepts and collaborative efforts with other providers, suppliers, and manufacturers is required. Advocating for environmentally conscious policies and guidelines contributes towards the broader cultural shift that is required, along with support of research and development that is focused on innovative eco-friendly dental technologies and practices.

Measuring sustainability impacts

- Healthcare systems account for approximately 5% of a country's carbon footprint (Pichler, 2019). Around 63% of dentistry's footprint comes from travel (Duane, 2024)
- The Life Cycle Assessment (LCA) is a tool that examines the life cycle of healthcare processes and products. It collects data such as air pollution, impact on fresh water quality, carbon emissions and its outputs can be translated into other measures such as human health consequences (disability-adjusted life years, DALYs)
- DALYs measure years of life lost due to premature mortality and disability, giving insights into the overall health implications of environmental factors
- Both the environmental ramifications of a healthcare system and the social consequences of manufacturing a healthcare product must be considered, from the perspective of people, profit, and planet (net zero carbon)

Areas of sustainability

Prevention

- This is the priority in sustainable dentistry, whether primary, secondary, or tertiary prevention
- Primary prevention includes measures such as water fluoridation, the most cost-effective, low carbon prevention process to date (Duane, 2022)
- Secondary prevention is to prioritize preventive interventions with lower environmental footprints such as bamboo toothbrushes
- Thirdly, emphasizing evidence-based preventive interventions such as fluoride varnish, free toothpaste where necessary during routine patient visits will enhance oral health outcomes and minimize the environmental impact associated with disease management
- Integrating environmental conversations into patient education, e.g. discussion on sustainable diet choices, oral health practices

Travel

- Dentistry has a large carbon footprint from both patient travel and staff travel. Patients may have to attend regularly and frequently, such as for orthodontic treatment
- Strategies to reduce travel may include: combining appointments, prioritizing evidence-based treatment, tele-dentistry for monitoring of conditions, encouraging walking, cycling or car-sharing

Energy, water use, biodiversity
- The contribution of energy to the dental carbon footprint is around 15% (Duane, 2024)
- Hospital and building estates teams can ensure sustainable infrastructure to minimize reduction of energy waste from heating and lighting, considering factors such as insulation, draught-proofing, double glazing and smart meters
- The environmental impact between new construction and retrofitting or upgrading existing ones should be considered
- Reduction of energy from devices should be considered. Consider high-energy devices (washer disinfectors, autoclaves, fridges), moderate energy and low-energy devices (curing lights). Appliances should be turned off when not in use rather than standby mode
- More environmentally-favourable energy sources such as wind, photovoltaic, should be used where possible
- Sustainable water drainage systems to combat floods and cope with droughts should be considered. The use of captured rainwater and recycled grey water for non-potable purposes is encouraged
- Greenspace areas (e.g. green roofs and walls) positively impacts biodiversity and emotional well-being

Procurement
- Within a dental setting, this contributes a potential 22% to the carbon footprint (Duane, 2024)
- A 'buy less, buy better' approach minimizes excess purchases, maintains more effective stock control, and allows partnerships with sustainability-focused suppliers. See Box 5.11 for features of sustainable products

Personal protective equipment (PPE)
- Consider alternatives to single-use items
- Source eco-friendly materials and manufacturing processes for PPE
- Financial considerations, such as exploring cost-effective reusable options and negotiating with suppliers for environmentally friendly options should be part of the decision-making process
- Proactively seek appropriate waste management contracts for effective PPE disposal and recycling

---

Box 5.11 Products that have sustainability features
- Fit for purpose
- Not fossil-fuel based
- Grown or locally processed
- Supplied in sustainable packaging
- Biodegradable into harmless elements
- Easy to clean and reuse
- Simple to recycle
- Transported with clean vehicles or locally
- Produced with renewable energy
- Manufactured in ways that do not involve labour abuse
- Involving suppliers with good environmental practices

Waste

- Ensure staff are familiar with the waste stream bin colour-coding system, ensuring proper disposal of different types of waste
- Implementation of the 'nudge theory' can encourage correct waste management without conscious decision-making (Wilmott, 2022)
- Carry out waste audits, involving weighing, emptying, re-weighing waste bins to help identify how waste is categorized and managed
- Recognizing barriers to adopting sustainable waste management (lack of understanding, perceived inconvenience, etc.) and implementing staff education, awareness initiatives, incentives to foster positive waste behaviour
- Developments in technology to change manufacturing processes to reduce waste, for example, aligner treatment currently generates a lot of waste as each aligner requires an upper and a lower model to be printed, for each stage of treatment. They currently cannot be recycled and therefore are discarded. The plastic aligners also cannot be remelted or remoulded. Developments to directly print aligners without the need for printing models will help reduce waste

Behavioural changes

- Nitrous oxide has a global warming potential 298 times that of carbon dioxide (Dahling, 2020). Techniques like capture and cracking may help mitigate emissions although more quantitative evidence on their effectiveness is needed (Dahling, 2020)
- General anaesthesia poses environmental challenges related to its resource-intensive nature, expensive drug use, impact of travel for the patient and considerable number of required staff members and the impact of disposable materials
- Intravenous sedation may require travel due to limited access to specific centres, additional chaperones may be required and there is waste from single-use instruments
- Preventive care, early intervention, and maximizing treatments per session can help reduce the need for additional behavioural support techniques
- Sustainability quality improvement processes (SusQI) analyse and measure each alternative approach to find carbon hotspots and reduce accordingly

References

Dahling S, Wennerhed F (2020). Nordic Know-How 2020: #1 Nitrous Oxide. Available at: https://nordicshc.org/images/Nordic_know-how_2020_Nitrous_Oxide_2.pdf.

Duane B, Lyne A, Parle R, Ashley P (2022). The environmental impact of community caries prevention—part 3: water fluoridation. Br Dent J, 233(4):303–7.

Net Zero Carbon. People Planet Profit. Available at: https://netzerocarbon.com.

Pichler P-P, Jaccard IS, Weisz U, Weisz H (2019). International comparison of healthcare carbon footprints. Environ Res Lett, 14(6):064004.

Susqi. Study the system. Available at: https://www.susqi.org/study-the-system

Wilmott S, Pasdeki-Clewer E, Duane B (2022). Responsible waste management: using resources efficiently. In: Duane B (ed) Sustainable Dentistry. BDJ Clinician's Guides. Springer, Cham. Available at: https://doi.org/10.1007/978-3-031-07999-3_10

Dental health tourism

Health tourism is when patients who live overseas travel to the UK to have treatment. This is permitted on a private basis and may be permitted for NHS treatment if the patient pays for the costs incurred. It is estimated that health tourism from unpaid bills costs the NHS per year approximately £300 million for medical treatment of European Economic Area (EEA) visitors and non-permanent residents, £1000 million for non-EEA visitors and £330 million for illegal migrants (data from migrationwatchuk.org).

The regulations place a legal obligation on trusts to establish if people to whom it is providing NHS services are not ordinarily resident in the UK. From April 2017, NHS hospitals in England were subject to a legal duty to charge overseas patients upfront for non-urgent care.

NHS charging regulations

The NHS (Charges to Overseas Visitors) Regulations 2015, SI 2015/238 have been made under s.175 National Health Service Act 2006 to provide a charging framework for those individuals not classed as ordinarily resident in the UK.

What does 'ordinarily resident' mean?

It means living in the UK on a legal, settled, and permanent basis, for the time being. Individuals are not automatically entitled to free NHS care just because of:

- UK nationality or passport holder
- Being registered with a UK-based GP
- Having an NHS number
- Paying National Insurance or taxes in the UK
- UK address or property ownership

The European Health Insurance Card (EHIC) entitles EEA and Swiss visitors who are insured through their own state healthcare system to access emergency NHS treatment free of charge.

Protection of the wider public

Certain conditions remain exempt from charges to protect the wider public. This list can change depending on global and national health circumstances. Examples of conditions include anthrax, botulism, malaria, measles, rabies, rubella, SARS, tuberculosis and HIV. The exemption still applies even if the outcome is a negative test result.

Who is responsible for identifying patients who are not entitled to free care?

Ultimately, all staff are. Many trusts will have an overseas visitor manager, who can be notified by frontline staff, clinicians, admission managers, nurses, etc. about patients who are not ordinarily resident.

Identifying overseas visitors

Trust staff should identify all patients who may be liable to charges. All patients accessing NHS services are asked the same baseline questions in order to establish whether they are ordinarily resident.

- Are you a UK/EEA national or do you have a valid visa or leave to enter/remain in the UK?
- Which countries have you lived in for the past 12 months?

Patients who are unable to demonstrate the right to live in the UK or have lived for more than 3 months in another country should be re-referred to the overseas visitor manager for an interview.

Going abroad for treatment

UK patients who wish to travel abroad for health treatment are advised to discuss with their GP or GDP in the first instance. The EHIC or UK Global Health Insurance Card (GHIC) does not cover travel for planned treatment; it only covers necessary unplanned treatment when travelling.

As the UK has left the EU, there are two routes to access treatment:

- The S2 (planned treatment) route—this is a direct funding arrangement between the NHS and healthcare provider of the EU country the patient wishes to access treatment in. Prior authorization from NHS England is required and the patient may be required to cover a proportion of the cost
- The EU directive route—the patient pays for the treatment upfront and then claims eligible costs back from the NHS on their return

Scenario—Overseas treatment

Your 25-year-old type-1 diabetic patient tells you that she plans to go to an Eastern European country for full-mouth veneers, as she cannot get this treatment for free on the NHS. She asks for your advice.

Published guidelines:

- The GDC and British Dental Health Foundation have produced a guideline
- The Oral Health Foundation guidelines

Considerations:

- Don't assume the worst. Many countries have experienced, highly trained, and skilled clinicians who could provide dental treatment of an excellent standard
- In some situations, patients can apply for prior authorization for funding for *medical* treatment before travelling abroad. But the NHS will not reimburse the cost of *dental* treatment abroad. Similarly, travel or accommodation expenses will not be reimbursed
- Travelling abroad to seek out high-quality dental care is not an issue but the treatment should be well-researched rather than focused on a holiday destination. Lack of clear information from the provider, pressure to commit to a decision fast and a discussion only about the benefits are all warning signs
- Health insurance—travel insurance may not provide cover for planned treatment abroad, so additional insurance may be required

Qualifications:

- It is important to research the qualifications and skillset of the treatment providers. Liaising with a UK GP or GDP for guidance is recommended, especially as patients may be unaware of medical credentials and qualifications. Does that country have a professional regulatory body and is it compulsory for dentists to register with them? Or can anyone carry out dental treatment. What are the standards enforced by the

regulatory body. Who can use the title 'specialist' and what, if any, additional qualifications are required
- Is it possible to meet the clinician first to establish a rapport and trust?
- Are there any language barriers? This is especially important when consenting for treatment and communicating risks

The treatment itself
- Most patients travelling abroad are doing so for more complex and higher cost procedures; by their nature, these are more likely to result in complications
- Is the treatment clinically necessary? Different countries have different standards for when to extract teeth versus restoring. It is advisable to get an opinion and treatment plan from a UK dentist/specialist first for comparison. Full-mouth veneers are always an option, but is there a less invasive option too?
  - Complete a comprehensive clinical assessment and provide a summary of your suggested treatment plan—are veneers her best option? Does she need any input from other dental specialities?
  - Provide copies of any relevant records, e.g. radiographs, history of previous restorations, dental study models/intraoral scans
- If the treatment is significantly cheaper than the UK, determine why the cost differences exist. Check are the materials of a comparable standard, have all the required radiographs been taken, are necessary pre-treatments being undertaken also
- Ask to see reviews and case photographs for patients who have had similar treatments
- Ensure adequate consideration is given to the patient themselves: past treatment, expectations, digital mock up or try-in of proposed result, patient's medical history, etc. In this scenario, a type-1 diabetic patient will require careful management, thus early morning flights and long treatment sessions may not be appropriate. Diabetes can have potential implications on periodontal health as well

Follow-up:
- What are the aftercare arrangements for suture removal, second stage of the procedure, etc. Will a UK GP or GDP be willing to take over treatment if needed. Many patients require multiple visits for adjustment of the occlusion post-cementation
- What is the arrangement in case of complications, e.g. sensitivity, loss of vitality, decementation of restoration, bleeding?
- What is the complaints process if treatment does not proceed as planned
- Consider additional costs: aftercare, extended trip if there are issues, changing flights, the need for repeat trips in the future

Getting It Right First Time (GIRFT)

The Getting It Right First Time (GIRFT) project is a national programme designed to improve medical care across the NHS by reducing unwarranted variations. The first speciality to be reviewed was orthopaedic surgery. This same model has been applied across 40 medical and surgical specialities, including oral & maxillofacial surgery (2018) and hospital dentistry (2021).

GIRFT consists of five key strands:

1. Data gathering and analysis—to obtain a detailed picture of the current national practice, outcomes, and related factors.
2. Direct clinical engagement between clinical specialists and individual trusts to examine individual trust behaviour in the context of the national picture. This enables the trust to understand where it is performing well and what it could do better.
3. National report—to identify opportunities for improvement across the relevant services.
4. Implementation phase—GIRFT team supports trusts, commissioners, and ICS to deliver the improvements.
5. Best-practice guidance and support—standardized and integrated patient pathways and elective recovery work in high volume/low complexity specialities.

GIRFT is an ongoing national project with regular updates to the various workstreams associated with it. The website is frequently updated: https://gettingitrightfirsttime.co.uk/

The Hospital Dentistry GIRFT

The Hospital Dentistry GIRFT was published in 2021:

- It found that 5% of dental care is carried out in secondary care
- The report focused on specialities linked to OPCS codes: oral surgery, orthodontics, restorative dentistry, and paediatric dentistry
- Oral medicine and special care dentistry were also considered
- The report made 21 recommendations
- Each recommendation is linked to actions, owners and a time scale
- Three overarching themes were identified:

1. Oral health and prevention

All healthcare providers should understand the role of good oral health in general health and well-being and be able to advise patients on how to achieve it.

2. Creating equitable access to treatment

Managed clinical networks involving primary and secondary care clinicians as well as commissioners would improve system design and enable a better patient experience.

3. Addressing the workforce challenge

Workforce planning should include provision for more general dental practitioners with enhanced skills to provide more care outside hospitals.

The recommendations are summarized as follows:

Cross-speciality: Understanding the work being done and who is doing it

1. Review of dental speciality and treatment function codes to enable quality improvement, workforce planning, and service redesign. The clinician responsible for care and the clinician who delivered the care should be identifiable.
2. Type of anaesthetic should be recorded and reported using OPCS4 procedure codes as part of the commissioning data set.
3. Primary and secondary diagnoses (comorbidities) recorded for all activity in an outpatient setting, to allow quality assurance.
4. Procedure code use reviewed to ensure clarity and consistent use.

Cross-speciality: Commissioning integrated dental pathways

5. Dental referrals should be part of an e-referral management system to ensure they are managed in a consistent and co-ordinated way.
6. All areas should have an MCN in each dental speciality. These should liaise with ICSs.
7. Workforce and training for each speciality should be reviewed. The clinical academic workforce is a priority to ensure that undergraduate/ postgraduate training programmes can be delivered.
8. Oral health is recognized as an essential part of general health and well-being: establish an integrated approach, with emphasis on hard-to-reach groups, across secondary care, primary care dentistry, medicine, and pharmacy, through ICSs and primary care networks.

Cross-speciality: Managing intra-trust referrals

9. Local commissioning should ensure that patients with complex medical conditions (e.g. oncology, haematology and cardiology) are seen in a timely fashion in the most appropriate setting. National guidelines should be developed to enable this.

Paediatric dentistry

10. All referrals for children requiring general anaesthetic for dental extractions should be accompanied by a treatment plan to avoid repeat admission. Non-specialists providing this must be aligned to a specialist-led paediatric dental MCN.
11. Waiting lists for children requiring exodontia must be reduced. Children at risk of oral infection should wait no more than 14 days from RTT and should not be prescribed multiple courses of antibiotics due to the wait.
12. Strategies from the Children's Oral Health Improvement Programme Board (COHIPB) should be implemented at provider and commissioner level. Oral health is treated as a high priority as part of the overall paediatric well-being agenda and included in the work of Paediatric Surgery Operational Delivery Networks (ODNs).

Oral surgery

13. Outpatient and day case prices for dental procedures should be reviewed to remove incentives for inaccurate recording. Specifically, a day case setting should only be used and recorded where clinically necessary, e.g. general anaesthetic (GA) or sedation requiring recovery.
14. Revised guidance from the Royal College of Surgeons on temporomandibular joint dysfunction to:
- Provide clarity on when to refer to secondary care
- Consider whether care could be provided by a level 2 service

- This should be supported by action to reduce barriers to treatment in primary care and embed the guidance into everyday practice

Oral medicine

15. Dental and non-dental hospitals and primary care should work together in regional oral medicine networks to manage referrals and deliver care to shared standards based on a hub and spoke model and clearly defined pathways as outlined in the commissioning standard.

Restorative dentistry

16. All head and neck cancer, cleft lip, and palate and hypodontia MDTs should have a consultant in restorative dentistry as a core member from the outset. Patients should move through treatment seamlessly, without delays that can cause iatrogenic damage. For children under 18, a paediatric dentist must be involved.

Orthodontics

17. Where orthognathic surgery or oral surgery is planned after orthodontic treatment has already begun, patients should not have to wait more than 18 weeks, so as not to extend orthodontic treatment times and increase the risk of iatrogenic damage.

18. The Peer Assessment Rating Index should be recorded for every completed orthodontic case with external audit of outcomes reported and reviewed through the MCN.

19. Trusts, general dental practitioners and community dental service (CDS) should provide coordinated dental care for people with special care needs, identifying and breaking down traditional barriers between settings as envisioned by NHS Long-Term Plan.

Procurement

20. Enable improved procurement of devices and consumables through cost and pricing transparency, aggregation and consolidation, and by sharing best practice.

21. Reduce litigation costs by application of the GIRFT programme's five-point plan:

- Clinicians/managers assess their position compared to the national average when reviewing the litigation cost per activity
- Clinicians/managers discuss with the legal department or claims handler to confirm claims are correctly coded to that department. Inform NHS Resolution of any claims incorrectly coded
- Once claims have been verified, clinicians/management to review claims to determine where patient care or documentation could be improved
- Claims should be triangulated with learning themes from complaints, inquests and serious untoward incidents (SUI)/serious incidents (SI)/ patient safety incidents (PSI). Undertake reviews where they have not been completed
- Findings should be shared with all frontline clinical staff in a structured format at departmental/directorate meetings (including MDT meetings, morbidity, and mortality meetings where appropriate)
- Where trusts are outside the top quartile of trusts for litigation costs per activity GIRFT, national clinical leads, and regional hubs to:
  - Support trusts in the steps taken to learn from claims
  - Share examples of good practice where it would be of benefit

Oral and Maxillofacial surgery GIRFT

The national report for oral and maxillofacial surgery (2018) made six main recommendations that have been endorsed by the British Association of Oral and Maxillofacial Surgeons (Table 5.7).

Table 5.7 Summary of the national oral and maxillofacial surgery GIRFT programme

Recommendation	Context/explanation	Response/subsequent actions
Data quality and data collection	Issues with coding to the correct speciality, be it oral surgery or oral and maxillofacial surgery as these codes had different tariffs associated	Publication of 'Outpatient activity coding in Oral Surgery' in 2023 to maintain a consistent approach to coding by NHS trusts and better data collection.
Perform dentoalveolar surgery in an appropriate setting	Dentoalveolar surgery made up most of the workload in oral and maxillofacial surgery (OMFS) departments. Services to be provided in primary care to reduce need for secondary care	Commissioning of tier 2 oral surgery services. MCN with oral surgeons/OMF surgeons acting as the chair of the network.
Improving efficiency by organizing care through networks	The use of hub and spoke models through local networks to optimize quality and efficiency, with a focus on complex care	These are being implemented for orthognathic surgery and head and neck cancer care.
Optimizing the secondary care pathway	Variation in the number of outpatient follow ups and readmission rates	Audits and quality improvement projects. More use of clinical networks.
Litigation	Set national benchmarks for litigation cases. Learn from cases which involved litigation	Triangulation of claims, learning from complaints, inquests, and serious incident reviews. Identify trusts which are outliers in this area.
Procurement	Improve procurement of devices and consumables	Procurement data (e.g. purchase price index and benchmarking tools to maximize cost-effectiveness). Look at national pricing and procurement.

References

Hospital Dentistry GIRFT Programme National Specialty Report, Elizabeth Jones February 2021.
NHS Staff Survey FAQ Update: 17 August 2023 Version: 5.
Oral and Maxillofacial Surgery GIRFT Programme National Specialty Report, Maire Morton 2018.

Role of the legal team

The general role of a legal team is to provide advice, representation, and assurance to the trust board, management team, and clinical teams. The specific role and composition of the legal team will vary between trusts and other organizations. The clinical team, in particular dental consultants should be aware of when they should consult with the team.

Roles within the legal team

The legal team may be composed of solicitors, barristers, paralegals, and other administrative staff. All legal teams will also access external legal advice and representation from external solicitors and barristers.

The following are the general roles within a trust:

- General counsel—A senior lawyer who provides strategic level advice and assurance to the trust board, of which they may be a member
- Solicitor—A qualified lawyer regulated by the Solicitors Regulation Authority (SRA) who provides advice and guidance. They are qualified to provide litigation services on behalf of the trust
- Barrister—A qualified lawyer regulated by the Bar Standards Board (BSB) who will provide advice and guidance. They are qualified to represent and provide advocacy services on behalf of the trust in all courts and tribunals in England and Wales
- Paralegals—Provide legal support services to the qualified lawyers
- Claims manager—Liaise with NHS Resolutions (NHSR), the trust, and external solicitors to manage any civil claims for compensation brought against the trust
- Inquests manager—Liaise with coroners and the trust to manage any coroner's investigations or inquests because of a death

Functions of the legal team

The legal team may be contacted by the dental clinical team for a range of reasons, they may provide advice or guidance on:

- Contracts and procurement
- Regulation (e.g. regulation of medicines and devices)
- Consent to treatment
- Mental Capacity Act 2005
- Mental Health Act 1983
- Parental responsibility
- Disputes regarding treatment
- Coroners and inquests
- Civil litigation (claims brought against or by the trust; for example, clinical negligence and personal injury, breach of contract)
- Criminal matters
- Intellectual property
- Planning and property
- Information Governance
- Safeguarding legislation

The legal team will also support (either directly, or by seeking external representation) with the following:

- Providing reports to the management committees and trust board of the legal functions within the trust

- Making applications to the court to determine what treatment is in a patient's best interests, where there is a dispute or uncertainty
- Preparing witness statements required for courts and tribunals
- Supporting witnesses who may be required to give oral evidence to a court or tribunal
- Managing civil claims to which the trust is a party, with NHSR and external solicitors and barristers
- Managing coroner's investigations and inquests
- Liaising with external solicitors where disputes (including safeguarding issues) require the involvement of the trust in legal proceedings

NHS Resolution

NHS Resolution is an arm's-length body of the Department of Health and Social Care. It supports NHS trusts to resolve disputes, and handles clinical negligence claims and other third-party claims against a trust by appointing external solicitors and paying any awards (agreed or court ordered) against a trust (subject to contributions).

Patient safety and risk management

What is patient safety?

The origins of patient safety can be traced back to the Hippocratic Oath which states, 'first, do no harm'. Healthcare delivery is a complicated system reliant on multiple individuals and processes. Many aspects of these systems have the potential for errors, which may lead to:

- Harm to the patient
- Harm to the care provider
- Loss of trust in the healthcare system
- Burden on the teams that work in these systems
- Fiscal cost

There is inherent risk in healthcare but errors can be reduced by following principles that mitigate this risk. There should be a constant preoccupation with patient safety and vigilance for the occurrence of adverse events.

Defining patient safety

Patient safety is more than just the absence of harm in healthcare. The World Health Organization (WHO) defines it as:

'A framework of organized activities that creates cultures, processes, procedures, behaviours, technologies, and environments in healthcare that consistently and sustainably lower risks, reduce the occurrence of avoidable harm, make error less likely and reduce its impact when it does occur.'

The WHO outlines the principles for maintaining patient safety:

- Engage patients and families as partners in safe care
- Achieve results through collaborative working
- Analyse data to generate learning
- Translate evidence into measurable improvement
- Base policies and actions on the nature of the care setting
- Use scientific expertise and patient experience to improve safety
- Instil a safety culture into the design and delivery of healthcare

NHS reports and policies

Several reports have been published on patient safety, quality, and learning from errors. Table 6.1 summarizes their impact and relevance to dentistry.

Table 6.1 A summary of NHS reports, their impact, and relevance to dentistry

Report	Summary and main findings	Response and impact	Dental aspects
An Organization with a Memory (Donaldson, 2000)	Introduction of a mandatory reporting system for adverse healthcare events, among other recommendations.	Introduction of NRLS and StEIS in 2003.	Dental hospital incident reports feed into these national databases.

Table 6.1 (*Contd.*)

Report	Summary and main findings	Response and impact	Dental aspects
High-Quality Care for All (Darzi, 2008)	More focus on quality in healthcare rather than speed of care. (See Chapter 5, quality and performance management)	Increased patient choice. Care Quality Commission (CQC) established in 2009.	CQC aims to ensure care services in England provide people with safe, effective, and high-quality care, and to encourage those providers to improve.
Never Events Framework (National Patient Safety Agency, 2009, with subsequent updates)	Originally, eight core Never Events (already considered to be serious incidents) were listed, including wrong site surgery, and retained instruments post-surgery. The list has evolved since the first edition.	Increased focus on error in healthcare and the use of root cause analysis. Never Event data published by NHS Improvement since 2015. Widespread use of surgical safety checklists.	Between 2015 and 2021, wrong tooth extraction was specifically included in the list of surgical Never Events.
Report on the Mid Staffordshire NHS Foundation Trust Public Inquiry (Francis, 2013; see chapter 1, The Francis and Berwick reports)	Commissioned after multiple patient safety failings at Mid Staffordshire NHS Foundation Trust 290 recommendations relating to healthcare delivery, primarily in hospitals.	Government responded by commissioning the Berwick report later the same year.	Introduction of Statutory Duty of Candour from 2014. General Dental Council (GDC) standards (2013) states that dental professionals must 'record all patient safety incidents and report them promptly to the appropriate national body'.

(*Continued*)

Table 6.1 (*Contd.*)

Report	Summary and main findings	Response and impact	Dental aspects
A promise to learn—a commitment to act. (Berwick, 2013; see chapter 1, The Francis and Berwick reports)	Several recommendations relating to patient safety, including: • Abandon blame as a tool • Focus on working with patients and carers to achieve health goals • Caution when using quantitative targets • Expect transparency • Responsibility for functions related to safety and improvement are established clearly and simply	Several initiatives including proposals for greater data transparency and changes to regulation. The NHS to become a system devoted to continual learning and improvement of patient care.	Further clarified the role of the CQC in regulation of dental care in hospitals and dental practices.
National Safety Standards for Invasive Procedures (NatSSIPs, 2015)	Aim to reduce the number of patient safety incidents related to invasive procedures where there is a risk of a Never Event occurring.	Focus on the use of checklists in surgery. Providers encouraged to develop their own standardized local procedures for safety.	Development of the LocSSIPs for Dentistry by RCS England (2016), providing dentists with a framework around which to base their own patient safety protocols and checklists.
NatSSIPs 2, 2023	*Organizational standards:* clear expectations of what trusts and external bodies should do to support teams to deliver safe invasive care. *Sequential standards:* procedural steps that should be taken where appropriate by individuals and teams, for every patient undergoing an invasive procedure.	Less emphasis on rare Never Events and 'tick box culture'. More focus on team structures and interactions.	Builds on the work developing checklists and standard operating procedures since the original NatSSIPs in 2015.

Science and theories of patient safety

Human factors

Human factors and ergonomics aim to understand the interactions between humans and the systems in which they work while acknowledging the innate fallibility of humans. Much of the work on human factors originates in the airline industry and other safety critical industries. Boeing is thought to have introduced the first safety checklist in 1935. In dentistry, human factors encompass every member of the team in every process.

Human factors and ergonomics have three domains:
- Physical: workplace environment and its impact on performance
- Cognitive: cognitive activities and characteristics of an individual, including communication, a factor in many patient safety incidents
- Organizational: psychosocial characteristics of people and organizational or structural policies and processes (also known as macro-ergonomics)

The 'Dirty Dozen' concept was described by George Dupont in 1993. It is a list of the 12 most common elements that can influence people to make mistakes. These are summarized in Table 6.2

Table 6.2 'Dirty Dozen' concept

Lack of communication	Distraction	Lack of resources	Lack of knowledge
Norms—workplace culture	Complacency	Lack of teamwork	Fatigue
Pressure	Lack of awareness	Lack of assertiveness	Stress

There are also two useful acronyms used to describe the circumstances in which staff might become unsafe. These are:

Hungry Angry Late Tired (HALT)

Illness Medication Stress Alcohol Fatigue Emotions (IMSAFE)

Situational awareness

Situational awareness is 'developing and maintaining a dynamic awareness of the situation and the risks present in an activity, based on gathering information from multiple sources from the task environment, understanding what the information means and using it to think ahead about what may happen next' (Martin Anderson, Human Factors 101).

In dentistry:
- During safety critical parts of a procedure, the 'sterile cockpit' model can be used—where there is silence in the theatre/treatment area, and focus is on the task at hand and nothing else
- Smartphones can be a source of distraction for clinicians especially when they are being used for personal communications in the workplace

Non-technical skills for surgeons (NOTSS)

NOTSS were developed by the Royal College of Surgeons of Edinburgh and the University of Aberdeen. They identified that surgical competence relies on:

- Appropriate clinical knowledge
- Good technical skills
- High standards of non-technical skills

Surgical and dental training is focused on the first two competencies. NOTSS aims to address the third aspect (see Table 6.3). The application of these skills can be used to provide feedback to surgical teams to improve their skills.

Table 6.3 The NOTSS taxonomy

Category	Elements
Situational awareness	- Gathering information, understanding information - Projecting and anticipating future state
Decision-making	- Considering options - Selecting and communicating options - Implementing and reviewing decisions
Communication and teamwork	- Exchanging information - Establishing a shared understanding - Coordinating team activities
Leadership	- Setting and maintaining standards - Supporting others - Coping with pressure

Patient safety models

The Swiss cheese model

The 'Swiss cheese model' (Reason, 1990) describes how adverse events or systems failures occur conceptually (see Figure 6.1).
- There are a series of safeguards, barriers, and defences in place that work in tandem to prevent these events from occurring
- Ideally, each defensive layer would be intact. In reality, they are like slices of Swiss cheese, with many potential holes in each layer of defence
- The presence of holes in one particular slice is unlikely to lead to an adverse outcome as the other layers will prevent its occurrence
- When accidents or incidents do occur, it is due to the 'holes' in each layer lining up so that a trajectory of accident opportunity opens up and therefore is highly likely to occur

This model may not always be applicable for health-related incidents:
- It is linear in nature and not always applicable
- It assumes that adverse outcomes can be identified and fixed, usually through compliance, standardization of process, and training
- There is an assumption that when errors occur, it is due to a deviation from standard, successful care

SUCCESSIVE LAYERS OF DEFENCES

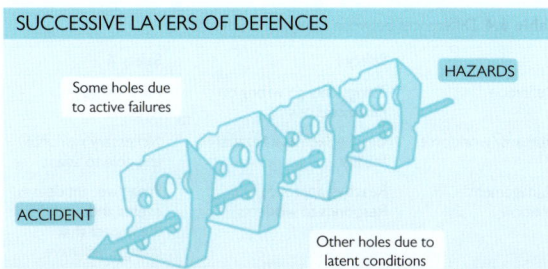

Figure 6.1 The Swiss cheese model. Reproduced from: Reason, J. (1990). Human Error. Cambridge: Cambridge University Press.

Organizational accident model

The organizational accident model considers
- Negative consequences of organizational processes, such as planning, forecasting, design, maintenance, strategy, and policy
- These latent conditions are transmitted along organizational and departmental pathways to the workplace—clinic, operating theatre
- They create the local conditions that promote errors and violations (e.g. high workload or poor human–equipment interfaces)
- Many unsafe acts are likely to be committed, but very few of them will penetrate the defences to produce damaging outcomes
- Engineered safety features, such as alarms or standard procedures, can be deficient due to latent conditions as well as active failures
- The model presents the people at the sharp end as the inheritors rather than as the instigators of an accident sequence

Safety I and Safety II

A 'Safety I' (see Table 6.4) approach to patient safety is concerned with studying events retrospectively and learning from these infrequent occurrences. Many situations are uneventful, or at least cause little or no harm, therefore it is sensible to focus on these as a source of learning.

Safety II aims to focus on why things go well and to examine the resilience in systems that are working effectively, acknowledging that the vast majority of outcomes are successful.

Table 6.4 Differences between Safety I and Safety II

	Safety I	Safety II
Definition	Things only go wrong on rare occasions	Most things go to plan
Humans/workforce	Can be seen as a hazard/liability	Necessary resource and able to adapt
Management principle	Reactive approach Responds to incidents	Proactive, anticipates events and considers the impact that changes will have
Purpose of investigation	Identify the causes of failings	Understand what works well in order to explain why things occasionally go wrong and make changes in advance of this
Risk assessment	Identify causes from investigations/contributary factors	Understands that performance variability in complex systems is difficult to monitor/control

Patient safety culture

A patient safety culture is one where safety is prioritized, resourced, and practised by the team and its leaders. The NHS Patient Safety Strategy (2019) encourages an engaged, visible leadership promoting openness and continuous improvement, valuing diversity and equality.

In a patient safety culture, safe care is delivered through:
- Continuous learning and mitigation of safety risks
- Supportive, psychologically safe teamwork
- Enabling and empowering all staff to speak up

Just culture

A 'just culture' aims to create an environment in which staff feel supported and empowered to raise concerns without fear or shame:
- Staff do not feel that they will be blamed for errors
- The focus is on what was responsible, not who is responsible
- The bigger picture is examined to see how events unfolded

Developed by NHS England, the Just Culture Guide aims to support consistent, constructive, and fair evaluation of the actions of staff involved in patient safety incidents.
- It acknowledges that the majority of incidents are due to deeper causes rather than the actions of one individual
- It includes the need for disciplinary or regulatory action, although this is rarely necessary

The CQC has used a Safety II approach to identify safety practices rated good or outstanding:
- Compassionate leadership, including:
  - Direction—shared purpose between all staff
  - Alignment—clear goals for staff and teams, aligned with the vision
  - Commitment—developing team trust and motivation
- Developing a team with psychological safety involves:
  - Civility—making personal connections with team members
  - Creating a leadership promise and behaviour framework that staff can sign up to
  - Appreciation of team members and granting them the permission and freedom to innovate

First and second victims

When incidents occur, the incident has an impact on the patient and their family; these are the first victims. The clinician or clinical team involved can suffer psychological harm; they are the second victims.
There is some criticism of the phrase 'second victim':
- It has led to more focus being placed on the clinician rather than on the first victim or their families
- Victims bear no responsibility or accountability; they elicit feelings of sympathy. This may mask underlying issues within a healthcare service that are causing actual harm to patients

A six-stage cycle is used to describe the aftermath of an event:
1. Chaos and accident response
2. Intrusive reflections

3. Restoring personal integrity
4. Ending the inquisition
5. Obtaining emotional first aid
6. Moving on

Emotional and psychological support can help second victims to progress through this cycle more rapidly. Some of the behaviours observed in those who are second victims include:
- Hypervigilance
- Stress and anxiety
- Shame and feelings of inadequacy
- Risk avoidance and self-doubt about knowledge and skills
- Insomnia and difficulty concentrating

The impact on clinicians, especially those in training, can be immense. It can increase the risk of future incidents if not properly managed. This can lead to underperformance and depression. Early intervention and support are recommended to minimize the long-term sequelae. Support is available from Practitioner Health in England.

The adoption of the NHS Just Culture Guide may help with managing those involved in safety incidents in a more supportive fashion while still highlighting areas of malpractice which do require intervention from an employer or regulatory body.

The patient safety incident response framework (PSIRF)

The PSIRF is a new framework which encourages engagement with everyone affected by patient safety incidents. It replaces the Serious Incident Framework 2015. It focuses on maintaining effective systems to respond to patient safety incidents, with a focus on learning and improving patient safety. It will be a contractual requirement for NHS trusts. Primary care settings may also wish to adopt PSIRF.

Patient safety culture in dentistry

Patient safety culture in dentistry appears to lag behind that in medical specialities, especially in general dental practice. This may be because:
- Dentistry is lower risk than medicine/surgery
- The outpatient nature of dentistry makes following up on complications and care-related issues challenging
- Data collection can be difficult due to variations in dental records
- Most dental care is carried out in dental practices which are run as businesses and reporting of harm may have a financial impact

Suggestions for improving the dental safety culture are below (see Box 6.1)

Project Sphere

This is a recent initiative by NHS England via the Office of the Chief Dental Officer to develop safety initiatives in dentistry and reduce the blame culture which is frequently cited. This is a result of perceived punitive consequences, such as litigation and regulatory action.

Never Events

Never Events are defined as serious incidents that are wholly preventable because guidance or safety recommendations that provide strong systemic

---

Box 6.1 Building a patient safety culture in dentistry

- Encourage an open culture where all members of the team feel empowered to speak up on issues
- Bring safety to the agenda during meetings
- Encourage incident reporting, even for incidents considered to be low harm or near misses
- Investigate safety incidents using a transparent process
- Learn from these investigations and adopt a 'Just Culture' and supportive processes for managing those involved
- Provide training for the team on Patient Safety and NOTSS
- Move from a reactive culture to a proactive one where systems are designed with safety in mind

---

protective barriers are available at a national level and should have been implemented by all healthcare providers.

Wrong tooth extraction was included in the NHS England Never Events Framework from 2015 to 2021.

- It was consistently the most frequent wrong site surgery event, accounting for 20–25% of Never Events
- It was removed from this list as the systemic barriers were not strong enough to prevent this from happening in all cases
- This decision cited that dental anatomy can be variable and previous dental interventions can change the anatomy of a patient

Dental Never Events

While there is no widely accepted list, the following have been cited as Dental Never Events.

- Failure to check past medical history
- Inhalation or swallowing of a crown or instrument
- Restoring the wrong tooth
- Oxygen and/or emergency drugs not being available
- Allergic reaction due to not checking medical history
- Extracting the wrong tooth
- Iatrogenic damage to an adjacent tooth
- Delay in routine referral
- Delay in urgent referral
- Using dirty instruments
- Treating the wrong patient

There is limited published data on these events in the literature and the frequency of such incidents is unknown. Some dental societies in the UK have developed reporting schemes in an attempt to more formally log, identify, and review the various types of adverse incidents that can occur in primary and secondary practice. Examples include the British Orthodontic Society (BOS) adverse event reporting tool.

Surgical safety checklists

- In 2009, the WHO introduced a 19-point checklist for surgical safety. This was adopted by the NHS and its use in operating theatres was mandated from 2010
- The use of these checklists was based on evidence that they improved patient outcomes
- Checklists have limitations in relation to their content, implementation, training, and how they are used in practice
- They should be frequently revisited

Checklists in theatre settings must adhere to the NatSSIPs 8. These are an evolution of the WHO checklist. There are two versions of these:

- Minor procedures—such as dental extractions under local anaesthetic
- Major procedures—such as oral/maxillofacial procedures under a general anaesthetic

NatSSIPs 8 for minor procedures:

1. Site marking required where relevant (the Palmer dental notation)
2. Team brief appropriate to context
3. Sign in
4. Time out can be combined
5. Implant checks should be performed where relevant
6. Count can be proportionate if site accessed via a needle or surface incision. If guidewires are used, they should be counted, for reconciliation of items
7. Sign out may be concise
8. Debrief if required

NatSSIPs 8 for major procedures:

1. Site marking required where relevant
2. Team brief with full team in attendance
3. Sign in
4. Time out should be completed separately
5. Implant checks should be performed where relevant
6. Full count procedure required and reconciliation
7. Sign out
8. Debrief should be carried out.

Further detail can be found on the Centre for Perioperative Care website: https://cpoc.org.uk/

Checklists in dentistry

WHO checklists have been modified to make them suitable for dental settings.

- These are the only interventions which have demonstrated an improvement in safety outcomes in dentistry
- They should be viewed as part of the armamentarium clinical teams use to maintain safety standards and to reduce risk

Checklists have evolved over time but the underlying principles remain:

- They serve as an aide-mémoire and should be based on existing processes rather than introducing new ones without proper justification
- The checklist promotes communication between team members
- There must be team engagement in the development of the checklist

- The whole team needs to understand its value, with senior members role-modelling its regular use
- Training must be provided to the team
- Patient involvement can enhance the effectiveness of the checklist

Examples of checklists used for invasive dental surgery in NHS trusts include:

- The checklist is used in conjunction with a whiteboard which is completed for every surgical procedure and is placed in a clearly visible place
- Biopsy checklists to ensure that samples are correctly processed
- Recording the removal of sharps from surgical trays to reduce sharps injury
- Clinicians are encouraged to use terms such as 'last tooth in arch' or to refer to the last tooth in a series as number 8 using the Palmer notation as this can avoid confusion. Supernumerary teeth should be carefully charted so that their position is known and described in relation to the rest of the dentition

Incident reporting

Incident reporting for serious incidents is mandatory in dental care settings. This process has CQC oversight. The term 'incident recording' is now preferred as it is thought to encourage more recording.

There are several benefits to incident reporting:

- Near misses are identified and actions can be taken to avoid these
- Incident reports can safeguard against poor quality clinical care
- Clinical teams can learn from incidents and barriers can be put in place to prevent them occurring again
- Reports can be used to identify trends and highlight system errors which need to be addressed
- They can be used to develop protocols based on risk management

It is acknowledged that there are also several barriers to incident reporting in healthcare, these include:

- Difficulties in accessing reporting systems
- Perceived poor processing of incident reports
- Inadequate engagement from professionals
- Insufficient visible actions from reports
- Fear of litigation or punitive consequences of reporting incidents

Incident reporting tools

The most common incident reporting tools in the NHS are the Datix and Ulysses systems. The systems ask for the following details:

- The type of incident, the date and time
- The directorate/service the incident reporter works for
- Description of the event
- Action already taken
- Who else was involved (witnesses, patients, employees)
- Whether this relates to safeguarding, use of CPR, controlled drugs, patient fall, pressure sore, or sharps incident
- An assessment of incident severity
- The reporter's details and line manager

The report is sent to the relevant staff/teams.

The introduction of 'learn from patient safety events' (LFPSE) (see page 170) will lead to some changes, with the nature and detail of questions becoming more specific. Reports will go straight to the national system, rather than stopping at a local level for agreement on levels of harm and context.

Incident reporting systems only detect a small number of adverse events. A low number of incident reports does not mean that incidents are not occurring. A recent initiative in the NHS, embedded in the Safety II approach, is to record, or report when good outcomes are observed. Some NHS trusts have developed a GREAT-ix system for reporting positive outcomes.

Serious incidents

Serious incidents (SI) are defined as: 'events in healthcare where the potential for learning is so great, or the consequences to patients, families, and carers, staff or organizations are so significant, that they warrant using additional resources to mount a comprehensive response. Serious incidents can extend beyond incidents which affect patients directly and include incidents which may indirectly impact patient safety or an organization's ability to deliver ongoing healthcare' (Serious Incident Framework, NHS England 2015).

There is no list of serious incidents as such, although Never Events are considered to be serious incidents.

Serious incidents are automatically reported through the LFPSE system. This is monitored by the CQC to monitor risks and incidents in clinical care. Once an SI has been reported, notification needs to be made to:

- Trust executive team
- Divisional director, general manager
- Risk management team
- Commissioning body

This list is not exhaustive and will vary depending on the hospital's management structure.

Potential courses of action following an SI may include:

- De-escalation if following investigation it is deemed to not be an SI and the situation has resolved
- Root cause analysis with a serious case review
- Deterioration of the situation requiring the trust's media team involvement or police action
- Involvement of the trust's legal team, who will report to the NHS litigation authority
- Learning and feedback

The patient safety incident response framework (PSIRF) sets out the NHS's approach to developing and maintaining effective systems and processes for responding to patient safety incidents for the purpose of learning and improving patient safety. It:

- Promotes a proportionate response
- Implements compassionate engagement for those affected
- Applies system-based approaches to aid learning

Medical devices

Adverse incidents involving medical devices, including those caused by human error, that pose (or have the potential to pose) a risk to the safety of patients, health and care professionals or others at risk must be reported to the medical device safety lead in the trust and the relevant national body:

- England and Wales—MHRA reporting adverse incidents
- Northern Ireland—Northern Ireland Adverse Incident Centre
- Scotland—Health Facilities Scotland online incident reporting

Investigating and learning from adverse incidents

Root cause analysis (RCA)

A RCA is a structured investigation to identify the true cause of a problem and actions needed to eliminate it (see Box 6.2). It seeks to understand the environmental context that led to it, rather than just focusing on the individuals concerned. It is an interdisciplinary impartial process designed to ask 'why' at each level.

Root cause analysis (RCA) has been criticised as it often looks for a single source of error leading to the incident. A systems approach may be more

> **Box 6.2 The process for conducting a RCA**
> 1. Identify the subject matter
> 2. Review relevant existing literature and protocols/guidelines
> 3. Plan the investigation
> 4. Carry out an investigation, either:
>   - Concise investigation (low level of harm)
>   - Comprehensive investigation (actual or severe harm)
>   - Independent inquiry (commissioned investigation if high public interest and serious event)
> 5. Outline the action plan required
> 6. Disseminate an action plan
> 7. Evaluate implementation of the new action plan

appropriate in healthcare. This can identify issues within an organization which can lead to safety lapses and therefore incidents.

An RCA is required if:

- There is an ongoing trend of low/medium level risks
- There is uncertainty as to why there is a continuing trend
- A high-risk incident or near miss has occurred

When an RCA is conducted:

- The principles of Just Culture should be followed and the investigation should be proportionate to the incident
- Caution must be exercised when carrying out such investigations to ensure that the causes are identified and addressed
- There should be engagement with the healthcare team
- The NHS Patient Safety website can be consulted for useful tools to help support those leading on patient safety investigations

After action review (AAR)

AAR is a method of evaluation used when the outcomes of an activity or event have been particularly successful or unsuccessful. Everyone involved in the event should attend the review, which is led by a facilitator. The group defines what the intended outcome was and what actually happened and determines whether this contributed to either the success/failure of the task. They aim to understand the differences between the intended and actual outcomes and what can be learned. Key learning points are disseminated to the wider team or organization.

Systems engineering Initiative for Patient Safety (SEIPS)

SEIPS is a form of systems modelling:

- Patient safety incidents result from multiple interactions between work system factors
- SEIPS describes how a work system can influence processes which subsequently shape outcomes
- It acknowledges that work systems and processes constantly adapt
- It looks for interactions rather than simple linear cause and effect
- When a learning response thoroughly examines the different work system components and their interactions, safety actions can focus on wider system issues, not individuals

Duty of candour

The duty of candour is a professional and statutory (legal) requirement to be open and honest with patients or families when something goes wrong with treatment or care which causes, or has the potential to cause, harm or distress (see Box 6.3). Its introduction as a legal duty was a recommendation of the Francis Report (see chapter 1; the Francis and Berwick reports).

Box 6.3 Common adverse incident terms

Adverse event: an event that could have/did result in harm.

Near miss: any adverse event which could have caused harm.

Significant adverse event: an adverse event which has led to major harm or death.

Never Event: an event which should never happen due to the availability of nationally agreed procedures, protocols, or guidelines to prevent it.

Minor harm: an incident where a patient required additional or prolonged monitoring after an event, or minor treatment.

Moderate harm: short term harm requiring additional treatment or procedures.

Severe harm: permanent or long-term harm to the patient.

There are two types of duty of candour:

1. A professional duty of openness and transparency for any incident which impacts the patient. This is overseen by regulatory bodies such as the GDC.
2. A legal duty to communicate with the patient if the incident appears to have caused or could lead to notifiable moderate or severe harm, prolonged psychological harm, or death. This is regulated by the CQC (see Box 6.4).

Box 6.4 Notifiable safety events

The CQC defines patient safety incidents and the threshold for duty of candour processes. Notifiable safety events are incidents that meet all three of the following criteria:

• It must have been unintended or unexpected
• It must have occurred during an activity which the CQC regulates
• In the reasonable opinion of a healthcare professional, the incident already has, or might, result in death, or severe or moderate harm to the person receiving care

In services other than an NHS trust or foundation trust, a notifiable event is one which resulted in, or requires treatment to prevent:

• Death of the person
• Sensory, motor or intellectual impairment that has lasted, or is likely to last, for a continuous period of at least 28 days
• Changes to the structure of the person's body
• Prolonged pain or prolonged psychological harm, or
• A shorter life expectancy for the person using the service

Where there is a legal duty, clinicians must:
- Tell the person face-to-face. The most appropriate team member will usually be the lead or accountable clinician (consultant)
- Apologize. This does not mean an admission of legal liability
- Provide a truthful account of what happened, explaining whatever is known at that point
- Explain to the relevant person what further enquiries or investigations you believe to be appropriate
- Follow-up by providing this information, and the apology, in writing, and providing an update on any enquiries
- Keep a secure written record of all meetings and communications with the relevant person

Throughout the process, 'reasonable support' should be given to the person, for example:
- Environmental adjustments for those with physical disabilities
- An interpreter for someone who does not speak English well
- Information in accessible formats
- Signposting to mental health services
- Support of an advocate

Patients expect to be told three things as part of an apology:
- What happened
- What can be done to deal with any harm caused
- What will be done to prevent someone else from being harmed

Senior clinicians

Consultants and senior clinicians have a responsibility to set an example and encourage openness and honesty in reporting adverse incidents and near misses.
- Actively foster a culture of learning and improvement
- Make sure that systems are in place to give early warning of any failure, or potential failure, in the clinical performance of individuals or teams (e.g. clinical audit, patient feedback, etc.)
- Ensure that any concerns about the performance of an individual or team are investigated and addressed quickly and effectively
- Ensure that the team is appropriately trained in patient safety and supported to openly report adverse incidents
- Work with others to collect and share information about patient experience and outcomes
- Ensure systems or processes are in place so that:
  - Lessons are learned from analysing adverse incidents/near misses
  - Lessons are shared with the team
  - Concrete action follows on from learning
  - Practice is changed where needed

Legislation

Each of the constituent nations in the United Kingdom have implemented recommendations regarding an organization's duty of candour, with some incorporating this into legislation.

England
- Health and Social Care Act 2008 (Regulated Activities) Regulations 2014. The CQC can prosecute for breaches of this regulation

Northern Ireland

Department of Health (Northern Ireland) Duty of Candour Policy proposals and a 'Being Open Framework' in April 2021, outlines:
- A statutory individual duty of candour (IDC) and a statutory organizational duty, both with criminal sanctions
- A statutory IDC without criminal sanctions. Individuals would be sanctioned by their employer, regulator, and professional body, and a statutory organizational duty with criminal sanctions
- A statutory IDC without criminal sanctions, and separate criminal sanctions for withholding, destroying, or providing false or misleading information, and a statutory organizational duty with criminal sanctions

Scotland
- The Health (Tobacco, Nicotine, etc. and Care) (Scotland) Act 2016 and The Duty of Candour Procedure (Scotland) Regulations 2018
- Organizations must publish an annual report on incidents when the duty has been applied. This includes the number of incidents, how the organization has implemented the duty and what has been learned or improved

Wales
- Duty of candour is a legal requirement for NHS organizations in Wales, outlined in the Health and Social Care (Quality and Engagement) (Wales) Act 2020. NHS providers are legally required to report annually on incidents

Why do incidents occur in dentistry?

Many of the patient safety incidents in dentistry relate to human factors, but they can also relate to system failures and patient factors. The areas of hospital-based dental care that are associated with risks to the patient and suggestions for mitigation are outlined below.

Lack of experience

- Junior members of the team and students 'don't know what they don't know'; this blind spot can affect patient outcomes
- This is especially relevant in a dental teaching hospitals
- Dentists with less experience are more likely to face litigation claims

Suggestions for mitigation

- Training and an open culture
- Standardized processes for safety critical aspects of patient care such as the surgical safety checklist
- Adequate supervision and support for junior members of the team
- Provide mentoring/personal tutors for junior team members, such as Educational Supervisors, student support, and pastoral care services
- Ensure that clinicians are practising within their own competence
- Appropriate trust and local induction processes

Poor communication

- Patients who have a limited understanding of the language being used
- Patients with learning disabilities and those who lack capacity
- Ineffective communication within teams
- Suboptimal handover communication
- Poor referrals e.g. ambiguity about the teeth requested for extraction

Suggestions for mitigation

- Use of interpreters and services such as Language Line
- Communicate with the patient's family and carers to provide the best treatment. It may be necessary to have a 'best interests meeting'
- Listen to and empower patients and their carers
- Examine team dynamics and make use of 'team briefs'
- Encourage team members to speak up
- Provide training in communication skills
- Investigate complaints thoroughly with a focus on themes
- Use established tools for handover such as SBAR—situation, background, assessment, recommendation
- Use of referral pro formas

Poor interpersonal relationships

Poor interpersonal relationships can have a negative impact on patient care. Clinicians may refuse to work with certain colleagues and patients may be denied the most appropriate care if they are not referred to the most appropriate colleagues.

Unhealthy levels of competition can also impact patient care.

Suggestions for mitigation

- Provide support for the team
- Multi-source feedback, which may be part of the appraisal process

- Report unsafe behaviours and concerns about clinicians
- Build a patient safety culture within the organization

Time pressures, tiredness, exhaustion, and fatigue/burnout

- Clinicians experiencing these feelings may pose a risk to their patients
- Overbooked clinics can be unmanageable and lead to adverse incidents
- Inadequate time can lead to clinicians taking 'shortcuts'
- Distractions during complex procedures can lead to errors

Suggestions for mitigation

- Psychological support for clinicians
- Appropriate workloads and sharing of responsibilities
- Adequate support from management
- Audits to demonstrate the overbooking of patients and appropriate changes to be made
- Rest time given to those who are working in shift patterns
- Use of the 'sterile cockpit' model in relation to surgery

Medical histories and comorbidities

- Many dental settings rely on patient-declared medical histories. This is a risk as patients may not understand the questions, or their memory of their health conditions may be unreliable
- Comorbidities are becoming more frequent as life expectancies increase. The dental side effects of many newer drugs may have an impact on patient outcomes
- Lack of knowledge in managing medical emergencies

Suggestions for mitigation

- Training to enable the team to take detailed medical histories
- Access to the patient's Summary Care Record—a short summary of the patient's GP and medication history available on some electronic notes systems
- Communicate with members of the patient's wider clinical team
- Continually update knowledge of medical comorbidities and pharmacology
- Ensure regular medical emergencies and resuscitation training as per national standards. Team training is also recommended

Misdiagnosis or lack of a diagnosis

Diagnoses are not always included in dental notes, or patients may be mis-diagnosed and then receive inappropriate treatment.

Suggestions for mitigation

- Conduct audits on note keeping
- Provide training/CPD
- Enable straightforward referral processes when clinicians are unsure of the diagnosis or management

Radiation safety

Suggestions for mitigation

- Ensure regular training and compliance with IR(ME)R 2017 regulations

Hierarchy and deference

Members of the team are reluctant to speak up when they see poor standards of clinical care or errors/omissions by senior staff.

Suggestions for mitigation

- Developing psychological safety, where individuals within the team feel safe to speak up, be open, admit mistakes, feel supported, and where vulnerability is valued
- Recognise that seniority does not necessarily equate to skill
- Develop leaders who practise open communication
- Provide mentorship to support clinical leaders
- Provide NOTSS training

Reluctance to report safety incidents

Fear of punitive action or detrimental effects on their careers may lead to clinicians feeling reluctant to report safety incidents.

Suggestions for mitigation

- Encourage a positive safety culture with openness where people feel comfortable talking about incidents and learning from them
- Avoid blame
- Regulator responses to patient safety incidents need to be proportionate
- Provide support for those involved in patient safety incidents (the second victim concept)

Delays in referrals/treatment

Delays in care can lead to patient safety issues. This may be due to delayed referrals or inappropriate management of missed, cancelled, or rearranged follow-up appointments. Examples include late cancer diagnosis or impacted canines causing resorption of adjacent teeth.

Suggestions for mitigation

- Ensure referral pathways are straightforward and accessible
- Liaise with managed clinical networks
- Work with management and commissioners to ensure that patients are seen within an acceptable timeframe
- Appropriate triage of referrals
- Audit against national standards for waiting times (18 week referral to treatment and 2 weeks for urgent referrals)
- Ensure appropriate administrative procedures so that follow-up appointments are booked and rearranged in an appropriate timeframe when clinics are cancelled
- Provide patients with contact details for the department—secretaries or clinical nurse specialists

Assumptions

- It may be assumed that a task has been completed when it has not
- The use of email for urgent communication about clinical matters is discouraged as there can be a dangerous assumption that once the email is sent, the contents have been read and acted upon. This also shifts the responsibility from the clinician sending the email to the one receiving it

Suggestions for mitigation

- Improve communication and encourage the use of checklists and standard operating procedures
- Use the telephone for urgent clinical matters. If email must be used, then follow-up with a further email or a telephone call to ensure that the information has been acted upon and allow proper dialogue

Use of electronic notes and templates

Electronic notes are now widespread in healthcare. They have several advantages over paper notes; however, the use of templates can lead to incorrect clinical information being recorded.

Suggestions for mitigation

- Ensure that the notes system is fit for purpose
- Ensure that the clinical team has appropriate access to the clinical notes. When passwords or access expires, there are processes in place to renew these in a timely fashion
- Use templates carefully and avoid the use of phrases such as 'NAD—nothing abnormal detected' in the template
- Templates can have a role in avoiding harm as they can be used as an aide-mémoire for clinicians when assessing a patient, this is especially useful for more junior members of the team

Risk management

A risk describes an event in the future which can adversely affect the trust, its patients, staff, and visitors.

- Risks can assume many forms, including clinical, financial, operational, information, and health and safety
- They differ from incidents, which are events that have happened

Risk management is a process designed to safeguard the safety of patients, staff members and visitors in the clinical setting (and beyond).

Trusts and dental departments must:

- Have systems in place to identify, analyse, and evaluate risks
- They must reduce the likelihood of them occurring and/or mitigate their adverse impacts
- Be proactive in identifying and prioritizing risks that could jeopardize their ability to meet their objectives
- High risks must be reviewed regularly (often monthly) to ensure their responses are appropriate and measured

Identifying risks

Risk reporting is the responsibility of all staff. Patients and visitors may also identify risks which should be reported. The use of checklists is often used by trusts to establish possible types of risk.

Potential sources of risk identification include:

- Serious incidents
- Near misses
- Quality improvement projects
- Patient and staff questionnaires
- CQC inspections
- Health and Safety Executive inspection reports

Risk assessment

Risk assessment is a tool used within the NHS and by organizations to understand how a particular risk should be managed.

- A risk assessment matrix (Table 6.5) is used, which categorizes the outcome and likelihood of a particular risk occurring into five levels
- A maximum risk score of 25 is possible through the multiplication of the outcome level with the probability level
- Risks awarded a score of 15 or more are considered 'high-risk' and are reviewed regularly (usually monthly) and are monitored at local risk management committees (LRMC) also termed risk action groups (RAGs)

Risk identification

1. Identify the risk

What is the nature of the hazard/risk? Who is affected (e.g. staff, patients, trust assets)

2. Assess and evaluate the risk

Using the risk assessment matrix (Table 6.5), ascertain the likelihood of the risk occurring and the potential impact it will have on the trust. Make a decision about how the risk should be managed. Outcomes can include

Table 6.5 Risk matrices and their status. Adapted from NHS Resolution

Liklihood Score	1	2	3	4	5
Descriptor	Rare	Unlikely	Possible	Likley	Certain
Expected Frequency	Not expected for years	At least once in the year	Up to once a month	At least weekly	Frequently

The RAG status for each risk:

Impact	Rare	Unlikely	Possible	Likley	Certain
5 **Catastropic** Severe harm or death	5	10	15	20	25
4 **Major** Severe harm, which is temporary, or moderate harm, which is permanent	4	8	12	16	20
3 **Moderate** Moderate harm, which lasts less than two months.	3	6	9	13	15
2 **Minor** Mild harm	2	4	6	8	10
1 **Insignificant** No harm	1	2	3	4	5

Table 6.6 The '4 Ts' response to risk. Adapted from NHS Resolution

Response	Action
Terminate	Changing how an activity is carried out or stopping it removes the risk in its entirety.
Tolerate	The risk scores low on the assessment matrix OR nothing can be done to mitigate the risk further. An example is using personal protective equipment (PPE) to reduce the risk of cross-transmission in the dental environment.
Treat	The risk can be mitigated through appropriate action. e.g locking controlled drugs in a secure location with keys only accessible by named members of staff.
Transfer	Transferring the risk to another named group or individual. e.g the secure storage of patient medical records by a recognized third-party group.

treatments and controls. A control refers to existing measures which are in place to mitigate risk. A treatment is further policy or strategy required to mitigate a risk if the level of risk is deemed too high after implementing controls.

3. Formulate a response

A response is formulated with the 4 Ts: terminate, tolerate, treat or transfer (see Table 6.6).

Risk register

Each trust will have a risk register, a log of all the risks identified within the trust. This register will vary in content by trust, but generally will contain:
- A title and description, date raised
- Directorate/team affected
- Details of the potential consequences
- Inherent risk—risk impact and likelihood without key controls
- Current risk—risk impact and likelihood with key controls in place
- Risk owner—individual or team responsible for managing the risk
- Key controls—actions already in place to mitigate the risk
- Actions in place should the risk become an issue
- Treatment plan/owner—strategies to develop and implement should the risk level be unacceptable after controls are applied
- Date by—plan completion date

The risk register is discussed monthly at the LRMC/RAG (see below).

Risk management roles

Senior management committees

Each trust will have several committees involved in managing risks within a hospital trust.
- Trust level—Audit and risk committee and/or risk management boards who monitor and review all aspects of governance and risk

management and ensure the provision of systems which manage risk in the Trust appropriately
- Local/Directorate level—LRMC, risk review groups, and health and safety committees. These are all involved in the identification and management of risks
- Other risk management teams include infection control, security, finance, clinical activity, and fire safety, etc.
- Certain risks are managed in specific job roles (e.g. radiation safety)

Consultants/clinical lead

Consultants will exercise risk management within and outside their service, supported by the risk management policy and teams as above. In a dental department this includes:
- Ensure local risks are appropriately identified, assessed, and evaluated—through undertaking and documenting risk assessments
- Identify inadequate risk controls and escalate to the responsible lead
- Work with allied specialities/teams to identify risk and manage risk
- Comprehensive trust and local induction and training with risks and mitigations identified
- Ensure a local risk register is available to all staff
- Encourage team members to openly discuss potential areas of risk
- Discuss incidents and risks at team meetings so that all staff are aware
- Arrange audits or quality improvement programmes to ensure mitigating actions are implemented
- Engage with the RAGs

Risk action group (RAG)

The RAG is a local committee at clinical service level and it is a key forum to discuss risks and incidents in the department and trust. These occur monthly. Attendees will vary by trust, but usually include:
- Clinical director and/or department clinical lead
- General manager and/or service manager
- Consultant representatives
- Lead nurse/matron
- Member of the patient safety or risk management teams

The group will review:
- Current and recently closed trust-wide serious incidents
- Identified trust-wide learning
- Incidents where that department is the main speciality involved
- Trust level risk register
- Dental department/speciality risk register

Morbidity and mortality meetings

Surgical morbidity and mortality (M&M) meetings discuss patient outcomes and mortality rates with the aim of achieving and maintaining high standards of care, quality control, and professional education. *Good Surgical Practice* published in 2014 by the Royal College of Surgeons (RCS) states that all surgeons should regularly attend M&M meetings as a key activity for reviewing the performance of the surgical team and ensuring quality.

Although the RCS has published a practical guide for setting up, running and participating in M&M meetings, their structure and content vary widely between teams and trusts.

Prescribing safety

Standards for prescription writing are outlined in the British National Formulary (BNF). It is important that:

- Any prescription is legible
- Doses, duration, and patient details are correct
- Cross through any blank areas on the prescription form to prevent other drugs from being added to the prescription
- A contact phone number must be provided to allow the pharmacist to communicate with the prescriber

Table 6.7 outlines prescribing issues that may arise in dentistry.

Prescribing resources for dentists:

- College of General Dentistry: Antimicrobial Prescribing in Dentistry (2020): https://cgdent.uk/antimicrobial-prescribing-in-dentistry/
- Scottish Dental Clinical Effectiveness Programme: Drug Prescribing for Dentistry (2021): https://www.sdcep.org.uk/published-guidance/drug-prescribing/
- British National Formulary: https://bnf.nice.org.uk/

Patient group directions

Patient group directions (PGDs) provide a legal framework that allows some registered health professionals to supply and/or administer specified medicines to a predefined group of patients, without them having to see a prescriber (such as a doctor or dentist).

Table 6.7 A summary of some of the issues that relate to prescribing in dentistry

Issue	Explanation
Adverse drug reactions	Dentists must have the appropriate medical emergency drugs to deal with anaphylaxis.
Interactions	Polypharmacy is becoming more commonplace. Dentists must: • Check for interactions before prescribing • Have a contemporary list of the medications that their patient is prescribed • Check the Summary Care Record provides this information from the patient's GP record • Adverse reactions can be reported to the MHRA using the yellow card scheme
Dosing/ dispensing errors	The importance of double-checking doses and expiry dates should not be overlooked.
Sedation	Sedative drugs including midazolam are controlled drugs and liaison with the pharmacy is essential to ensure that these are managed according to national standards. Flumazenil must be available wherever midazolam is being used.
Antibiotic overuse	This is a societal problem which dentistry also contributes to. The principles of antibiotic stewardship should be followed when prescribing.

PGDs can be used by dental hygienists and dental therapists in:
- NHS practices in England, Wales, and Scotland and their equivalents in Northern Ireland
- Private dental practices in England registered with the CQC
- Private dental practices in Wales, provided the individual dentists are registered with Health Inspectorate Wales
- Private dental practices in Northern Ireland registered with the Regulation and Quality Improvement Authority
- Private dental practices in Scotland registered with Health Improvement Scotland

The Human Medicines Regulations 2012 require a PGD to be signed by a dentist and a pharmacist. The expiry date of a PGD should 'not exceed 3 years from the date the PGD was authorized'.

The dental hygienist and dental therapist:
- Should be trained and competent to perform the procedure
- Are professionally accountable for their actions or omissions
- Should also ensure they have adequate indemnity arrangements in place

Requirements

PGDs need to contain the following:
- The period when the PGD will be in effect
- The description or class of medicinal product it relates to
- The clinical situations when medicinal products of that description or class can be used
- Whether there are any restrictions on the quantity of medicinal product that can be sold or supplied on any one occasion—and if so, what those restrictions are
- The clinical criteria under which a patient is eligible for treatment and whether anyone is excluded from treatment under the PGD
- The circumstances in which further advice should be sought from a doctor or dentist
- The pharmaceutical form or forms in which the medicinal products of that description or class are to be administered
- The strength or maximum strength at which the products can be administered, the applicable dosage or maximum dosage, the route and frequency of administration and the minimum or maximum period of administration
- Relevant warnings
- The circumstances in which any follow-up action is needed
- Referral arrangements for medical advice
- What records should be kept of the supply, or the administration, of products

Measuring patient safety

Patient safety is measured at national and local levels. The requirement to record incidents is regulated by the CQC.

National

The collection of national data about patient safety began in 2003.
- Learn from Patient Safety Events (LFPSE) was introduced in 2023 and replaced both the National Reporting and Learning System (NRLS) and Strategic Executive Information System (StEIS)
- These systems collect data on patient safety incidents in England
- Data from Datix and Ulysses reports feed into them and reports are issued by NHS England based on this data. These reports can be used at a local level to highlight aspects of patient care and safety
- Patients can also report incidents using the system, although uptake of this has been limited
- Patients are not always aware that incidents have occurred as they may not have caused a noticeable injury

This LFPSE system is:
- Capable of machine learning from incidents
- Aims to be more efficient and responsive when identifying risks
- Has more focus on 'minor harm' incidents which if not addressed can lead to further harm to patients
- Better at aggregating data and allowing thematic analysis

Locally/within an institution

There are several ways in which safety can be measured in a dental hospital or department:

Adverse event reporting
- Learning and sharing reports with those involved and the wider team raises awareness of what can go wrong
- This can be useful in preventing similar incidents in the future

Audits
- These can be used to demonstrate compliance with patient safety initiatives such as surgical safety checklists
- Procedural audits, where processes are observed in real time, identify where potential safety risks are
- Data should be collected over a period of time in order to examine trends and potential deviations from standard care

Patient reported measures
- Identify areas of good practice and areas where there is room for improvement (see also section on 'Measuring performance')

Trigger tools
These are case note reviews that look for a defined event (trigger) which may indicate that an adverse event has taken place.
Triggers suggested for dental care include:
- Use of flumazenil during conscious midazolam sedation which implies that the patient was over-sedated
- Failed implants

- Post-surgery complications—pain, infection, etc.
- Soft tissue or nerve injury
- Dental extraction following endodontic treatment/crown/restoration
- Allergy, toxicity, foreign body
- Aspiration/ingestion of foreign body

Peer review

Various tools exist for checking the safety of clinical teams. The NatSSIPs documents include templates including qualitative interview tools on aspects of the psychological safety of a clinical team. Multidisciplinary teams can visit clinical areas as observers. This can provide:

- Quantitative data, such as whether processes were followed or whether there were any incidents observed
- Qualitative data, including interviews with team members and questions relating to the safety culture in the department
- The discussion of these findings in an open culture will encourage positive patient safety behaviours

Assess whether care is safe now

The NatSSIPs guidelines highlight questions that can be asked of any clinical team:

- What is the composition of the clinical team?
- Who are the patients and what are their clinical needs and their views on safety?
- Is the team able to complete the required tasks?
- Does the team have the tools and the equipment needed to complete the tasks?
- Is the environment conducive to safety?
- What is the team's culture and its members' views on safety?

Safety thermometer

- This is used to measure and convey the idea of 'harm-free care', that is, the percentage of patients who did not have any of the common harms expected in a clinical area
- The data can be displayed on a ward or outpatient department as a visual representation for both patients and staff
- This data can be collected via review of clinical notes, or interviewing patients. Examples in dentistry could include:
  - Incidence of dry socket
  - Patients returning to theatre
  - Incidence of postoperative infection
  - Management of pain

Scenario—Patient safety 1—teeth or knees

A 28-year-old patient attends the day surgery unit for removal of his impacted third molars. The oral surgeon is doing their ward round and they find that the patient is being consented for a knee arthroscopy by the orthopaedic registrar.

Immediate actions taken

- The patient details should be checked using the wristband and clinical notes to confirm he is listed for removal of impacted molars

- The orthopaedic registrar should apologize to the patient
- The correct consent by the oral surgeon/team should be taken
- Establish with the orthopaedic registrar if there was a specific reason that led to the error, which could be repeated and that should be rectified immediately and highlighted to staff e.g. incorrect bed name/numbers on the board, communication issues (hearing difficulty, language barrier/need for interpreter)
- Check that other patients due to have operations that day have been appropriately consented and escalate immediately to theatres, orthopaedic consultant, and discuss at the team brief

Actions taken to prevent similar issues

- This is a near miss. A Datix/Ulysses should be raised. This will be sent to the risk management team and patient safety team
- Inputting the directorate/service information will ensure that the report is sent to the responsible clinicians (clinical lead/ward matron)
- These individuals should assess whether there is an immediate patient safety risk and action taken as required
- If not, the incident will be raised by the risk management team at the next RAG meeting. The details of the incident will be discussed, an individual responsible for managing the incident will be identified and an appropriate plan of action determined
- Consider auditing a cohort of patient notes to ensure that all planned procedures are adequately and clearly recorded
- Sometimes it is appropriate to complete a consent form at a previous appointment and then ask the patient to confirm consent and re-sign it on the day of the procedure. This allows the patient further time to reflect on the consent process and potential benefits vs. risks

If this is an isolated incident:

- The incident should be discussed at clinical governance/departmental meetings and clinicians should be reminded to check patient identities before clerking them for surgery. The importance of the patient stating their name and date of birth should be emphasized
- Raise awareness of the impact that anxiety can have on the behaviour of patients on wards prior to surgery

The risk manager at the RAG highlights a similar incident report that was submitted a month prior. What would you do?

This may indicate a systemic concern or pattern of behaviour. More information is needed to identify the cause(s):

- Speak with clinicians involved, including other individuals in your department who take consent, the ward/admin staff, members of other surgical specialities and service managers. Ensure that all consent processes are overseen by appropriate senior members of staff
- Review previous incidents: the risk management team and RAG would have oversight and knowledge of other reports within and outside your department and this may help identify the issue
- Clinical audit or quality improvement programme
- Peer review
- A formal RCA
- Review of PROMs/PREMs—this may identify patient concerns regarding the environment

The issue should be placed on the risk register. It would be the responsibility of the service manager and a senior clinician (consultant) to investigate and identify issues, with the aid of the risk management team.

The cause may relate to an individual, the ward environment or department and appropriate remedial steps should be taken. Examples include:

- A specific clinician struggling with workload (see Staff Management, chapter 7)
- A trainee working beyond their capacity (see Trainee Management, chapter 9)
- The ward environment—which may be chaotic, understaffed, or under-resourced. This may justify a review of working patterns, skill mix, level of clinical activity or a business case to increase capacity (see Running a Department, chapter 5)
- Poor handover or lack of communication within a team. This can be reviewed, with the creation of pro formas or additional training

Other considerations

- Patients in hospital beds can feel disempowered and anxious and may agree to interventions without knowing what they are signing up for
- There can be high levels of trust between patients and clinicians, the patient signed the consent form as they believed that this must be the right operation for them as the orthopaedic registrar said that it was
- The patient details were not adequately checked before the consent was discussed with the patient

Scenario—Patient safety 2—missed diagnosis

A 13-year-old child is seen at the orthodontic clinic for treatment planning and initial records. Lateral cephalometric radiographs and an orthopantomograph are taken. These are taken at the end of the consultation and briefly checked but not reported on by the postgraduate student who ordered them.

The child starts a course of orthodontic treatment. 18 months later, during a review appointment, a large radiolucency in the right mandible is noted on the baseline radiographs. This had not been picked up before this appointment. The patient is asymptomatic.

Immediate actions

- Patient safety is the priority; refer to oral surgery. Obtain a radiology report/update radiographs as required
- The senior clinician (consultant) should apologize to the patient and their parent, outlining what has happened, the onward referral and the steps to prevent recurrence. If the patient or parent is unhappy with this response and would like to make a complaint, you should signpost them to Patient Advice and Liaison Service (PALS)
- Complete a Datix/Ulysses to be reported to the LFPSE (and CQC)
- The incident should be investigated, discussed at the RAG and if appropriate added to the risk register
- The Duty of Candour should continue to be followed and a letter should be sent to the parent within 10 working days to outline the circumstances of the incident and the measures the team is taking to mitigate the impact of this incident

Medium-term actions and other considerations
- Radiographs should always be checked by the clinician ordering them. When students or trainees are involved in a patient's care, the senior clinician should review all notes and investigations
- Given that this involves a trainee, their educational supervisor should be informed. It may be appropriate for additional support (academic or pastoral) to be provided

The following measures may be taken to prevent similar issues:
- A standard operating procedure may be introduced for checking radiographs
- Radiographs should not be taken 'on the way out' of the clinic as this can lead to omissions. Patients should return to the clinic after having radiographs taken, so that the findings can be explained to them
- Templates for the electronic notes system encourage recording of radiographic findings. There are systems available that will not allow the clinician to progress to the next part of the notes until they have completed the previous part, this can be used in digital checklists to ensure compliance

Additional patient safety scenarios

The following scenarios should be managed in a similar fashion as scenario 1 and 2. Each reflects variations in the immediate steps or later steps in management.

A 23-year-old patient attends for the extraction of his upper right third molar under local anaesthetic due to it causing buccal trauma. He has been consented for the procedure at an earlier clinic appointment and had the upper left third molar removed the previous year.

A student is carrying out the extraction under supervision. The checklist for dental extractions has been completed up to the 'time-out' phase. The student starts the extraction without asking the supervisor to check that they are about to extract the correct tooth. The supervisor walks past and realizes that the student is removing the healthy, un-restored upper right second molar.

Immediate actions
- The student should be asked to stop the procedure, patient safety is the priority; a gauze should be placed
- The senior clinician should explain what has happened to the patient and apologize to them
- As the upper right second molar has not been fully removed, the injury is considered to be a lateral luxation. Splint the tooth and book a follow-up review appointment. The upper right third molar should be removed at a later date
- Record the situation in the patient's notes
- The student should be taken to a quiet place for a discussion about what has happened. The nurse should stay with the patient
- Implement the duty of candour process and complete a Datix/Ulysses

Additional considerations
- If they wish to make a complaint, signpost them to PALS

- The patient may consider claiming damages from the trust due to the experience and the unnecessary injury to the healthy tooth, in particular as this tooth may require endodontic treatment
- In such a situation the cost is covered by the hospital's Clinical Negligence Scheme for Trusts (CNST), although the student/consultant may have their own indemnity and should consult with them
- The standard operating procedure for tooth extraction was not followed
- The student may have carried out a 'time-out' with the nurse, but was then distracted by having to top up the local anaesthetic. When the student returned to the forceps, they were placed on the wrong tooth
- All members of staff and students should be reminded about the importance of following the protocol for tooth extraction and the need for students to have the tooth for extraction checked by the supervisor before starting the procedure

You are an orthodontic registrar and you are undertaking a debond of an appliance and notice the bur in the handpiece has fractured during use.

Immediate steps
- Stop the procedure
- Establish if the bur is visible in the mouth, if so, ask the patient to turn their head to one side to encourage the object to fall into the cheek rather than the oropharynx. Use forceps or high-volume suction to remove it
- Alternatively, encourage coughing to remove the object
- If the item is not retrieved, establish whether there are any signs that the object has been inhaled (such as choking or coughing) or ingested (such as difficult or painful swallowing)
- If the object is not retrieved, the patient should be sent to A&E
- If there are any signs of airway difficulty, you should call the hospital emergency number (2222) and follow basic life support (BLS) protocol

The object is recovered immediately, what steps would you take?
- Explain to the patient what has happened
- Confirm whether they are happy to continue or would like to delay the remainder of the treatment (if safe to do so)
- If continuing, establish what has happened before restarting
- If it reflects technique, then seek advice from the supervisor
- If the instrument is faulty, test a replacement bur/handpiece outside of the mouth before continuing
- If another bur is faulty, you should inform the supervisor immediately. They will inform any clinicians who may be using the same bur/batch and find alternatives
- An incident report should be submitted, if a recurring fault is suspected, the:
  - Manufacturer should be informed (to arrange a product recall if faulty)
  - The MHRA should also be informed
  - The incident may be reported using the British Orthodontic Society incident reporting form

You are a consultant oral surgeon and a 24-year-old, single mother has attended your department for a six-monthly review of right-side facial discomfort, which was initially diagnosed as temporomandibular joint dysfunction (TMD) by a previous dental core trainee 1 (DCT1) colleague. You are on a busy, overbooked clinic, which is running 45 minutes late. The patient arrives frustrated, and she says the clinic always runs late. She mentions her symptoms have deteriorated, and that a small swelling in front of her left ear, which was present at the last appointment, has increased in size. You assess the patient and take a panoramic radiograph which shows a moth-eaten area, and irregular radiopaque changes affecting the right glenoid fossa and condyle. What are the issues surrounding this scenario?

Diagnosis
- Review the diagnosis at each visit, especially if it is a chronic condition
- Always consider the risk of 'availability bias' when a patient presents with typical symptoms of a common condition that has previously been diagnosed as such by former colleagues. In this situation, the risk is that you continue with the same diagnosis already made as it would seem to be the obvious diagnosis. Changing the diagnosis would mean potentially overruling another colleague's diagnosis. In addition, a busy list may make it easier to conform to a previous diagnosis
- Consider senior review if symptoms are deteriorating or atypical

Clinic capacity and waiting time
- If a clinic is running late, inform reception to notify patients
- Staff may feel under pressure to 'get through the list', reducing time to conduct thorough examinations and formulate diagnoses. If there is an ongoing clinic capacity issue escalate it to the service manager
- Patients who are waiting for prolonged periods should be acknowledged individually or via PALS
- Overbookings should only be authorized by named staff members

Next steps
- Initiate urgent oral and maxillofacial surgery (OMFS) referral
- The patient has come to harm as they have had their diagnosis delayed and misdiagnosed. A Datix is required. The case is a learning tool for other trainees to spot red flag signs for more harmful pathologies which can disguise themselves as common conditions
- As part of duty of candour requirements, inform the patient

Further reading
- A Just Culture Gude (2021) NHS England. Available at: https://www.england.nhs.uk/wp-content/uploads/2021/02/NHS_0932_JC_Poster_A3.pdf
- Academy of Medical Sciences. Available at: https://acmedsci.ac.uk/policy/policy-projects/methods-of-evaluating-evidence
- After action review 2015 NHS England. Available at: https://www.england.nhs.uk/improvement-hub/wp-content/uploads/sites/44/2015/08/learning-handbook-after-action-review.pdf
- BAOS patient safety webpage. Available at: https://www.baos.org.uk/patient-safety2/
- Black and Bowie in 2017: Black, I., Bowie, P (2017). Patient safety in dentistry: development of a candidate 'never event' list for primary care. *Br Dent J*, 222:782–8.
- Great-ix reporting. Available at: https://greatix.org/

- Human Factors 101. Situation Awareness: Making Sense of the World. Available at: ℘ https://humanfactors101.com/topics/situation-awareness/
- Kalenderian E, Lee JH, Obadan-Udoh EM, Yansane A, White JM, Walji MF (2022). Development of an inventory of dental harms: methods and rationale. *J Patient Saf*, 18:559–64.
- NatSSIPs 2 document. Available at: ℘ https://www.england.nhs.uk/patient-safety/natssips/
- NHS England Patient Safety resources. Available at: ℘ https://www.england.nhs.uk/patient-safety/
- NHS England. Learning from patient safety events: https://www.england.nhs.uk/patient-safety/learn-from-patient-safety-events-service/
- NHS Patient Safety. Project Sphere. Available at: ℘ https://www.england.nhs.uk/primary-care/dentistry/leading-the-change/patient-safety/
- NHS training package for clinicians/managers. Available at: ℘ https://www.e-lfh.org.uk/programmes/patient-safety-syllabus-training/
- RCSEd NOTSS. Available at: ℘ https://www.rcsed.ac.uk/professional-support-development-resources/learning-resources/non-technical-skills-for-surgeons-notss
- Scott SD, Hirschinger LE, Cox KR, McCoig M, Brandt J, Hall LW (2009). The natural history of recovery for the healthcare provider 'second victim' after adverse patient events. *Qual Saf Health Care*, 18:325–30.
- SEIPS quick reference guide and work system explorer Version 1, August 2022 NHS England. Available at: ℘ https://www.england.nhs.uk/wp-content/uploads/2022/08/B1465-SEIPS-quick-reference-and-work-system-explorer-v1-FINAL.pdf
- Sujan M, Pickup L, Bowie P, Hignett S, Ives F, Vosper H, Rashid N (2021). The contribution of human factors and ergonomics to the design and delivery of safe future healthcare. *Future Healthc J*, 8(3):e574–9.
- The NHS Patient Safety Incident Response Framework. Available at: ℘ https://www.england.nhs.uk/patient-safety/incident-response-framework/
- Vincent C (2010). *Patient sSafety*. 2nd ed. Chichester: Wiley-Blackwell Publishing Ltd.
- WHO patient safety resources. Available at: ℘ https://www.who.int/teams/integrated-health-services/patient-safety
- World Health Organization. Global Patient Safety Action Plan 2021–2030. Available at: ℘: https://www.who.int/teams/integrated-health-services/patient-safety/policy/global-patient-safety-action-plan

Capacity

Every patient should legally be able to give valid consent before medical or surgical intervention. Failure to obtain consent is considered battery and is punishable by law.

- At 18 years, a person is presumed to have capacity unless evidence can reasonably prove otherwise
- The Family Law Reform Act 1969 extends this to 16 and 17-year-olds making decisions regarding surgical or medical interventions
- Capacity can change over time. Lack of capacity can be temporary, so the clinician must not presume a patient's capacity based on a single interaction
- Some patients will have the capacity to make some decisions while lack the capacity to make others. For example, a patient may allow clinical examination of a painful tooth but lack the capacity to understand the risks of removing the same tooth

The Mental Capacity Act

The Mental Capacity Act (MCA, 2005; England and Wales only) ensures support for individuals lacking capacity and prevents excessive control over them. It balances their right to make decisions with the need for protection from harm. Professionals working with such individuals must adhere to the MCA code of practice:

- Chapter 4—Assessments of capacity
- Chapter 10—Independent mental capacity advocates (IMCAs)

An IMCA is mandatory for individuals lacking support. They are required in various scenarios, such as serious medical treatment proposals (see Table 6.8) and advocacy services are available under the Act, provided by the local authority.

The MCA sets out principles which form the basis of decision-making for a person aged 16 and above:

1. A person is assumed to have the capacity and the ability to make decisions themselves unless one can reasonably prove otherwise.

Table 6.8 The role of the IMCA

Advocate can:	Advocate will not:
Listen to the person's views and concerns	Give their personal opinion
Help the person explore their options and rights (without pressuring them)	Solve problems and make decisions for a person
Provide information to help the person make informed decisions	Make judgements about a person
Help the person contact relevant people, or contact them on their behalf	
Accompany and support the person in meetings or appointments	

2. All practical steps must be taken to support a person to make a decision.
3. Patients should not be deemed to lack capacity because they make an unwise decision.
4. Any decision for a patient not deemed to have capacity should be made in their best interests.
5. Any treatment for a person deemed to not have capacity should be carried out in the least restrictive way of that person's basic rights.

Assessment of capacity

Capacity is assessed through a two-stage process:
- Stage 1—Does the person have an impairment of their brain or mind that impairs their function? Is it permanent or temporary?
- Stage 2—If so, does this impairment render the person unable to decide at this point in time? This can be determined by asking:
  - Does the person understand the information being relayed to them?
  - Can the person retain the information long enough to make a decision?
  - Is the person able to communicate their decision (verbally, written, or by any other means)?

Where decisions about care are complex, a multidisciplinary approach to care should be sought, incorporating other relevant specialities e.g special care dentistry and IMCAs.

Assessment of capacity for adults in Scotland follows the same principles, underpinned by the Adults with Incapacity (Scotland) Act [2000]. In Northern Ireland, the Mental Capacity Act (Northern Ireland) [2016] applies, again with similar principles.

Consent

Consent refers to the agreement by a patient to accept a medical examination or intervention.

Valid consent

Valid consent must satisfy three requirements: competence, voluntariness, and knowledge.

Competence refers to a patient being able to understand the proposed information and procedure and make a decision about the treatment. The term is often used interchangeably with 'capacity'.

Voluntariness refers to patients being able to make their own decisions without coercion. Involving family members or trusted individuals in care decisions is vital, however the final decision for a person with capacity rests with them.

Knowledge refers to patients being given enough information to make an informed decision. The legal stance on how much information should be provided was tested in the Sidaway case and, more recently, in the Montgomery Supreme Court ruling.

Patients can appoint a Lasting Power of Attorney (LPA), a legal document, to make healthcare-related decisions on their behalf if they lose capacity.

Montgomery Ruling 2015

The Montgomery Ruling stipulated that patients should be aware of any material risks applicable to their treatment and of any suitable alternative treatments. The ruling says that 'the test of materiality is whether, in the circumstances of the particular case, a reasonable person in the patient's position would be likely to attach significance to the risk, or the doctor is or should reasonably be aware that the particular patient would be likely to attach significance to it (Montgomery vs. Lanarkshire Health Board 2015).'

Clinicians must:
• Spend time understanding issues central to the patient's condition and tailor the consent process to the patient's circumstances
• Complex treatment plans should be discussed and documented with an adequate 'cooling-off' period for the patient to consider their options

It can be challenging to ascertain the patient's level of understanding and values they would assign significance to.
• Document the conversation and provide the patient with information leaflets
• A two-stage consent process may be more appropriate, where the patient returns another day for a further conversation
• This is required for high risks procedures or those with serious consequences

Children and consent

A clinician can treat a person under 16 years without a parent or legal guardian being present if the person is deemed to have sufficient understanding. The term 'Gillick competent' is used to describe such individuals, often interchangeably with 'Fraser competent'.

Patients aged 16 or 17

For patients aged 16 or 17 who are deemed to lack capacity, the decision to proceed with an investigation or treatment is different in England, Wales, and Northern Ireland, compared with Scotland.

- In England, Wales, and Northern Ireland, someone with parental responsibility can give permission for an investigation or treatment that is in the best interests of the patient
- In Scotland, a 16- or 17-year-old without capacity is considered an adult without capacity

In a hospital setting, protracted courses of treatment (e.g. orthodontics) and complex surgery in children (e.g. management of impacted teeth under general anaesthetic) should always be discussed and performed in the presence of a parent or legal guardian.

Consent from one parent is sufficient, except for the following circumstances:

- There is a known disagreement between parents
- Cases involving immunization or circumcision
- The local authority has parental responsibility
- For non-therapeutic, innovative, or controversial treatment

In an emergency, to prevent death or serious harm, treatment can be carried out without consent. However:

- An attempt should be made to contact a parent
- Thorough documentation should be recorded in the patient's notes
- Liaising with the hospital legal team is advised
- In some cases, an urgent court authorization may be possible

Treatment without consent is permitted to manage the immediate emergency, any further ongoing treatment requires consent.

> ## Implied and expressed consent
>
> Express consent—Consent given orally or written for a specific examination or intervention.
> Implied consent—A patient has not given express consent, but their actions imply permission to examine their mouth when opened. Examination does not necessarily give consent to other more invasive tests such as percussion or sensibility tests.

Consent forms

The GDC Standards stipulate that any procedure involving conscious sedation or general anaesthetic must be carried out with written consent. Written consent forms in NHS hospitals are specific to age and capacity.

Consent forms do not replace discussions and interactions with patients. A patient's signature on the consent form does not act as a substitute for permission to proceed with treatment. Consent is an ongoing and dynamic process; withdrawal can occur at anytime.

If consent forms are being used:

- Lay terms should always be used
- Abbreviations should always be written in full initially

In hospital settings, it is often the case that the person completing the consent form is not the person carrying out the procedure. Whoever is completing the consent form must have had appropriate training to take consent and possess knowledge about the proposed intervention and be able to understand the risks involved. Advocates and interpreters should sign in the designated area on the consent form. If an intermediary service is being used (e.g. Language Line), then the reference number for the encounter should be recorded on the consent form.

Scenario—Consent/capacity 1

Mr Peters, a 50-year-old male has been referred to your department by the cardiothoracic team with pain from an unrestorable lower right first molar (LR6). He has infective endocarditis and is due for an urgent valve replacement. The cardiothoracic team has asked that any acute foci of infection are managed prior to his cardiac surgery.

A radiograph shows apical changes consistent with a chronic apical infection of the LR6.

You explain to Mr Peters that the tooth requires extraction; however, he does not want the tooth extracted. He uses this tooth to chew, and does not want to lose it.

What are the main considerations in this scenario?
- A patient requires urgent intervention for a life-threatening condition. It appears that they are refusing treatment to a procedure which may affect the long-term prognosis or success of their underlying condition
- Any patient above the age of 18 years must give valid consent before intervention takes place
- Capacity to make a decision must be established before a decision is made regarding treatment. There is always a presumption of capacity, and a capacity assessment should only be made if there is doubt about their capacity
- Patients with capacity have the right to refuse treatment, even if it may affect their life, endanger their life, or appear objectively unwise
- There is a presumption of capacity, and capacity assessment should only be undertaken if there is doubt about their capacity

What do you do if the patient refuses extraction of the tooth?
- An adult patient with capacity can withhold consent to any procedure, even if it endangers their life
- The patient does not have to give a reason for refusing treatment, even if it seems irrational and illogical to the treating team
- Patients may refuse treatment due to misconceptions about what the treatment may entail. The risks and benefits of the treatment must be outlined to the patient including the risk to cardiac health
- Offer a second opinion
- Ensure the patient is supported in their decision by other senior healthcare professionals, friends, and trusted individuals

What else must you consider?
- Thoroughly document your discussions as soon as possible
- Ensure patients know that they can change their mind
- Discussions with other medical teams can be helpful

- Patients admitted with urinary tract infections (UTIs) and other acute presentations may present with fluctuating degrees of capacity

Which legal cases set precedent or are considered reference cases for the decision made?
- Montgomery v Lanarkshire Health Board [2015]
- King's College Hospital NHSFT v C & V [2015] EWCOP 80
- Case B (adult refusal of medical treatment) [2002] 2 All ER 449

Scenario—Consent/capacity 2

You are an oral surgery consultant. Dexter is a 15-year-old medically healthy patient who has been referred for surgical removal of a palatally impacted upper left permanent canine (UL3). Dexter's primary complaint is wanting his teeth to be 'straighter'. He has clearly said that he does not want surgery although his parents are keen for surgery. The upper left deciduous canine (ULC) is fully erupted, non-mobile, and exhibits incisal edge tooth-surface loss. He has attended with his father.

What is the legal position on Dexter's refusal of treatment?
- The patient is under 16 years therefore a judgment needs to be made on whether they are 'Gillick competent' i.e. does the child have sufficient understanding and intelligence to enable them to understand fully what is proposed?
- The clinician must decide whether the child has understood the proposed treatment and consequences of refusing treatment. In this case, refusal of treatment is likely to severely compromise any fixed orthodontic treatment, eventual loss of the deciduous canine, compromised aesthetics, and the potential pathological sequelae of leaving an ectopic/impacted tooth in situ (e.g. cyst formation and resorption of the neighbouring roots). Alternative treatment options must be discussed, even if deemed a compromise
- If the child still refuses treatment, and the clinician is satisfied that the child is of maturity and possesses the understanding to make such a decision, it would be unwise to force such care on them
- The courts can overrule this decision. They are unlikely to do so where this is for aesthetic reasons but may do so if the treatment was necessary to save the child's life or to prevent serious deterioration in their quality of life
- However, if a child who is judged to be competent refuses treatment, this can be overruled by a person with parental responsibility, if doctors think it is in their best interest

How should this issue be approached?
- Explore why the child is refusing treatment
- Involve the parents and the patient in your discussions. Discuss all the alternative options and allow time for consideration
- Involve the wider team, such as a clinical psychologist to aid decision-making
- See the patient jointly with the referring orthodontic clinician to alleviate concerns

Does a father always hold parental responsibility for the child?
- The father has parental responsibility if he is married to the child's mother at the time of conception or birth, has acquired it through a court order, or if he is named on the child's birth certificate

Further reading
- Dungarwalla MM, Bailey E (2020). Consent in oral surgery: a guide for clinicians. *Dental Update*, 47(2):92–102.
- GMC Decision-making and consent. Available at: 🔗 https://www.gmc-uk.org/-/media/docume nts/gmc-guidance-for-doctors---decision-making-and-consent-english_pdf-84191055.pdf
- NHS. Mental Capacity Act. Available at: 🔗 https://www.nhs.uk/conditions/social-care-and-support-guide/making-decisions-for-someone-else/mental-capacity-act/)

Cross-infection and dental aerosols

The transfer of microorganisms from contaminated surfaces or from person to person is known as cross-infection. Healthcare workers have a legal and ethical obligation to comply with regulations to minimize the risk of cross-infection in the dental environment. Infection Prevention and Control forms a core part of the clinical governance structure within NHS trusts.

Control of Substances Hazardous to Health Regulations

The Control of Substances Hazardous to Health Regulations (COSHH) (2002) stipulate that employers must risk assess and protect their employees and other relevant users through the control of exposure to hazardous substances. These substances include both chemicals and biological agents.

- A biological agent is defined as a microorganism, cell culture, or human endoparasite, whether or not genetically modified, which may cause infection, allergy, toxicity, or otherwise create a hazard to human health
- The use of chemicals in confined spaces, particularly where there is a reaction between them and human products, can be problematic leading to respiratory complications

Any staff member joining a trust (who is working in a clinical area):
- Will undertake mandatory infection control training as part of induction, this usually requires an annual update
- Will undergo scrutiny through the occupational health department to:
  - Review immunization status
  - Carry out health assessment screening to determine suitability and fitness to undertake their job roles. This is also an ideal time to address the requirements of consideration of 'reasonable adjustments' in those with medical conditions likely to be deemed a disability under the Equality Act (see Chapter 7)

Staff working in clinical areas must:
- Take reasonable precautions to protect their patients from communicable diseases
- Follow the NHS immunization & vaccination trust framework which complements the 'green book' to ensure compliance with the Health & Safety at Work Act (HSWA) 1974
- Apply trust infection control policy when working in the clinical environment
- Report failures in enacting the infection control policy to the infection control lead (e.g. lack of suitable personal protective equipment (PPE), or repeated instances of failure to maintain good hand hygiene)

Responsible clinicians (consultants) and managers in a dental department have delegated responsibility for implementing COSHH and infection policies within their departments. This includes:
- Bringing appropriate policies to the attention of their team
- Compiling an inventory of hazardous substances and conducting a written risk assessment
- Ensuring COSHH assessments are professionally performed, reviewed, and are accessible to the staff using hazardous substances

- Ensuring the team has appropriate information, instruction, and training before using hazardous substances and are familiar with how to use any control measures
- Control measures should follow the 'hierarchy of controls'. Where the risk cannot be otherwise avoided, select the correct type and specification of PPE where the assessment indicates that it is needed and appropriate
- Carrying out or arranging appropriate exposure monitoring and/or health surveillance in conjunction with occupational health where required

Hand hygiene

Hand hygiene remains a cornerstone of good cross-infection control. This includes:
- Keeping nails short and cleansable
- Avoiding nail varnish
- Covering cuts with waterproof dressings
- Removing wristwatches
- Not wearing rings with stones
- Being bare below the elbows
- Washing systematically with soap and water when in a clinical environment

Alcohol-based hand rubs are useful adjuncts for hand hygiene when liquid soap, water, and sink facilities are unavailable. They are unsuitable when hands are soiled and ineffective against *Clostridium difficile* and norovirus infection.

Hand-hygiene audits are used to ensure that all staff present in clinical areas are complying with the trust infection control policy.

They must be conducted systematically (usually monthly with a minimum number of hand-hygiene observations per week) with a designated infection control lead responsible for the collection and reporting of data. Failure to comply will trigger an action plan to ensure that satisfactory hand hygiene is taking place.

Universal precautions

All patients should be treated without discrimination with the assumption that they may unknowingly be carrying potentially infectious microorganisms. As such, *universal precautions* are used when treating all patients in a clinical environment.

In addition to hand hygiene, other infection control measures include:
- Assessing patients for their infection risk
- Use of PPE
- Managing equipment used in clinical environments
- Management of linen, body fluids, and blood
- Safe disposal of infectious waste and sharps
- Appropriately managing exposure to potentially infectious agents

The use of PPE controls the exposure of hazardous substances to the clinical team. Commonly used PPE in dentistry includes plastic aprons, surgical face masks (type IIR), goggles with side protection, gloves (commonly nitrile-based to prevent latex allergy reactions).

The main routes of infection are transmission through contact (direct or indirect), parenteral, aerosols, and contaminated waterlines.

Coronavirus Disease (COVID-19)/Severe Acute Respiratory Syndrome Coronavirus 2 (SARS-CoV-2)

The biggest threat to modern dentistry was the arrival of the COVID-19 pandemic and the cessation of all dental activity in the United Kingdom (except for limited sites). The pandemic was not the first novel coronavirus to affect dental activity, with the Severe Acute Respiratory Syndrome (SARS) 2003 epidemic resulting in the closure of Hong Kong's dental school.

Aerosol-generating procedures (AGPs) with particles less than 5 μm present an increased risk of respiratory infection transmission. Guidance published at the pandemic's peak recommended:

- Use of high-volume suction
- Rubber dam
- Measured fallow-time between treatments

Face masks

Several types of masks are available for use in the clinical environment. The most common masks are type IIR and fit-tested filtering facepiece 3 (FFP3) masks. Respirator hoods are available for individuals who do not sufficiently fit into an FFP3 mask. Masks are quantified based on their bacterial filtration efficiency (BFE).

Type IIR are four-ply masks which provide a fluid-repellent barrier, offering protection from saliva and blood during treatment. They can often be combined with a visor which provides suitable eye protection.

FFP3 masks are filtered masks designed to filter 98% of airborne particles with less than 2% leakage reported. They must be appropriately fitted before use.

Current guidelines

At the time of writing, the current guidance from the UK government states that staff who have symptoms of a respiratory illness and are unwell should stay away from the workplace. There is no requirement to take a lateral flow test.

Staff can return to work if they are feeling well enough and are not in contact with patients who are severely immunocompromised.

For healthcare workers providing direct patient care to those who are immunocompromised with symptoms of a respiratory illness and high fever it is required is to take a lateral flow device test as soon as possible. If the test is positive, the healthcare worker should not attend work for 10 days.

COVID-19 is still prevalent within the community, and testing is no longer routine. Therefore, all patients should be asked regarding respiratory symptoms (such as a persistent new cough), and consideration should be given to delaying elective/non-urgent dental treatment.

Where urgent care is required, consider the following:

- Book the patient at the end of the day in a closed room
- Use PPE consisting of a disposable gown, gloves and fit-tested filtering facepiece (FFP3) mask
- Following an AGP, a downtime of at least 10 minutes is advised in an environment with a suitable number of air exchanges

Where a patient does not exhibit respiratory symptoms, a disposable apron, gloves and standard type IIR surgical mask should be used with a visor/goggles. It is no longer advised to routinely use FFP3 masks for AGPs.

Ventilation of dental surgeries allows the replacement of potentially contaminated air with fresh air.

- Ventilation can be naturally achieved (e.g. windows, doors and vents), while mechanical ventilation uses fans to extract the air
- Current guidance stipulates that treatment rooms should have at least ten air changes per hour

Further reading

- Department of Health and Social Care (2021). Immunization against infectious disease— 'The Green Book'. DoH, London. Available at: ℛ http://www.dh.gov.uk/en/Publicationsandstatistics/Publications/PublicationsPolicyAndGuidance/DH_07991
- GOV.UK. Managing healthcare staff with symptoms of a respiratory infection or a positive COVID-19 test result. Available at: ℛ https://www.gov.uk/government/publications/covid-19-managing-healthcare-staff-with-symptoms-of-a-respiratory-infection/managing-healthcare-staff-with-symptoms-of-a-respiratory-infection-or-a-positive-covid-19-test-result#healthcare-staff-with-symptoms-of-a-respiratory-infection-including-covid-19-or-a-positive-lfd-test-result
- Health & Safety at Work Act (HSWA) 1974—Section 7—Health & Safety Executive.
- HSE (2000). *Management of Health and Safety at Work Regulations 1999 L21*. HSE Books, Sudbury. Available at: ℛ http://www.legislation.gov.uk/uksi/1999/3242/contents
- HSE (2002). *Control of Substances Hazardous to Health Regulations 2002 (as amended). Approved Code of Practice and Guidance*, 5th edn, L5. HSE Books, Sudbury. Available at: ℛ http://www.legislation.gov.uk/uksi/2002/2677/contents/made
- NHS Education for Scotland. Ventilation Information for Dentistry. Available at: ℛ https://www.sdcep.org.uk/media/mavp4zzt/sdcep-ventilation-information-for-dentistry.pdf
- NHS Immunization & Vaccination Trust Framework Version 2.0 NHS England.
- SDCEP. Rapid review of AGPS. Rapid review of AGPs. Scottish Dental Clinical Effectiveness. Available at: ℛ https://www.sdcep.org.uk/published-guidance/covid-19-practice-recovery/rapid-review-of-agps/

Sharps injuries

Sharps injuries are a known risk within the dental clinical environment. A department should have the necessary safeguards to reduce this risk, and staff should be aware of the process for managing a sharps injury.

The risk of a sharps injury may be reduced through:
- Correct sharps management
- Correct attire
- Appropriate disposal

A sharp is defined as something which can pierce a yellow clinical waste bag. Extracted teeth are considered 'sharps' and should be disposed of in a sharps bin unless they contain amalgam.

The safe management of sharps is the responsibility of all those involved in clinical work and waste disposal.

It is the operating clinician's responsibility to account for the disposal of all sharps during a procedure in an outpatient setting. Theatre will have individual counts for this. Off-site facilities often manage instruments, and individuals may encounter sharps inadvertently left on the instrument trolley.

Blood-borne viruses

In a clinical setting, a percutaneous (sharps) injury may lead to exposure to blood-borne viruses (BBVs).

While most infectious diseases can be spread via this route, the main pathogens of concern are hepatitis B, C, and HIV. Some trusts also test for HTLV (Human T-cell lymphotropic virus) at the time of a sharps injury.

The risk of transmission from a sharps injury is approximately as follows:
- Hepatitis B—1 in 3
- Hepatitis C—1 in 30
- HIV—1 in 3000

The risk of contracting hepatitis B is minimal as all healthcare workers in the UK should have been vaccinated against it.

There is no vaccination for hepatitis C, due to the various genotypes and subtypes of the virus. The potential sequelae (liver failure/cirrhosis and hepatocellular carcinoma) are life-threatening.

Sharps injury process

After a sharps injury has occurred:
- Immediately stop the procedure
- Ensure the patient is safe
- Encourage the wound to bleed
- Wash the area with soap, avoiding alcohol-based products
- Do not scrub the wound, cover the wound with a dressing

The patient involved should be immediately informed of the situation, explaining that a sharps injury has occurred.
- In line with national guidance, obtain permission for taking a blood sample from the patient. Advise the patient of the protocol (which is derived from national policy) used to establish the risk of transmission of communicable diseases
- Explain to the patient that you will be testing for HIV, hepatitis B, and hepatitis C

- Consent must be obtained before bloods can be taken and a patient can refuse this request
- Sharps sustained while the patient is under IV sedation or general anaesthetic must be treated in the same way although a blood sample must not be taken until it is established that the patient has capacity
- The supervising clinician, consultant, or head nurse should be informed
- Report to the occupational health department and if out of hours discuss with the on-call microbiologist and report to the emergency department for blood tests
- Postexposure prophylaxis (PEP) will be given on a risk-assessed basis by the consultant microbiologist. It should be administered as soon as possible (within hours) where possible
- Report the incident to the trust's incident reporting system and also document in the patient's notes. Support should be provided for staff members as it may be their first time experiencing a sharps injury
- The incident can be difficult for both the clinician and patient, support should be provided to both as required

Once the sharps injury has been managed and the patient has safely been discharged, the standard process for learning and preventing further incidents should be followed. Additional measures that a department may implement include:

- Ensuring only clinicians who have used sharps are responsible for their disposal
- Use devices which protect the user from sharps (e.g. Ultra Safety Plus Twist Local Anaesthetic Injection, Septodont, France; BD Nexiva Cannulae, BD, USA)
- Ensure sharps bins are easily accessible in the clinical area and kept away from where they can cause harm to others
- Ensure that sharp burs and ultrasonic tips are removed immediately after their use
- Avoid re-sheathing needles
- Use retractors (instead of fingers!) when operating and using blade removal devices

Healthcare workers living with blood-borne viruses

The UK Advisory Panel for Healthcare Workers Living with Blood-borne Viruses (UKAP) has published guidelines for when clinicians may perform exposure prone procedures (EPPs).

These are defined as:

- Procedures where there is an opportunity for healthcare worker -to-patient transmission of BBVs
- This includes procedures where the worker's gloved hands may be in contact with sharp instruments, needle tips or sharp tissues inside a patient's open body cavity (including oral cavity), wound, or confined anatomical space where the hands or fingertips may not be completely visible at all times
- Dental procedures are considered EPPs

The trust and department should foster a supportive and non-stigmatizing environment which encourages healthcare workers (HCW) to access occupational health support and protect confidentiality.

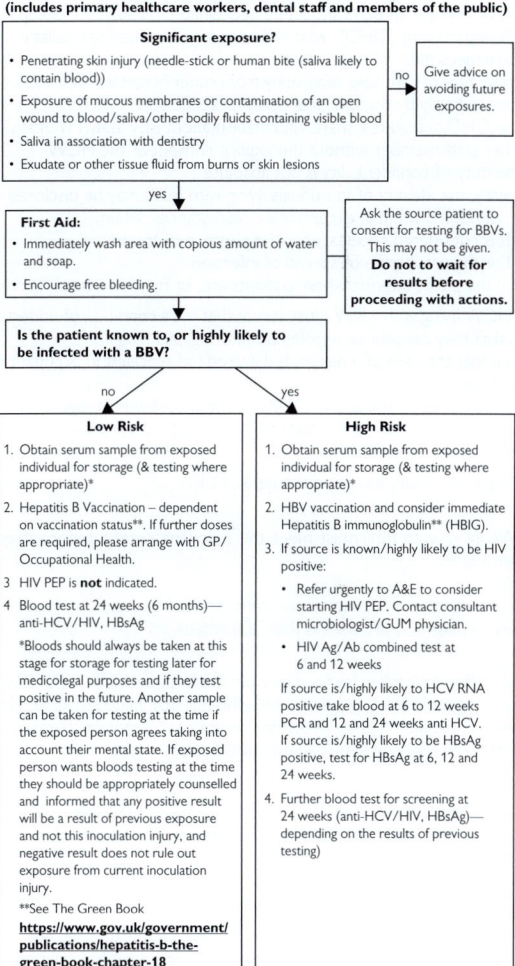

Management of Exposure to Blood Borne Viruses
(includes primary healthcare workers, dental staff and members of the public)

Significant exposure?

- Penetrating skin injury (needle-stick or human bite (saliva likely to contain blood))
- Exposure of mucous membranes or contamination of an open wound to blood/saliva/other bodily fluids containing visible blood
- Saliva in association with dentistry
- Exudate or other tissue fluid from burns or skin lesions

no → Give advice on avoiding future exposures.

yes ↓

First Aid:
- Immediately wash area with copious amount of water and soap.
- Encourage free bleeding.

Ask the source patient to consent for testing for BBVs. This may not be given. **Do not to wait for results before proceeding with actions.**

Is the patient known to, or highly likely to be infected with a BBV?

no ↓   yes ↓

Low Risk

1. Obtain serum sample from exposed individual for storage (& testing where appropriate)*

2. Hepatitis B Vaccination – dependent on vaccination status**. If further doses are required, please arrange with GP/Occupational Health.

3 HIV PEP is **not** indicated.

4 Blood test at 24 weeks (6 months)—anti-HCV/HIV, HBsAg

*Bloods should always be taken at this stage for storage for testing later for medicolegal purposes and if they test positive in the future. Another sample can be taken for testing at the time if the exposed person agrees taking into account their mental state. If exposed person wants bloods testing at the time they should be appropriately counselled and informed that any positive result will be a result of previous exposure and not this inoculation injury, and negative result does not rule out exposure from current inoculation injury.

**See The Green Book
https://www.gov.uk/government/publications/hepatitis-b-the-green-book-chapter-18

High Risk

1. Obtain serum sample from exposed individual for storage (& testing where appropriate)*

2. HBV vaccination and consider immediate Hepatitis B immunoglobulin** (HBIG).

3. If source is known/highly likely to be HIV positive:
   - Refer urgently to A&E to consider starting HIV PEP. Contact consultant microbiologist/GUM physician.
   - HIV Ag/Ab combined test at 6 and 12 weeks

   If source is/highly likely to HCV RNA positive take blood at 6 to 12 weeks PCR and 12 and 24 weeks anti HCV. If source is/highly likely to be HBsAg positive, test for HBsAg at 6, 12 and 24 weeks.

4. Further blood test for screening at 24 weeks (anti-HCV/HIV, HBsAg)—depending on the results of previous testing)

Figure 6.2 Summary of the process of managing a sharps injury in a dental environment.

All matters arising from and relating to the training and or employment of HCWs living with BBVs should be coordinated through the occupational health department (OHD), who will have an accredited specialist in occupational medicine.

- These records are held separately from other hospital notes and can be accessed only by occupational health practitioners
- The OHD should not share information about BBV status with any other staff member without the explicit consent of the HCW
- The duty of confidentiality is not absolute
- Legally, the identity of individuals living with BBVs may be disclosed with or without consent in exceptional circumstances, when:
  - It is considered necessary for the purpose of treatment
  - For the prevention of spread of infection
  - In the public interest where patients are, or may have been, at risk

The HCW living with a BVV must accept that it is a condition of undertaking EPPs that they consent to ongoing monitoring, including:

- Be under the care of a designated accredited specialist in occupational medicine
- Be registered on the UKAP-OHR, a central confidential register
- Release of viral load test results to the accredited specialist in occupational medicine

The regulations vary based on the type of BBV.

HIV

HCWs living with HIV must meet the following criteria before they can perform EPPs:

Either

- Be on effective combination anti-retroviral therapy and
- Have a plasma viral load less than 200 copies/ml

Or

- Be an elite controller (defined as a person living with HIV who is not receiving antiretroviral therapy and who has maintained their viral load below the limits of assay detection for at least 12 months, based on at least three separate viral load measurements)

And

- Be subject to plasma viral load monitoring every 12 weeks
- Be under the joint supervision of an accredited specialist in occupational medicine and their treating physician
- Be registered with UKAP-OHR

Hepatitis B

HCWs living with hepatitis B must show their viral load does not exceed 200 IU/ml at least one year after cessation of treatment before a return to unrestricted working practices can be considered.

They must have their plasma viral load tested every six months. Table 6.9 summarizes the actions taken based on this result.

Hepatitis C

HCWs who have active or current infection (those who are HCV RNA positive), are restricted from carrying out EPPs.

Table 6.9 Summary of the monitoring arrangements for HCWs living with HIV and Hepatitis B (HBV)

Viral load (copies/ml)		Action taken
HIV	HBV	
<50	<60	No action.
≥50 but <200	≥60 but <200	Occupation health to advise on case-by-case basis. Retest after 10 days.
≥200 but <1,000		A second test should automatically be taken 10 days later. If maintained above 200 copies/mL, cease EPPs, until less than this in two consecutive tests no less than 12 weeks apart.
>1,000	≥200	The HCW should cease conducting EPPs immediately. A second test on a new blood sample 10 days later. If viral load remains above this, a full risk assessment to determine risk of patient transmission.

HCWs who have antibodies to HCV and are confirmed as having a sustained viral response (those who are HCV RNA negative), following treatment are allowed to perform EPPs,

Patient notification exercise

UKAP should be consulted for advice on undertaking a Patient Notification Exercise (PNE).

The need for a PNE should be determined on a case-by-case basis taking into consideration:

- A risk assessment of the HCW's practice and probity in relation to the risk of BBV transmission to EPP patients
- The relative infectious window period
- Significance of any viral load 'blip'

Further reading

- Department of Health and Social Care (2021). *Immunization against Infectious Disease— 'The Green Book'*. London: DoH. Available at: ℘ http://www.dh.gov.uk/en/Publicationsandstatistics/Publications/PublicationsPolicyAndGuidance/DH_07991
- Integrated guidance on health clearance of healthcare workers and the management of healthcare workers living with blood-borne viruses (hepatitis B, hepatitis C and HIV) UK Advisory Panel for Healthcare Workers Living with Blood-borne Viruses (UKAP). Available at: ℘ https://assets.publishing.service.gov.uk/media/65423f21d36c91000d935b8f/integrated-guidance-for-management-of-bbv-in-hcw-november-2023.pdf

Remote dentistry

Technological advances supporting more efficient delivery of dentistry have been embraced by the dental profession, supporting remote consultation and monitoring of treatment particularly in orthodontic care. Digital technology has also increased options for remote peer-to-peer training, diagnosis, treatment planning, and mentorship. Although technology has rapidly evolved to increase remote care capability, including across different jurisdictions; the regulatory and legal framework globally remains relatively immature. Guidance and restrictions can vary between countries and even within states of the same nation. Consequently, clinicians must consider how existing standards and legislation may apply to the remote delivery of care. Some of the issues relevant to the delivery of remote care in the UK are considered below.

Regulatory and legal framework

Remote provision of care

This area is not specifically addressed by the GDC "Standards for the Dental Team" or associated guidance, however it should be considered that the same standards apply irrespective of how care is delivered. Ultimately, remote models of care should not compromise care and ideally should enhance it.

In response to growth in direct-to-consumer orthodontics, the GDC published a statement confirming these services fall within the legal definition of dentistry and so could only be performed by registrants. Although specific to direct-to-consumer orthodontics, it is reasonable to apply these general principles to other models of remote care.

- A physical, clinical examination is necessary to confirm suitability
- The GDC registrant prescribing treatment is responsible for complying with GDC Standards
- The treating dentist must make and retain full patient records, including reasons for deviating from established practice and guidance
- Direct interaction is essential as part of the consent process. The term 'direct' includes remote interaction between the patient and treating clinician

Remote prescribing

GDC Guidance states that dentists should only prescribe medicines for dental patients remotely 'if there is no other viable option and it is in their best interests'. Outside of the COVID-19 pandemic, these situations would ordinarily be rare in a dental setting.

The High-Level Principles of Remote Consultation and Prescribing document was co-authored by multiple UK regulators during the pandemic to support safe delivery of remote care. This document does not override existing GDC regulatory and professional standards guidance.

Remote prescribing and remote consultation should only be considered when it is appropriate and safe to do so. To minimize risk, consider:

- Limiting remote care to existing and known patients and where identification can be confirmed
- Avoiding remote care for potentially vulnerable patients e.g. children

- Ensuring patient consent for remote care is valid and documented. Patients should understand the limitations and be able to decline remote care
- That full assessment of presentation/symptoms is possible and a clear diagnosis can be made
- Limiting remote care to cases where the clinician has access to previous records, radiographs, and medical history
- Ensuring a face-to-face appointment can be promptly arranged

Care quality commission (CQC)—England

The CQC confirmed the provision of orthodontic aligners, even where the patient has taken their own impressions, to be a regulated activity. Providers of these regulated activities based in England are therefore required to have CQC registration. Other regulators in the UK (HIS, HIW, and RQIA) have to date not provided specific guidance.

Indemnity

Indemnity/insurance is usually limited by jurisdiction and might not automatically include remote work. Clinicians providing services outside the UK should ensure their indemnity/insurance satisfies laws in other countries.

Data protection

Records relating to remote care must be securely stored and accessible, in accordance with the Data Protection Act 2018. If digital technology is used to support remote diagnosis and planning, it is important that clear protocols are in place to ensure that all parties using or providing information are fully compliant with data protection requirements for storage, access, and sharing data; this should be established in any contract with a service provider.

Medical device regulations

Medical device regulations still apply to remote supply of medical devices. A registrant importing appliances manufactured outside of the UK is responsible for ensuring the manufacturer or authorized representative complies with the regulations.

Other considerations for remote care

The following additional controls should be considered when providing remote care:

Cross-border care

Providing care across different jurisdictions introduces additional legal and regulatory challenges:

- Where is the 'dentistry' being practised and does the clinician need to be registered in another country?
- In which country would a claim be brought; has the clinician appropriate indemnity that meets local requirements?
- Management of emergencies—if a patient needs urgent care, can a clinician make an immediate referral? This may be further compounded with time zone differences and lack of local knowledge
- Who is responsible for other aspects of the patient's dental care and how will information be communicated?
- What are the restrictions on the prescribing, sale, and supply of medicines?

Peer-to-peer remote diagnostic and planning services
- Ensure patient consent is valid for sharing information in accordance with data protection legislation
- Quality assurance; records shared must be comprehensive and of sufficient quality to allow full assessment and ensure that treatment proposed is appropriate and justified
- Establish written protocols specifying the parameters of the relationship, the role and responsibility of each party and arrangements in place for data protection, quality assurance and complaint handling
- Each party should establish the qualifications/training and current registration and indemnity of the other party

Remote monitoring tools
- Identify independent evidence to support the efficacy of the remote monitoring system and outputs
- Develop clear protocols establishing how often a patient should be seen face-to-face and in what circumstances remote appointments should not be offered
- Where remote monitoring tools transmit data to the practice—clarify what action must be taken in specific circumstances, by whom and in what timeframe
- Determine liability when errors arise due to failure of equipment and whether this lies with the system supplier. This may depend upon compliance with manufacturer's instructions and maintenance of the system by the user

Further reading

- Care Quality Commission. Dental mythbuster 39: Direct-to-consumer orthodontics. Available at: ℘ https://www.cqc.org.uk/guidance-providers/dentists/dental-mythbuster-39-direct-consumer-orthodontics
- Dental Protection. COVID-19 and remote consultations—how we can help. Available at: ℘ https://www.dentalprotection.org/uk/articles/covid-19-and-remote-consultations-how-we-can-help
- Dental Protection. Teledentistry—Additional complications. Available at: ℘ https://www.dentalprotection.org/uk/articles/teledentistry-additional-complications

Managing complaints

A complaint is an expression of dissatisfaction with an aspect of a service. This may be verbal or written via letter, email, or social media.

The following legal framework underpins complaint management:

- The National NHS complaints policy
- The individual trust's complaints policy
- The NHS Constitution which outlines the patient's right to complain
- The NHS Complaints Regulations 2009

Complaint handling

- All staff are responsible for taking concerns and complaints seriously and trying to resolve them wherever possible
- A complaint should be acknowledged properly. Reassure that it will be addressed; often, saying the phrase 'I am sorry that you are unhappy and I will look into this for you' will help defuse the situation in the immediate moment
- Aim for local resolution where possible/appropriate
- Signpost how issues can be escalated to a senior manager or PALS and the complaints team who offer confidential advice and support to patients and families
- The complaints team assesses the complaint (see Figure 6.3). They:
  - Grade the complaint (using the risk management matrix, see Table 6.5)
  - Establish if there are any immediate safety or safeguarding issues
  - Establish whether the duty of candour process is required
  - Consider whether consent should be sought
  - Establish which directorate/service should lead the investigation
  - Determine the likely timeframe
  - Consider whether external NHS bodies should be involved
  - Register the complaint onto Datix/Ulysses
- Based on the level of risk, an investigation is undertaken by the clinical lead, or higher management such as the directorate lead or escalated directly to executive level
- The complaints team assesses the response timeframe based on:
  - Complexity of the complaint
  - Number of teams/specialities involved
  - Timespan of the events complained about
  - Whether the complaint is associated with a serious incident
- There are no specified timeframes (NHS complaints regulations)
  - Timescales are agreed in consultation with complainants
  - They usually range between 25 and 60 working days
  - If exceeding 6 months, a written explanation should be sent
- The internal investigation is proportionate to the level of the complaint, this may involve staff interviews or internal/external RCA
- The complaint response is drafted by the complaints team, reviewed by governance teams, and sent to the CEO, who is responsible for approving and signing final complaint response letters
- Staff involved in a complaint should be provided with well-being support and advice
- Details of a complaint should not be filed in the patient's medical notes, as this could compromise future care for them
- A separate complaints log should be maintained

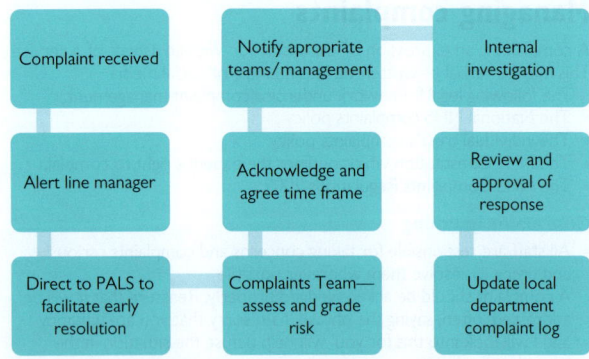

Figure 6.3 The complaint process in an NHS trust.

Redress

The redress for a complaint will be tailored to each individual case. This may range from:
- Apology, explanation, acknowledgement of responsibility
- Remedial action—change in protocol, decision, training/supervision
- Financial compensation if justified

The patient may choose to appeal the result:
- Internal appeal—the clinical director will investigate in conjunction with the medical director
- External appeal, the Parliamentary Health Service Ombudsman may investigate and decide the final outcome, which may be:
  - Patient's complaint is upheld or
  - No case to answer/there was no compromised care
- If a solution is not reached at that stage, there may be involvement from the CQC/NHS England

Learning from complaints

Having a robust complaint system will support staff in handling complaints and also support the complainant.

Learning from complaints can help improve patient care and reduce further complaints in the future. It will also highlight any trends and indicate if systems need reforming or the patient pathway improved. Learning from complaints may take various approaches:
- Disseminate reports to departments/people involved with local meetings or risk register
- Conduct audits to identify complaints and determine whether the trend is improving and if the issues that were raised have been addressed
- Weekly and monthly risk action meetings, which may involve PALS, the complaints team, legal team, risk management team

- Action log to prevent further occurrences, for example by involving the hospital improvement team or clinical governance or facilitating local training in dispute resolution
- A specific training requirement that is required for a staff member may be facilitated by the line manager or educational supervisor
- Trust, divisional, or speciality meetings for high level complaints
- Compilation and monitoring of quarterly or annual reports

Safeguarding patients

Safeguarding children, young people, and adults with support needs is everyone's responsibility. It involves the dental team, health and social care teams, and the local authority.

Legal and ethical requirements

The General Dental Council (GDC) Standards outline the obligations for dental care professionals in relation to safeguarding:

- Principle 8 highlights that professionals must raise concerns and take appropriate action if patients are at risk
- Principle 9 highlights the prevention of risk through maintaining appropriate professional boundaries and relates to safe staff recruitment

It is the responsibility of the healthcare professional to keep up to date with and follow their respective nation's legislation and guidance (Table 6.10, 6.11). Each employer will have local safeguarding policies and procedures which clinicians should familiarize themselves with.

Table 6.10 Legislation and guidance on safeguarding adults with care and support needs in the devolved nations

Nation	Legislation	Guidance	National legislation
England	Care Act 2014 Safeguarding Vulnerable Groups Act 2006 The London multi-agency policy and procedures to safeguard adults from abuse finalized February 2016	Care and Support Statutory Guidance	Domestic Abuse Act 2021 Modern Slavery Act 2015 Mental Capacity Act 2005 Equality Act 2010 Mental Health Act 1983
Wales	Social Services and Well-being (Wales) Act 2014	Working Together to Safeguard People	
Northern Ireland	The Protection of Children and Vulnerable Adults (2003) Order	Adult Safeguarding: Prevention and Protection in Partnership	Commissioner and transparency in Supply Chains (Modern Slavery Act 2015) Section 75 Northern Ireland Act 1998 (Equality)
Scotland	Adult Support and Protection (Scotland) Act 2007	Adult Support and Protection: Multi-Agency Guidelines August 2013	Commissioner and transparency in Supply Chains (Modern Slavery Act 2015) Equality Act 2010 Mental Health Act 2003

Table 6.11 Legislation and guidance on safeguarding children in the devolved nations

Nation	Legislation	Guidance	National legislation
England	Children Act 1989 (Section 17 &47) 2004 (Section 11) Children and Social Work Act 2017	Working Together to Safeguard Children 2023 Promoting the Health of Looked After Children Statutory Guidance 2015 National Service Framework for Children and Young People and Maternity Services 2004	Sexual Offences Act 2003 Female Genital Mutilation Act 2003 Modern Slavery Act 2015 Counter Terrorism and Security Act 2015 Forced Marriage Act 2007
Wales	Children Act 1989 (Section 17 &47) and 2004 (Section 11)		
Northern Ireland	The Children (Northern Ireland) Order 1995	Co-operating to Safeguard Children and Young People in Northern Ireland	Sexual Offences Act 2003 Female Genital Mutilation Act 2003
Scotland	Children (Scotland) Act 1995 The Children & Young People (Scotland) Act 2014	Getting it Right for Every Child (GIRFEC) 2015	Sexual Offences Act 2003 Prohibition of Female Genital Mutilation (Scotland) Act 2005 Forced Marriage, etc. (Protection and Jurisdiction) (Scotland) Act 2011

Key stakeholders

A robust safeguarding system in a trust will have features such as:

- Staff have knowledge and skills to know how to identify maltreatment of a child or adult with care and support needs
- Staff recognize and take account of an adult's or child's care plan
- If staff have suspicions of maltreatment, they approach the relevant people for advice or make a prompt onward referral
- Understand the principles of information sharing and risk and harm prevention
- Contemporaneous and accurate record-keeping

NHS trust safeguarding team

Safeguarding is a legal duty for each NHS trust. It must appoint a safeguarding team and named individual, to:

- Provide advice regarding the assessment of safeguarding concerns and undertaking treatment for children at risk or under care orders
- Help with legal aspects, e.g. raising concerns and completing required documentation
- Provide training to staff

- Work in close liaison with the clinical governance, legal and adult/children's services teams

Hospital social work service

Some NHS trusts will have an in-house social work service, who:
- Advocate on a child's behalf
- Provide practical support and advice to the family
- Coordinate complex discharge plans when psychosocial needs are present
- Work alongside medical teams and the local authority to identify and respond to child safeguarding concerns
- If a child is deemed to be at risk, they will coordinate an assessment of the child's needs, the parent's capacity to keep them safe and to decide if any other action is needed to protect the child and prevent harm

Local statutory safeguarding adults boards

Multi-agency statutory boards responsible for providing strategic leadership and oversight in preventing, detecting, and protecting adults. They oversee implementation and quality assurance of local guidance and procedures for safeguarding adults.

Multi-agency public protection arrangements (MAPPA)

The police have a shared responsibility for the management of sexual offenders and violent offenders when they are released from prison. This is managed in partnership with probation staff, prison staff, and agencies such as social services, housing, and health.

Local authority children's services team

This team has the responsibility to ensure a proper investigation of suspected abuse in liaison with the hospital team or local social work service.

Local safeguarding children partnerships (LSCP)

LSCPs are a multi-agency response led by three statutory safeguarding partners: local authorities, police and integrated care boards.

They coordinate the activity of the relevant bodies to safeguard and promote child welfare, such as holding a child protection enquiry. The local authority has a duty under Section 47 of the Children Act 1989 to make enquiries to decide if a child is suffering, or is likely to suffer, significant harm.

Emergency duty team

This team receives and responds to referrals out of hours.

Supporting organizations for safeguarding children

Other organizations that may be involved in safeguarding children include:
- ADCS
- Article 39
- Barnado's
- BSPD
- CAFCASS
- Childnet International
- Childrens Commissioner
- Children's Rights Alliance for England
- NICE
- NSPCC
- UNICEF

Serious case review (SCR)

SCRs were established under the Children Act 2004. They are carried out when a child dies or comes to serious harm and abuse or neglect is suspected. By learning lessons, they are designed to prevent similar occurrences in the future. SCRs have highlighted:

- How serious harm and death can occur if safeguarding information is not shared between organizations
- How individually, the child's school, healthcare clinic, carers, social work team, etc. may have had concerns but as these concerns were not voiced and shared sufficiently between all the involved parties, no action was taken to escalate and resolve it

Working Together to Safeguard Children (2018) outlines how these services should work together, with emphasis on the responsibility of local authorities, local commissioning groups, and police.

Safeguarding adults with care and support needs

The duty of adult safeguarding (Box 6.5 and Box 6.6) applies to those aged 18 or above who:

- Exhibit care and support needs, irrespective of whether the local authority is addressing them
- Encounter or are at risk of experiencing abuse or neglect
- Are unable to shield themselves from the risk or experience of abuse and neglect due to their care and support needs
- An adult with temporary or permanent care and support needs

The individual's inability to protect themselves must arise from their requirements for care and support.

Local authorities must investigate if they suspect abuse or neglect of an at-risk adult. A healthcare professional may initiate the enquiry. Discussions involving the adult or their representative may precede a formal Section 42 investigation, leading to a multi-agency plan.

Section 42 Enquiries

- Ensure the safety of the adult by considering their preferences (obtained through discussions with relatives, friends, or advocates if required) regarding the level of risk for abuse or neglect
- Establish the facts
- Assess the level of risk and the adult's needs for protection, support, and resolution, while exploring potential solutions

---

Box 6.5 Adult safeguarding as defined by the Care Act 2014

'Protecting an adult's right to live in safety, free from abuse and neglect. It is about people and organisations working together to prevent and stop both the risks and experience of abuse or neglect, while at the same time making sure that the adult's wellbeing is promoted including, where appropriate, having regard to their views, wishes, feelings and beliefs in deciding on any action. This must recognise that adults sometimes have complex interpersonal relationships and may be ambivalent, unclear or unrealistic about their personal circumstances.'

> **Box 6.6 Adult safeguarding terminology**
> - Adult(s) with care and support needs *previously* adult(s) at risk/vulnerable adult(s)
> - Safeguarding adult reviews (SAR) *previously* serious case reviews
> - Safeguarding concern *previously* alert/referral
> - Enquiry *previously* Investigation
> - Planning discussion/meeting *previously* strategy discussion/meeting
> - Safeguarding plan *previously* protection plan

- Determine the necessary actions regarding the individual or organization responsible for harm
- Assist the adult in achieving resolution and recovery

An enquiry should proceed without consent if:
- The adult lacks mental capacity, despite efforts to maximize this
- It is in the best interests of the adult to conduct the enquiry
- There's an overriding public interest, such as when others are at risk

The Mental Capacity Act (MCA)

The Mental Capacity Act may be of relevance, and is detailed on page 178.

The deprivation of liberty safeguards (DoLS)

DoLS protects the rights of adults lacking capacity in care homes or hospitals in England and Wales. DoLS authorization is necessary when their care deprives them of liberty. This process ensures the deprivation is lawful and allows individuals to challenge it in court. In other settings or for individuals aged 16 or 17, the commissioner or local authority must seek court authority for deprivation of liberty.

Types of abuse

There are many types of abuse a vulnerable adult may be subjected to. These are summarized in Table 6.12.

Radicalization

PREVENT is part of the UK's counter-terrorism strategy to reduce the risk of people (including patients and staff) becoming involved in or supporting terrorism. The Counter-Terrorism and Security Act (2015) places a duty on statutory bodies to have 'regard to the need to prevent people from being drawn into terrorism'.

Healthcare workers should be trained to:
- Recognize signs that someone has/is being drawn into terrorism
- Locate available support such as the Channel programme

Preventing someone from being drawn into terrorism is comparable to safeguarding in other areas, including child abuse or domestic violence (Home Office 2019).

Deprivation, bullying, and adolescence may lead to a child feeling isolated and having a void in their life. They may become vulnerable to radicalization.

Table 6.12 Types of abuse in adults

	Definition/Causes
Physical	• Being hit, slapped, pushed, or restrained • Being denied food or water • Not being helped to go to the bathroom • Misuse of medicines • Inappropriate physical sanctions
Sexual	• Indecent exposure • Sexual harassment, or inappropriate looking or touching • Sexual teasing or innuendo • Sexual photography • Being forced to watch pornography or sexual acts • Being forced or pressured to take part in sexual acts • Rape, attempted rape, sexual assault
Psychological	• Emotional abuse • Threats to hurt or abandon • Being stopped from seeing people • Humiliating, blaming, controlling, intimidating, harassing • Verbal abuse • Cyberbullying and isolation • Unreasonable withdrawal of services or support networks
Domestic	Typically, an incident or pattern of incidents of controlling, coercive, or threatening behaviour, violence or abuse by someone who is/has been, an intimate partner or family
Discriminatory	Harassment, slurs or unfair treatment against protected characteristics under the Equality Act (see chapter 7)
Financial	• Stealing money or other valuables or inappropriate use of money by someone appointed to look after it • Coerced to spend money in a way they are not happy with • Internet scams and doorstep crime
Neglect	• Not being provided with enough food or the right kind of food, or not being properly cared for • Failure to help to wash or change dirty or wet clothes • Not arranging medical advice/treatment when needed • Not making sure they have the correct medication
Modern Slavery	• Human trafficking • Forced labour or debt bondage • Domestic servitude • Sexual exploitation
Self-Neglect	• Inability to avoid self-harm • Failure to meet health and social care needs • Lack of personal health or personal safety • Failure to maintain personal hygiene, health, or surroundings

Children are often radicalized during adolescence. Non-definitive signs may include:
- Isolating themselves from friends and family
- Talking as if from a scripted speech
- Unwillingness or inability to discuss their views
- Sudden disrespectful attitude towards others
- Increased levels of anger
- Increased secretiveness, especially around internet use

Discussing safeguarding concerns:
The following should be considered when discussing safeguarding concerns with an individual:
- Consider safety. Is it the right time, setting, and circumstance?
- Ensure the individual's safety remains a priority
- Ensure the individual's privacy, ideally use a closed room or private space
- Refrain from addressing concerns with accompanying persons
- If safe, work to separate the individual from accompanying adults
- Use an independent advocate or translator if needed, avoid using family members/carers
- Once the individual is alone and safe, consider asking relevant questions about living and working conditions
- Address the individual's wishes for help and support
- Reiterate that healthcare settings are a safe and confidential place to disclose any concerns. They will be heard, believed, and have access to independent support and help
- Arrange follow-up, ideally without the knowledge of accompanying persons
- Thoroughly and contemporaneously document the consultation with the objective reasons for your concerns that the individual is a potential victim of abuse and the actions taken

Escalating concerns for adult safeguarding
Each organization will have local policies on how to make a referral.
- When escalating concerns always ensure your own safety
- If you suspect a patient is at risk of being abused or has been abused, immediate action should be taken to ensure that they remain as safe as possible
- It is advisable to keep the patient's views, wishes, and desired outcomes documented whenever possible
- If the adult at risk or abuser has a responsibility or contact with children that are at risk, then you would need to follow the safeguarding children procedure in the first instance
- Figure 6.5 demonstrates how to escalate concerns if a staff member is suspected and Figure 6.6 if there are adult safeguarding concerns
- Discuss with your line manager or senior colleague. Any suspected abuse can be referred by the Office of the Public Guardian (OPG) to the appropriate adult social services by making a Safeguarding Adults At Risk referral (SAAR)
- Consent is required when sharing information for an adult with capacity beyond the immediate clinical team, with certain conditions. Consider the potential victim's capacity according to the MCA

- If the patient attends the emergency department or is admitted to the hospital and there is abuse suspected within their usual place of residence, then they must not be discharged until a protection plan is agreed
- The trust's incident reporting tool is used if the concern relates to an incident that occurred during the patient's treatment or the concern is about the organization itself
- There are some important considerations before sharing information (see Figure 6.4)

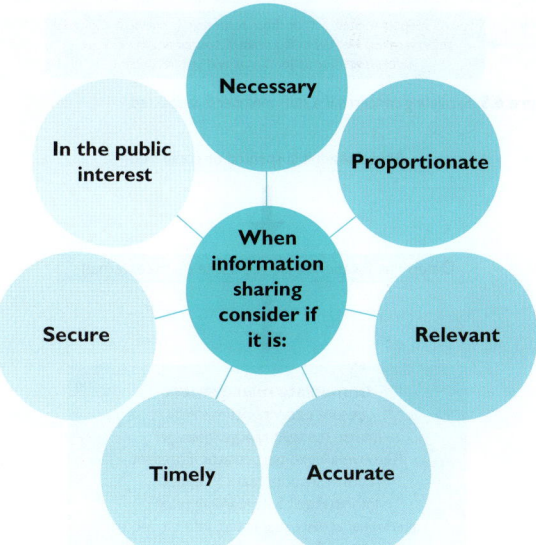

Figure 6.4 Considerations with information sharing.

Whom to contact
- During hospital working hours, advice can be sought from your line manager, supervising consultant, and the adult safeguarding team
- Out of hours, most trusts have a site manager
- If a crime is suspected, it can be reported to the police
- For safeguarding adults, the investigation can initially be undertaken by the NHS trust
- The LA takes the lead in coordinating the multi-agency approach
- The most closely involved agency is usually best placed to lead
- The LA will agree on investigations through its strategy meeting and discussion process, so police investigations are not compromised
- The investigation may be undertaken by the OPG where it has statutory powers under the MCA

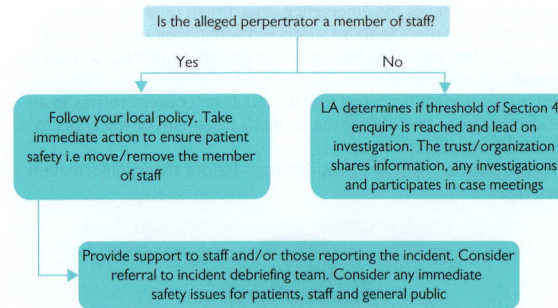

Figure 6.5 Escalating concerns if a staff member is suspected.

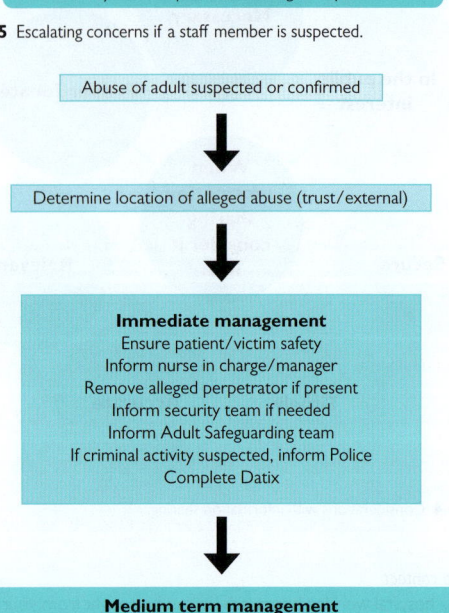

Figure 6.6 Escalating concerns for suspected abuse in adults.

Safeguarding children

Child protection is part of the safeguarding process. It focuses on protecting individual children identified as suffering or likely to suffer significant harm. This includes child protection procedures which detail how to respond to concerns about a child.

While working with children in a healthcare setting, a child-centred approach should be adopted (Box 6.7):

- Involve children and their families in the decision-making process
- Put the child's needs first when managing safeguarding concerns

Adverse childhood experiences (ACEs)

These are stressful or traumatic events that occur in childhood or adolescence in isolation or over a prolonged period that breaches their safety, security, trust, or bodily integrity (Table 6.13).

Harm

Maltreatment of children is an act by an individual in a caring role that has the potential to cause or does cause serious harm. Serious harm includes abuse or neglect resulting in, but not limited to:

- A potentially life-threatening injury

Box 6.7 Definition of safeguarding children

The Children Act 1989 and National Society for the Prevention of Cruelty to Children (NSPCC) define safeguarding children as: "The action that is taken to promote the welfare of children and protect them from harm, including:

- Protecting children from abuse and maltreatment up to their 18th birthday, or 19th if they have a disability
- Preventing harm to children's health or development
- Ensuring children grow up with safe and effective care
- Taking action to enable all children and young people to have the best outcomes"

Table 6.13 Adverse childhood experiences and the protective factors that help to reduce their impact (Young Minds, 2022)

ACEs	Protective Factors
Maltreatment	Trauma-informed policies and systems
Violence and coercion	Early intervention
Adjustment	Compassionate, attuned, and supportive responses from professionals
Prejudice	Acquisition of practical problem-solving skills
Household or family adversity	
Inhuman treatment	Ability to regulate emotions and manage emotional distress
Adult responsibilities	
Bereavement and survivorship	Access to supportive wider community
	Safe mutual relationships with peers

- Serious and/or likely long-term impairment of physical or mental health, or physical, intellectual, emotional, social, or behavioural development

The common assessment framework (CAF)

Low-level concerns, or those not meeting child protection thresholds, can be addressed through a collaborative approach involving multiple agencies to prevent escalation. Consent from the family is required for this early intervention. This approach is recommended when:

- There are concerns about a child's overall progress, including health, welfare, behaviour, learning, or other aspects of well-being
- The child, parent, or another person has raised a concern
- The needs are unclear or extend beyond the scope of your service
- A common assessment would help identify the child's needs and involve other services to address them

Processes may vary by region, and clinicians should be familiar with local procedures. CAF meetings involve all relevant parties to address unmet needs, with progress tracked against an action plan.

Social background

Child in need

The Children Act 1989 (Sect. 17) defines a child as being 'in need' if:

- They are unlikely to achieve or maintain, or to have the opportunity of achieving or maintaining a reasonable standard of health or development without the provision of services by a local authority
- Their health or development is likely to be significantly impaired or further impaired without the provision of such services
- They have a disability

Child in need of protection

A child is defined as being in need of protection if: 'there is reasonable cause to suspect that a child is suffering, or is likely to suffer, significant harm', Children Act 1989 (Sect. 47).

The definition of significant harm was amended under the Adoption and Child Act 2002 (Sect. 120) to include: 'impairment suffered from seeing or hearing the ill treatment of another'.

Looked after child (LAC)

A child that has been under the care of their local authority for 24 hours or more. The local authority arranges for the child to live somewhere other than at home.

A court may have granted a *Care Order* to place a child in care or there has been voluntary parental agreement. The child may stay in a children's home, with other family members or foster parents.

Looked after children are at greater risk of having mental health and behavioural problems as well as developmental or learning problems. Their outcomes may be attributed to:

- Previous neglect and abuse
- Frequent address changes and healthcare providers
- Inconsistent access to a trusted adult for support and guidance
- Poor communication between professionals and local authorities

Accommodated child

The parents retain parental responsibilities but there is a voluntary arrangement between them and the local authority for the child to stay elsewhere.

Notifications

Some organizations expect notification of attendances to be sent to the local safeguarding team or directly to children's services. It is important to follow the local safeguarding children or 'was not brought' policy with respect to non-attendance.

Private fostering arrangement

An arrangement between families/households, excluding local authority involvement, for the care of a child under 16 (or under 18 if disabled) by someone other than a parent or close relative (close relatives being parents, step-parents, siblings, aunts/uncles, and grandparents) for 28 days or more.

Private foster carers and those with parental responsibility must notify children's social care under 'The Children (Private Arrangements for Fostering) Regulations 2005' before privately fostering a child or in case of an emergency fostering situation.

Was Not Brought policy

Children who do not attend appointments should be referred to as 'was not brought' (WNB) rather than did not attend (DNA) to acknowledge that it is rarely the child's fault.

If a child or young person does not attend an appointment:
- Contact the parent/carer to establish the reason for the non-attendance and, where necessary, ensure that the parent/carer fully understands that the non-attendance could be perceived as a sign of neglect
- Document the reason for not attending in the child's clinical record
- Inform the child's GP, health visitor, school nurse, and lead professional if involved
- If the child/young person is subject to a Child Protection Plan or is Looked After, the social worker must also be informed immediately

A useful reference guide for implementation of this process can be found in *Implementing 'Was Not Brought' in Your Practice* by the British Dental Association.

When a child is not brought to health appointments, it is the responsibility of the clinician to review the records and decide if the non-attendance adds to ongoing concerns that would indicate a referral to children's social care needs to be made.

Junior clinicians should inform the responsible supervising consultant.

Recognition of abuse

Children are regarded as a vulnerable group as they can be neglected or subjected to abuse from those around them. There are various forms this can take, and these can overlap (Table 6.14):

Other forms of abuse to be aware of:
- *Online abuse*—Any type of abuse that happens online, whether through social networks, playing online games, or using mobile phones. Children and young people may experience cyberbullying, grooming, sexual abuse, sexual exploitation, or emotional abuse

Table 6.14 Types of abuse in children (Child protection and the dental team, DoH)

	Causes	Signs

Physical	Deliberately causing physical harm to a child:
	• Hitting
	• Shaking
	• Throwing
	• Poisoning
	• Burning
	• Scalding
	• Drowning
	• Suffocating
	• Causing or fabricating symptoms or deliberately inducing illness
	• Female genital mutilation (see below)
		• Bruising of face, ears, abrasions, lacerations, burns, bites, cord marks around neck, hair pulling, bony fractures, dental trauma, frenal injuries
		• Non-accidental injury sites: ears, eyes, triangle of safety on neck, forearm, groin, inner aspect of the thigh, soles of the feet
		• Injuries that do not match the explanation
		• Delays in presentation, untreated injuries, injuries to soft tissue with particular patterns
		• Conditions that may be confused for physical abuse:
		  • Birthmarks (haemangiomas)
		  • Mongolian blue spots
		  • Infections (scabies, impetigo)
		  • Bleeding disorders
		  • Osteogenesis imperfecta

Emotional	Persistent emotional ill-treatment resulting in severe and persistent adverse effects on the child's emotional development, e.g. inappropriate expectations, overprotection, witnessing ill treatment of another, exploitation, radicalization.	• Poor growth • Aggression • Challenging behaviour • Attention difficulties • Developmental delay • Attachment disorders • Anti-social behaviour • Self-harm • Substance misuse • Depression
Sexual	Forcing or enticing a child or young person to take part in sexual activities including prostitution or producing/engaging with sexually explicit material. Child sexual exploitation involves receiving gifts, money, or affection in return for sexual activities. Online grooming and trafficking can also occur.	• Direct allegations • Pregnancy (under 13 is unlawful) • Clear difference in power or mental capacity of young person's partner • Non-consensual concerns • STIs (intraoral warts/papillomas) • Trauma • Emotional behavioural signs, such as inappropriate sexual behaviour, self-harm, depression, drug abuse, soiling, or wetting NB: The age of consent for sexual activity is 16 in the UK. Under 13s can never consent to sexual activity

Table 6.14 (*Contd.*)

	Causes	Signs
Neglect	Persistent failure to meet a child's basic physical and/or psychological needs, likely to result in the serious impairment of the child's health or development. This includes dental neglect.	Child: • Inappropriate clothing • Failure to thrive or short stature • Inadequate supervision leading to frequent injuries • Failure to access medical care or treatment (headlice, dental caries after education) • Withdrawn or attention seeking behaviour due to lack of affection Parent/Carer: • Indifferent to the child • Seems apathetic or depressed • Behaves irrationally or in a bizarre manner • Is abusing alcohol or other drugs
Dental Neglect	Failure to respond to known significant dental problems.	When parents/carers have been educated in oral health practices for their children and have the means to maintain this but still present with: • Irregular dental attendance (multiple 'was not brought') • Repeated general anaesthesia for dental extractions • Repeated pain appointments

• *Bullying*—Behaviour that hurts someone else such as name calling, hitting, pushing, spreading rumours, threatening or undermining
• *Female genital mutilation (FGM)*—All procedures that involve partial or total removal of the external female genitalia, or other injury to the female genital organs for non-medical reasons. The practice has no health benefits for girls and women. There is a legal mandatory duty to report known cases of FGM in girls under the age of 18 to the police. Possible signs of FGM:
  • Depression, anxiety
  • Reluctance to undergo medical examinations
  • Difficulty walking, sitting, or standing
  • Change in behaviour
  • Absence from school with menstrual or bladder problems
  • Longer or more frequent trips to the toilet
• *Grooming*—When someone builds an emotional connection with a child to gain their trust for the purposes of sexual abuse, sexual exploitation, or trafficking
• Criminal exploitation
• Radicalization
• Domestic abuse and modern slavery/trafficking

When child maltreatment is suspected consider the following approach:
1. Listen and observe
2. Seek an explanation
3. Document the above
4. Consider, suspect, or exclude maltreatment

Record-keeping

Provide necessary dental care and keep full clinical records. Document factually and objectively all concerns and any referrals made. Arrange a follow-up appointment and document the following:
1. Basic personal information
2. Who accompanied the child
3. Observations of behaviour
4. Summary of discussions with the child or parent
5. Record observations and reasons given for seemingly trivial injuries
6. Diagrams as well as written descriptions or clinical photographs
7. Clearly state the difference between the facts and your opinion
8. Keep administrative notes such as attendance, non-attendance, cancelled appointments

Escalating concerns

Concerns should be raised in an appropriate way, and the following instances are indicative of safeguarding flags:
- Children in whom fabricated or induced illness or perplexing problems are confirmed or suspected
- Injuries in children without adequate explanation
- Injuries or risk of injuries in children under 12 months
- Cases involving children with concerns that are likely to result in civil or criminal proceedings
- Those where despite single or multi-agency support, the child is continuing to suffer significant harm and where there is interagency conflict on how the case should be progressed
- All unexpected child deaths
- Cases where sexual abuse is perpetrated by a child
- Sexual activity in children under 13 years of age
- Domestic abuse cases where the victim or perpetrator is under 16
- Cases where a member of staff belonging to the trust or to an external organization is alleged to have harmed a child
- Cases where a child is already looked after by the local authority (LAC) and has experienced additional harm

Consult colleagues

Concerns can be discussed or raised with the following:
- Responsible or supervising consultant
- Designated safeguarding lead in the department
- Safeguarding lead
- Child protection nurse
- Safeguarding team
- On-call consultant paediatrician
- Social worker, health visitor, local authority

Making a referral

If concerns remain about the child's welfare, then a referral should be made to the local children's services team via a pro forma stating your concerns and action points from the appointment.

- Consider whether further medical examination is required via the local emergency department
- Confirm receipt of the referral within 48 hours
- The GMC's 0–18 years guidance advises that 'you will be able to justify raising a concern, even if it turns out to be groundless, if you have done so honestly, promptly, on the basis of reasonable belief and through the appropriate channels'

Consent when referring

When a referral is made, the person with parental responsibility should be informed to obtain consent. Child In Need (CIN) referrals require consent. Consent for child protection referrals is recommended, unless:

- The patient will be at greater risk due to delays in obtaining consent
- The suspected perpetrator is the person with parental responsibility
- Discussion will impede police investigations

GDPR should not be seen as a barrier to sharing information, it is a framework for sharing to take place fairly and proportionately. The ICO would not penalize an organization for sharing personal data to protect a child. Any information should be shared securely.

Outcomes of a referral

The meetings and processes involved in determining outcomes following a child safeguarding referral are summarized in Table 6.15 and Figure 6.7.

Section 47 enquiries

If concerns remain, enquiries under Section 47 are conducted within 45 days of referral. The outcomes are as follows:

- Concerns not substantiated but are categorized as CIN, so a plan is agreed with the family and other practitioners to ensure future safety and welfare
- Concerns are substantiated but the child is not suffering or is not likely to suffer significant harm. Lead practitioner decides whether to convene a child protection conference (CPC)
- Concerns are substantiated and the child is at risk, a CPC is held within 15 days. If confirmed, a protection plan is initiated; otherwise, a safety plan is devised with the family and practitioners

Child protection conference (CPC)

When a child has suffered actual (or is likely to suffer) significant harm then a child protection conference (case conference) takes place. The local authority social care makes a child the subject of a child protection plan (CPP). This:

- Consists of a lead practitioner supported by a core group
- The CPP is outlined within 10 days of the CPC
- A multi-agency assessment is completed, the core group may commission further specialist assessments as necessary
- They provide or commission the necessary interventions for the child and their family
- A review conference is arranged within 3 months of the initial CPC

Table 6.15 Summaries of processes and outcomes in referral meetings

Outcome	Meeting	Process
Concerns about the child's immediate safety	*Emergency protection plan meeting*	• Immediate strategy discussion with children's social care, health and the police, and the NSPCC, if involved • Decision made regarding requirement for immediate protection • Legal advice and record outcome • Decision on immediate action and the sequence of information sharing • Relevant agency meets with the child and delivers the outcome of the meeting
No pressing concerns Does not require immediate protection and does not meet threshold for child in need (CIN)	*Team Around the Child (TAC) meeting:* Multi-agency meeting tasked with supporting a child or young person, and, where appropriate, parents/carers to identify unmet needs and produce package of support/interventions.	No local authority children's care involvement, but other action may be necessary, such as • Early help assessment • Help from universal and targeted services
Concerns remain Does not require immediate protection but does meet threshold for CIN. Family and other practitioners agree a plan.	*Professionals meeting:* Agencies discuss and share information where children are deemed to be in need and to decide a plan of support aimed at safeguarding the welfare of the child/children in the family	• Initial assessment within one working day • Full assessment within 45 working days + and inform referring agency of outcome • Child has not suffered and is likely not to suffer significant harm—no local authority intervention • Children's social care support required: communication with family and coordination of provision of services • CIN plan/CPP in place within 45 days • Review of plan and child outcomes for referral to: non-statutory services, Section 47 enquiry or closes case

Table 6.15 (*Contd.*)

Outcome	Meeting	Process
Child has suffered actual (or is likely to suffer) significant harm	*Case conference:* Multi-agency meeting led by children's social care to review information and consider whether the threshold has been met to make a child the subject of a child protection plan.	Strategy discussion outcomes: • Police investigation if criminal nature • No local authority involvement • Assessment under Section 17 (child in need) • Enquiries under Section 47 (child protection)

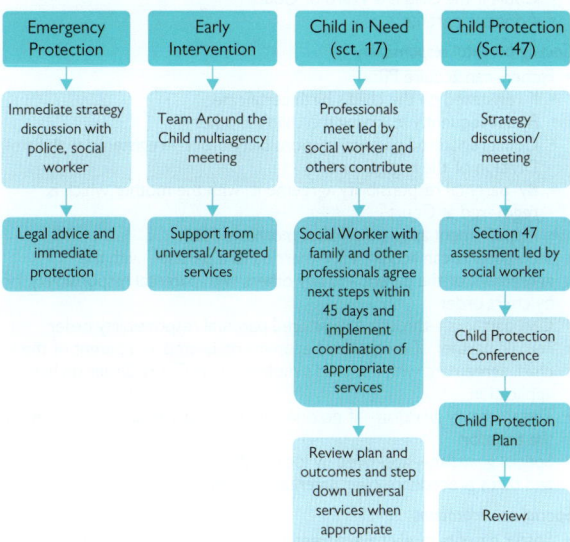

Figure 6.7 Overview of pathways for child safeguarding intervention.

- If there are no ongoing concerns about significant harm, the child is removed from the CPP. Further support is put in place as required
- If there are ongoing or further concerns, the child remains the subject of a revised CPP which is reviewed 6 months after the initial review

If concerns remain at 6 months, consideration is given to further protection, move to care proceedings, and decisions regarding parental responsibility.

Parental responsibility (PR)

Defined by the Children Act 1989 as: 'all the rights, duties, powers, responsibilities and authority which by law a parent of a child has in relation to the child and his property'.

The rights include:
- The right to consent to treatment if the treatment is in the child's best interests
- The right to disclose healthcare information about the child
- The right to access the child's healthcare and education records
- Parental responsibility can be held by more than one person, but is automatically held by:
  - Birth mother
  - Father if married to mother at the time of birth (not lost if subsequently divorced) or listed on the birth certificate
  - Court if the child is a Ward of Court
  - Adoptive parents

Gaining parental responsibility
- Fathers can acquire PR:
  - If registered on the child's birth certificate
  - By subsequently marrying the child's mother
  - Court registered parental responsibility order—registered with Family Division of the High Court
  - By 'parental responsibility agreement' with the mother which is registered at Court
  - Appointment as guardian after mother's death
- Step-parents can acquire PR if married to a parent—with the agreement of the parent and any others with parental responsibility, or by court order
- Civil partners—through a registered parental responsibility order
- Female partner of mother by becoming registered as a parent of the child, agreement with the child's mother or by Court Order on her application
- Testamentary guardian—if no one with parental responsibility survives the testator
- Special guardian—approved by local authority or endorsed by Court and takes precedence over parental responsibility

Special considerations
- Foster parents rarely have parental responsibility. This usually lies with the local authority
- Parental responsibility is maintained if the person is in prison, injures the child, or is sectioned under the Mental Health Act
- Consent is required from all persons with PR for circumcision, immunizations, and end-of-life decisions
- If the clinical team believe that a person with PR is not acting in the child's best interest they should engage with the trust legal team for application to Court. This is usually indicated in instances to preserve life and prevent deterioration
- For 'looked after' children, persons with PR hold this jointly with the LA, who can overrule non-consent if treatment is deemed in the child's best interest as recommended by their dentist or doctor

Agreements
- Care Order—LA share PR with parents. Court decides where child lives
- Supervision Order—LA do not share PR with parents. Child remains living with parents
- Emergency Protection Order—LA temporarily has PR for child. Short term order to remove a child in immediate risk of harm to allow the local authority to investigate
- Section 20 Agreement—LA do not share PR with parents. Parents agree for their child to be accommodated by local authority
- Special Guardianship Order—Special Guardian shares PR with parents, but their PR overrides that of the parents. Child lives with Special Guardian

Expectations for safeguarding training

The intercollegiate competency framework from the Royal College of Nursing outlines the training required for safeguarding in relation to the dental setting for both NHS and private providers.

When recruiting to new posts, organizations must ensure that a minimum of 30 minutes of mandatory safeguarding induction training is completed within 6 weeks. Table 6.16 outlines the safeguarding training that healthcare staff are required to complete.

Staff recruitment checks

When recruiting, the NHS trust must identify individuals who may pose a risk or are unsuitable to work with patients. This includes:
- An accurate job description and person specification which can be matched to the application form during the short-listing process
- Discrepancies can be identified and clarified at the stage
- Offers are subject to satisfactory references, verification of identity, professional registration, and right to work in the UK

Table 6.16 Safeguarding training requirements for staff working in healthcare settings (Adult safeguarding: Roles and competencies for healthcare staff, 2018)

Safeguarding training	Staff group	3 Yearly training requirements
Level 1	Frontline staff: All (clinical and non-clinical) staff in healthcare services	≥ 2 hours + annual competency review
Level 2	Dentists & dental care professionals: All (clinical and non-clinical) staff who: • have contact with children, young people and/or their carers • engage with adult patients, their families/carers or the public	≥ 4 hours + annual competency review
Level 3 (locally agreed based on need and risk)	• Consultants and specialists • Clinical staff in specialist services: • Special care • Paediatric dentistry • Orthodontics • Departmental safeguarding leads	≥ 8 hours + annual competency review
Level 4 & 5	Named and designated professionals	≥ 24 hours + annual competency review

Table 6.17 Staff requirements for disclosure and barring service (DBS) checks

	Types of Checks	Time Taken	Staff Group
Disclosure and barring service (DBS)	Standard	~ 2 weeks	Staff providing non-regulated activities e.g. receptionists or cleaners
	Enhanced	~ 4 weeks	All dental healthcare professionals including trainees
	Enhanced with barred list	~ 4 weeks	Individuals who have declared a new conviction/caution for a serious offence or a prior referral to DBS by an employer
Protecting Vulnerable Groups (PVG) Scheme, Disclosure Scotland	Standard/enhanced disclosure	~ 2 weeks	Staff providing non-regulated activities e.g. receptionists or cleaners
	Scheme record	~ 2 weeks	All dental healthcare professionals including trainees
	Scheme record update		Existing PVG member undertaking regulated work
Access Northern Ireland	Access NI basic	~ 1–2 weeks	Non-healthcare staff
	Access NI standard	~ 1 week	Staff not working with children or vulnerable adults
	Access NI enhanced	~ 4 weeks	All dental healthcare professionals including trainees

Table 6.18 The organizations and process of the safeguarding checks

	Organization	Process
England and Wales	Disclosure and barring service (DBS)	Pre 2014—employer requests new DBS certificate. Post 2014—employer checks certificate is up to date via DBS update service online
Scotland	Protecting Vulnerable Groups (PVG) scheme, Disclosure Scotland	Employees asked to register with PVG scheme and employers get notified of employee's record for the duration of their employment
Northern Ireland	Access Northern Ireland	Employers request new certificate that relates to the specific role/job and cannot be reused for later roles/jobs

New starters directly involved in patient care must undergo checks to identify any criminal convictions and ensure they are not barred from working with children, young people, or adults with support and care needs (Table 6.17).

Clinical dental staff are required to undergo enhanced checks when their work involves a regulated activity. The process varies by nation (Table 6.18).

Further reading

- BDA (2023). Working Together to Safeguard Children: A guide to multi-agency working to help, protect, and promote the welfare of children HM Government. Available at: ℘ https://www.bda.org/advice/patient-care-and-safety/assessment-and-safeguarding/safeguarding-patients/
- DoH. Child protection and the dental team: an introduction to safeguarding in dental practice Published by the Committee of Postgraduate Dental Deans and Directors (COPDEND). Available at: ℘ https://www.east-ayrshire.gov.uk/Resources/PDF/C/Childprotectionandthedentalteam-v1-4-Nov09.pdf
- GDC Guidance on child protection and vulnerable adults. Available at: ℘ https://www.youngminds.org.uk/professional/resources/understanding-trauma-and-adversity
- Information Commissioner's Office. Sharing data to safeguard children FAQs. Available at: ℘ https://ico.org.uk/for-organisations/uk-gdpr-guidance-and-resources/data-sharing/sharing-data-to-safeguard-children-faqs/
- NHS England. E-learning portal. Available at: ℘ https://www.e-lfh.org.uk/
- NICE (2009). Child maltreatment: when to suspect maltreatment in under 18s (CG89). Available at: ℘ https://www.nice.org.uk/guidance/cg89
- NSPCC. Safeguarding and child protection. Available at: ℘ https://learning.nspcc.org.uk/safeguarding-child-protection/
- NSPCC Learning (last updated 2022, 20 May 2022). Safeguarding children with special educational needs and disabilities (SEND). Available at: ℘ https://stateofchildhealth.rcpch.ac.uk/evidence/injury-prevention/accidental-injury/
- Royal College of Nursing (2018). Adult safeguarding: Roles and competencies for healthcare staff. Available at: ℘ https://www.rcn.org.uk/Professional-Development/publications/rcn-adult-safeguarding-roles-and-competencies-for-health-care-staff-011-256
- World Health Organization (2023). Female genital mutilation. Available at: ℘ https://www.who.int/news-room/fact-sheets/detail/female-genital-mutilation

Scenario—Safeguarding 1

You are a paediatric dentistry senior registrar. A child, aged 8, attends with an 'aunt' who looks after them. The child presents with poor oral hygiene, untreated caries and signs of malnutrition. You also observe the child flinching away from routine examinations and appearing anxious when asked about their home life.

What are the issues raised, and what are your short, medium and long-term management strategies for this patient?

Terms of reference +/– issues raised
- Children Act, 1989
- Private fostering arrangements
- Social worker involvement
- Parental responsibility & consent
- Neglect
- Clinical urgency

Key people/organizations
- Persons with parental responsibility
- Other responsible adults involved in the child's care, e.g. the 'aunt' they attended with
- Senior colleagues

- Other medical professionals involved in the child's care, including the GP and GDP
- Safeguarding team/social worker
- Local authority (children's services/social worker) and child's school

Short term
- Document observations and concerns factually in the clinical record
- Initiate a private chaperoned conversation with the child to build trust and gather additional information, ensuring a safe and comfortable environment
- Engage with the child's caregivers in a non-confrontational manner to discuss observations and offer support on oral hygiene and nutrition
- Gather information about persons with parental responsibility, does the aunt have parental responsibility?
- Seek immediate advice from your supervising consultant/senior member of staff and the safeguarding children team
- Contact children's social care to establish if they are already known to the private fostering team/have a CPP
  - If they are not, it is a statutory requirement to make a referral to children's social care to notify them of the private fostering arrangement
  - You should inform the parent/carer and child (if age appropriate) that you are undertaking this referral unless you feel that this will place the child, or another, at risk of harm
- Notify local children's social care services if neglect is suspected and complete an appropriate safeguarding referral form (CIN/CAF)
- When a referral is made you should confirm receipt of the referral and follow up within 48 hours to check the outcome
- Check any history of safeguarding concerns, e.g. via GMP/'SystemOne'- the safeguarding team may do this
- If the child is at immediate risk or 'imminent danger' of harm, e.g. not safe to return home, the police will need to be involved. A Police Protection Order can be arranged (for up to 72 hours) and then an emergency protection order (through the courts)
- Provide emergency treatment in the best interests of the child as required
  - You can only treat without parental consent if it is immediately necessary to preserve the child's life or to protect a child from irreversible harm such that there is no time to obtain consent from someone with parental responsibility or obtain consent from the court
  - These situations will be very rare, but even if there is a matter of hours, you can obtain an order from the court
- A social history will also need to be taken, to assess if there are any other children at home that may be at risk of harm. This would be followed up with the safeguarding team

Medium term

- Collaborate with other healthcare professionals involved in the child's care, such as school nurses or general practitioners, to share concerns and gather information about the child's well-being
- Conduct follow-up appointments to monitor oral health progress and assess changes in behaviour or living conditions
- Offer educational resources and support to the child and their family on proper oral hygiene practices and access to dental services
- Advocate and attend multidisciplinary safeguarding/multiagency risk assessment meetings involving social workers, educators, and healthcare providers to develop a holistic plan of action for the child's well-being

Long term

- Ensure continuous monitoring of the child's oral health and overall well-being through routine dental visits locally and maintain open communication with the child and their family while they are under your care
- Provide education to empower the child and their family in maintaining good oral health habits and overall wellness
- Advocate for wider team learning and implement systemic changes in policies and procedures within the team to enhance identification and response to child safeguarding concerns
- Participate in statutory and mandatory training and continuing professional development opportunities to stay informed about best practices in child safeguarding and welfare

Scenario—Safeguarding 2

A 45-year-old patient with Down's syndrome presents with poor oral hygiene, untreated dental decay, and signs of physical injuries, such as bruises and scratches. The patient appears withdrawn and hesitant to communicate during the appointment. What are the issues raised, and what are your short, medium and long-term management strategies for this patient?

Terms of reference +/− Issues raised

- Social worker involvement
- Physical abuse
- Neglect or self-neglect
- Clinical urgency
- Consent
- Mental Capacity Act

Key people/organizations

- Senior colleagues
- Medical professionals involved in the patient's care
- Safeguarding team
- Local authority (adult services/social worker)
- Office of the Public Guardian

Short term

- Document all observations and concerns factually in the patient's records, ensuring accuracy and confidentiality
- Ask the patient how the injuries were acquired

- Seek advice from your supervisor/safeguarding adults team
- Assume patient has capacity unless assessed otherwise. Consider an IMCA
- Initiate a private chaperoned conversation with the patient to establish trust and gather additional information, using clear and simple language adapted to their communication needs
- Assess the patient's immediate safety and well-being, providing support and reassurance as needed. Liaise with medical teams/A&E staff to arrange assessment and documentation of injuries
- Establish if children are involved; if so follow the safeguarding children pathway
- Consider contacting the local adult safeguarding team or social services to report suspicions of abuse or neglect and seek guidance on appropriate next steps
- Provide emergency treatment if required, if the patient gives consent. If they are assessed to lack capacity, a best interests decision may be made
- If the patient is in imminent danger, contact security and the police

Medium term

- If appropriate, collaborate with the patient's primary caregiver or support network, such as family members or care providers, to discuss observations and address concerns in a sensitive and non-confrontational manner
- Conduct follow-up appointments to monitor oral health progress and assess any changes in behaviour or physical condition
- Offer educational resources and support to the patient and their caregivers on proper oral hygiene techniques and strategies for promoting oral health in individuals with special care needs
- Advocate for multidisciplinary meetings involving healthcare professionals, social workers, and caregivers to develop a comprehensive care plan tailored to the patient's specific needs and circumstances

Long term

- Continuously monitor the patient's oral health and overall well-being during routine dental visits, maintaining open communication and ongoing support
- Provide ongoing training opportunities for the team to enhance their awareness and understanding of safeguarding issues and best practices in caring for adults with additional support and care needs
- Advocate for wider team learning and implement systemic changes in policies and procedures within the team to enhance identification and response to adult safeguarding concerns
- Collaborate with local community resources and support organizations to ensure ongoing support and advocacy for adults with additional support and care needs, promoting their health, safety, and well-being in the long term

Chapter 7

Staff management

Dental department staff

The dental team in a secondary care environment comprises:

1. Clinicians
2. Nurses
3. Dental technicians
4. Administrative staff
5. Auxiliary staff

Each of these staff groups has an independent line management structure. This has relevance for conflict management and escalation of concerns, with employees advised to raise issues within this structure initially. For more complex resolution of issues, there may be cross-over between different line management structures.

Although there is a 'banding' structure for clinician seniority, grade should never be a barrier to raising concerns, particularly if patient safety could be compromised. The hospital staff structure exists to signpost the correct manner to raise concerns, to indicate where responsibility lies and from what level staff performance is appraised.

All staff should follow the hospital trust's policies and regulations, available on the hospital's intranet.

Clinicians

- All practising dental clinicians will hold the relevant qualification: dental degree, dual qualified dental and medical degree for most oral and maxillofacial surgery and oral medicine consultants in the UK and degrees/diplomas for dental therapists, hygienists, orthodontic therapists, and clinical dental technicians
- Consultants hold ultimate accountability and responsibility for clinical care and for any doctors/dentists under their supervision (see Figure 7.1). They have both a clinical and managerial role involving mentoring and training more junior staff members and liaising with service managers, clinical leads, and other hospital departments such as human resources and finance
- Non-consultants may either be in training grades or non-training grades, dependent on whether they are on a UK training pathway with a national training number (see Chapter 9, Trainee management). Non-training grade doctors are either associate specialists (if they have completed dental speciality training) or staff grades if they have no additional specialist qualifications

Speciality trainees

- Trainees on a specialist pathway are termed speciality trainees
- Speciality trainees who have completed their specialist training and gained their certificate of completion of specialist training (CCST) may be in higher training positions, to become consultants. They are termed senior speciality trainees or post-CCSTs. Previously they were titled 'fixed-term training appointments' (FTTAs)
- Pre-CCST are 'junior' speciality trainees who are in training positions working towards their specialist accreditation

- Dentists working in the department who have not yet entered a specialist training pathway are dental core trainees. Further information on the specialist and training pathways is provided in Chapter 9, Trainee management
- The term junior doctor/dentist was used to describe qualified doctors/dentists who are either currently in postgraduate training or gaining experience, to become consultants, GPs or specialists. This has now formally changed to resident doctors/dentists and includes speciality trainees and dental core trainees

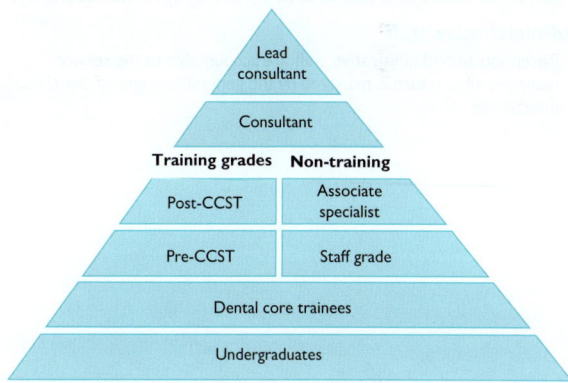

Figure 7.1 Pyramid of clinicians and experience level.

Honorary contracts

An honorary contract is distinct from a substantive contract of employment.
- It gives a doctor formal status with an employer
- It can provide opportunities to undertake paid work and access appropriate expenses, but it does not provide a salary or regular employment
- An honorary contract with an NHS employer might be held by a doctor who works primarily in an academic institution but remains clinically active

Academic staff

Academic staff are employed by both a university and NHS organization: one on a substantive basis and the other honorary.

The appraisal, disciplinary and reporting arrangements for NHS and university staff should follow the recommendations of the Follett Report (2001). The Universities and Colleges Employers Association (UCEA) provides advice and guidance on employment and matters relevant to the UK higher education sector.

Nursing

- The senior dental nurse is responsible for all the dental nurses within the department. They are then accountable to the matron. Junior/trainee nurses should first raise any concerns with the senior nurse

Dental technicians

- Some dental departments will have their own dental laboratory, led by the laboratory manager
- They will oversee any number of dental technicians, depending on the size of the department (see Chapter 11, Managing a dental laboratory)

Administrative staff

- Reception and administrative staff are accountable to the service manager, who in turn is managed by the general manager of the clinical directorate

Recruitment

The recruitment of dental staff, follows a set process (see Figure 7.2). Training grade dental recruitment is managed by Health Education England (HEE) via their local structures (see Chapter 9).

Consultant appointments are governed by the:
- NHS (Appointment of Consultants) Regulation Good Practice Guidance 2005 and the NHS Appointment of Consultant Regulation 1996 (see Figure 7.3)
- It is a legal requirement that all employing authorities in England and Wales comply with these regulations. Foundation trusts are exempt, but in practice, they too follow these guidelines
- There are nationally agreed policies and procedures from the Department of Health and Social Care (DHSC), Royal College of Surgeons (RCS), and NHS Employers

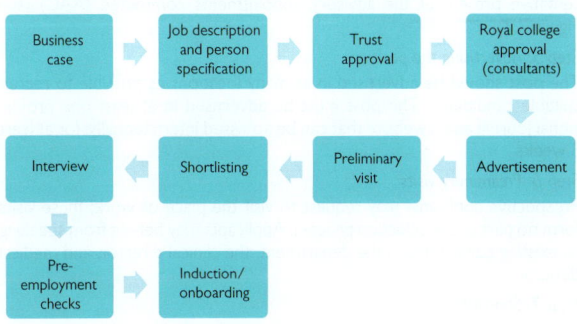

Figure 7.2 The recruitment process in an NHS trust.

Recruiting an NHS consultant

Step 1: Business case

A business case (see page 92) indicates the requirement for the position, the clinical objectives, the cost-benefit analysis and extra support required (secretarial, nursing, or administrative). The service needs must include clinical aspects but also consider additional roles such as teaching, training, supervision of junior staff, research and continuing educational requirements.

Step 2: Defining the post; job description and person specification

A job description (JD) and person specification (PS) are drawn up for approval at trust senior management level.

The job description includes information about the clinical services, key roles and responsibilities of the post, an outline of the job plan (including supporting professional activities (SPA) and direct clinical care (DCC)), teaching, and research roles. Trust values and relevant terms and conditions of service including pay are outlined.

The person specification is based on the job description and outlines:

- The essential and desirable qualifications, knowledge, skills, and experience
- How these attributes will be assessed
- The minimum entry criteria

Step 3: Hospital approval of job description and person specification

The JD and PS are forwarded to the service/operational manager or divisional director for the speciality, who will then obtain approval from the hospital management board. The human resources (HR) department must also approve these and following this, medical co-director approval is sought.

Step 4: Royal College of Surgeons approval

Once the JD has been approved by the trust, it is sent to the RCS regional advisor. All consultant JDs ideally should have RCS approval and a representative present at the advisory appointments committee (AAC) (see Figure 7.3).

Step 5: Advertising the position

The post should be advertised in as many locations as possible to recruit suitable candidates. The post must be advertised in at least one professional journal and a website that can be accessed internationally, for at least 3 weeks.

Step 6: Preliminary visits

Prospective applicants may request to visit the place of work; these visits form no part of the selection process. Applicants may benefit from speaking to existing consultants in the department, the clinical director, and medical director.

Step 7: Shortlisting

Applicants are compared to the person specification in an objective manner. Candidates who meet the shortlisting requirements will be invited to interview.

Step 8: Interview process

The AAC panel is convened, with mandatory internal members: chief executive, medical/dental director, consultant speciality representative and lay chair (trust non-executive director). External members include the RCS representative and a university representative, if an academic post. The panel confirms with the successful candidate immediately after the decision. The trust board confirms ratification of the appointment.

Step 9: Pre-employment checks

Checks are completed such as identification documents, professional registration, background checks, and occupational health.

Step 10: Induction/onboarding

A trust and local (department) induction should be carried out to outline: key policies and procedures, statutory requirements, etc.

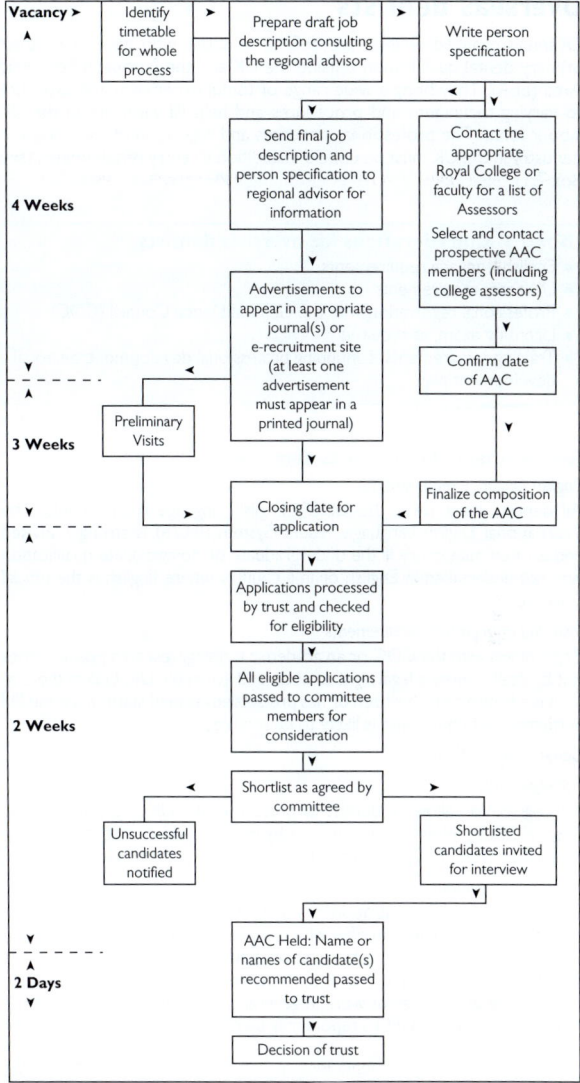

Figure 7.3 Steps in setting up an Appointments Advisory Committee. From: The National Health Service (Appointment of Consultants) Regulations Good Practice Guidance January 2005.

Overseas dentists

Overseas-qualified dentists are defined as those who have taken their primary dental qualification outside the UK and the European Economic Area (EEA). They bring a wide range of useful experience and exposure to varying techniques and procedures and help fill vacancies in the UK labour force. The professional standards and regulation of medicine and dentistry in the UK must be upheld in addition to entry requirements (see Box 7.1).

> **Box 7.1 Considerations for overseas dentists**
> - English language requirements
> - UK entry requirements
> - Professional registration with the General Dental Council (GDC)
> - Licensing exam, as required
> - Training requirements, continuing professional development, personal development plan

Requirements for overseas dentists

English language requirements

All dentists must meet the GDC's English language requirements. The International English Language Testing System (IELTS) is strongly advised and is often mandatory if the undergraduate or postgraduate qualification was not undertaken in English or in a country where English is the official language.

Visa and immigration requirements

Registration with the GDC or an academic training/research position does not by itself convey a legal right to enter and live in the UK. Unless the clinician is a British or Irish citizen or has pre-settled/settled status from the EU Settlement Scheme, a visa is likely to be required.

General Dental Council

Full registration

Full registration allows a dentist to practise in the UK in a practice or a hospital setting. However, it does not by itself allow a dentist to work as a performer in an NHS general practice, nor entitle them to a job.

Temporary registration

Dentists without full registration may be eligible for temporary registration, once they have received an offer of a supervised post for training, teaching, or research within an NHS hospital or dental school. This registration is linked to the position and thus is for a defined time period not more than 5 years. The dentist cannot work in general, private practice or in community dental service. An IELTS report may be required.

The Overseas Registration Examination (ORE) or the Licence in Dental Surgery Exam

Dentists from outside the EEA whose qualifications are not recognized for full GDC registration are required to pass the ORE. The ORE (formerly called the International Qualifying Examination) is organized by the GDC and consists of two parts. It is necessary to have a minimum of 1,600 hours of clinical dental experience prior to applying for the exam.

The Licence in Dental Surgery (LDS) examination is awarded by the Royal College of Surgeons of England (RCS England). Since June 2022, it consists of three separate parts.

The National Advice Centre for Postgraduate Dental Education (NACPDE) provides information for qualified dentists about working in the UK or studying for postgraduate dental qualifications in the UK. Candidates are advised to contact the appropriate bodies (e.g. GDC, RCS England) for the most contemporaneous information.

Training requirements

After passing the ORE, dentists may be required to complete one year of foundation training in order to work for the NHS. It is necessary for them to be listed on the NHS England's Performers list.

UK ENIC (The European National Information Centre for the UK) is the national agency for providing information and expert advice on international qualifications and skills. Previously called UK NARIC, it changed to UK ENIC, following the UK's exit from the European Union. UK ENIC can evaluate international qualifications and compare them to the UK education system; a statement of comparability is generated.

Rota management

The pay and conditions of junior doctors/dentists were revised in 2016. Full details may be found in:
- Terms and Conditions of Service for NHS Doctors and Dentists in Training (England) 2016 and Updated Version 11 (2023)
- Junior doctor handbook on the 2016 contract, British Medical Association (BMA)
- The Good Rostering Guide 2018

Doctor and dentist in training pay

Doctors/dentists are paid on national pay scales that are set each year. The pay scale is comprised of five nodal points, linked to the stage of training. Dental core trainees start at nodal point 3.

The doctors and dentists review body (DDRB) receives evidence from the BMA, the UK Health Departments, and NHS Employers. The DDRB then reports to the Secretary of State for Health and their equivalents for Scotland, Wales, and Northern Ireland with their recommendations on how to set the pay scales for the year. Each government makes its own final decision on whether to implement the recommendations in each of the four nations.

Rota design

A generic work schedule must be provided to a doctor at least 8 weeks before they start a placement. It should feature intended learning outcomes, scheduled duties, time for quality improvement and patient safety activities, periods of formal study, and the doctor's contracted hours.
- Rota—template working pattern design
- Roster—rota populated with specific details including staff names and dates

A roster is used to:
- Forecast the staffing levels and duties required to maintain the safe running of a service
- Facilitate the training and professional development of staff
- Allow for full leave entitlements to be taken

The design of a roster will consider factors such as: clinical patient needs, staff needs, trust needs, staffing levels, skills required to deliver a service, provision of training, quality improvement and general workforce availability/rota gaps.

Exception reporting

This is the process for a junior doctor/dentist to report any individual variations from the actual work schedule, on a per shift basis.
The purpose of exception reporting is to:
- Assess how common the issue is
- Determine how the doctor will be compensated
- Ensure prompt resolution and/or remedial action to ensure that safe working hours are maintained
- Educational opportunities are obtained in accordance with those stipulated in the work schedule

An exception report should be submitted when:
- A clinician is required to start earlier or leave later than their allocated shift time
- Additional shifts have been added to the day-to-day rota which do not appear on the rota template
- A junior doctor/dentist is unable to take a break on 25% of occasions over a 4-week period
- A doctor in training is unable to attend education/training sessions including clinics, theatres, and teaching on a regular basis due to service requirements in the department
- The training opportunities for doctors in training detailed in the work schedule are not provided

Guardian of safe working

An NHS Trust must appoint a guardian, to provide assurance that junior doctors/dentists are working in compliance with the safe hours requirements. They receive exception reports and escalate concerns to executive directors. They also intervene in urgent situations, such as if an exception report indicates that there is an immediate and substantive risk to the safety of patients or the clinician. They levy and distribute financial penalties for safe hours breaches.

Further reading

NHS Employers (2018). Good rostering guide. Available at: ℬ https://www.bma.org.uk/media/7509/pay-and-conditions-circular-md-4-2023-final_0.pdf

Consultant job planning

A job plan is an annual prospective agreement that sets duties, responsibilities, and objectives for the coming year. It is a requirement of a consultant and speciality doctor contract of employment.

It is an ongoing process, and a job plan may be reviewed sooner than a year if duties or needs have changed or there are concerns about whether objectives can be met. Although job planning and medical appraisal inform each other, they should be separate processes.

Components of job plan

A job plan should include all the work the consultant does for the trust, where and when it is undertaken. This includes:
- Timetable of activities
- Summary of all the programmed activities (PAs)
- On-call arrangements
- University work, for clinical academics
- Agreed flexible working arrangements and additional PAs
- Additional responsibilities such as clinical governance/audit lead, undergraduate/postgraduate dean, trade union duties, etc.
- Details of regular private work

Principles of job planning

The overriding principle should be to apply the 2003 Consultant Contract fairly and consistently. The job planning process should be collaborative and cooperative, a job plan should not be imposed. Where there is disagreement, this should be resolved through mediation.

Programmed activities (PAs)

PAs are blocks of time, usually equivalent to four hours, in which contractual duties are performed. A doctor working full-time will work 10 PAs or sessions per week. There are four basic categories of contractual work:
- Direct clinical care (DCC) - any work that involves the delivery of clinical services and administration directly related to them
- Supporting professional activities (SPAs)
- Additional responsibilities
- External duties

Supporting professional activities (SPAs)

SPAs underpin clinical care and contribute to ongoing professional development as a clinician. This includes activities such as:
- Teaching and training including clinical supervisor roles
- An assigned Educational Supervisor (AES) which may be approximately 0.25 SPA per trainee
- Medical education and continuing professional development
- Appraisal and revalidation
- Research, agreed in advance
- National roles (specialist societies, Royal Colleges)

For consultants, there is some national variation:
- Model contracts for England and Northern Ireland state that job plans will typically include an average of 7.5 DCC and 2.5 SPAs

- Scottish consultant terms and conditions set out the same split
- The Welsh model contract recommends three sessions of SPA
- The Academy of Medical Royal Colleges estimates that 1 to 1.5 SPAs per week is the minimum to meet the needs for continuing professional development (CPD)
- Consultants on locum or fixed-term contract consultants are routinely appointed on contracts with 1–1.5 SPA (assuming a 10 PA post), given the reduced responsibilities they have for service development. Doctors and dentists employed under the specialist, associate specialist, and speciality doctor (SAS) contract are entitled to a minimum of one PA or session of SPA time

The RCS recommends that there should be a job plan review for every new appointee within 6–12 months of starting their post, so that additional SPA time can be allocated should any additional activities have been undertaken by the appointee.

Academic staff

A clinical academic should have a single, integrated job plan. It should be jointly agreed between the substantive employer, the honorary employer, and the clinical academic outlining the academic and clinical roles and management and accountability arrangements for both.

Academic staff may have flexible timetabling of commitments over a period to help meet varying service needs; for example, part of the year focused on intensive research with fewer or no clinical commitments. There is flexibility in the honorary contract to agree a different DCC to SPA ratio for individual clinical academics.

References

British Medical Association guidelines on job planning. Available at: ℘ https://www.bma.org.uk/pay-and-contracts/job-planning/job-planning-process/an-overview-of-job-planning

NHS Improvement (2017). Consultant job planning: a best practice guide Available at: ℘ https://www.england.nhs.uk/wp-content/uploads/2022/05/consultant-job-planning-best-practice-guidance.pdf

NHS Employers (2013). Guidance notes for the employment of consultant clinical academics (England). Available at: ℘ https://www.nhsemployers.org/system/files/2021-06/clinical-academics-guidance-notes-2013.pdf

RCS (2016). *RCS Guidance and Checklist on NHS Surgical Consultant Job Descriptions*. London: RCS

Private practice

Consultants may offer private services within their NHS trust or externally, provided no conflicts of interest exist. Consultants should disclose details of regular private practice commitments as part of the annual job planning process. This includes the timing, location, and broad type of activity. NHS consultants should be appraised on all aspects of their practice, including private practice.

Key principles

The DHSC has published a code of conduct for consultants providing private services.

- NHS consultants and NHS trusts should work on a partnership basis to prevent any conflict of interest between private and NHS work
- The provision of services for private patients should not prejudice the interests of NHS patients or disrupt NHS services
- With the exception of the need to provide emergency care, agreed NHS commitments should take precedence over private work
- NHS facilities, staff, and services may only be used for private practice with the prior agreement of the NHS employer

Provision of Private Services alongside NHS Duties

As per the 2003 contract, employers may offer up to one extra PA per week to consultants who undertake private practice.

Information for NHS Patients about Private Treatment

- Consultants should not initiate discussions about providing private services for NHS patients
- Where an NHS patient seeks information about the availability of, or waiting times for, NHS and/or private services, this may be given
- Any information provided should be accurate and up-to-date
- Except where immediate care is justified on clinical grounds, consultants should not during their NHS duties make arrangements to provide private services, unless the patient is to be treated as a private patient of the NHS facility concerned
- Other NHS staff should not initiate discussions or make arrangements on behalf of a consultant

Referral of private patients to NHS lists

Private patients may seek to change their status and seek treatment as an NHS patient. These patients:

- Are entitled to NHS services on exactly the same basis of clinical need as any other patient
- They should not be treated on a different basis from other NHS patients
- Patients referred for an NHS service following a private consultation or treatment should join any NHS waiting list at the same point as if the consultation or treatment were an NHS service
- Their priority on the waiting list should be determined by the same criteria applied to other NHS patients
- Should a patient be admitted to an NHS hospital as a private inpatient, but subsequently decide to change to NHS status before having

received treatment, there should be an assessment to determine the patient's priority for NHS care
- A patient cannot be both a private and NHS patient for the treatment of one condition during a single visit. NHS and private care should be delivered separately

Seeing private patients in NHS facilities

The NHS trust can decide whether its facilities, staff, and equipment may be used for private patient services. NHS consultants may not use these facilities for the provision of private care without the agreement of their NHS trust, even if these services are being carried out in their own time, during annual or unpaid leave.

Where the trust has agreed to this use:
- The trust will determine the charge for the use of its facilities
- Any charge will be collected by the trust
- The charge will take full account of any diagnostic procedures used, the cost of any laboratory staff that have been involved and the cost of any NHS equipment that might have been used

Reference

GMC (April 2013). Financial and commercial arrangements and conflicts of interest. Available at: ℘ https://www.gmc-uk.org/-/media/documents/gmc-guidance-for-doctors---financial-and-com mercial-arrangements-and-conflicts-of-interest_-58833167.pdf

Further reading

DoH (2004). A Code of Conduct for Private Practice: Recommended Standards of Practice For NHS Consultants. Available at: ℘ https://www.nhsemployers.org/system/files/2021-06/cons ultants-code-of-conduct-private-practice-guide.pdf
Medical Protection Society (2022). Conducting private work in the NHS. Available at: ℘ https:// www.medicalprotection.org/uk/articles/conducting-private-work-in-the-nhs#:~:text=You%20 should%20only%20attempt%20to,not%20prejudice%20NHS%20service%20provision

Performance management

Performance management describes the arrangements that employers use to maintain and improve the performance of their workforce so that the organization achieves its goals. Measuring the performance of the service is covered in Chapter 5. Staff management is a pillar of clinical governance in the NHS.

Other processes in the department will also give an indication of staff performance, in relation to how the dental department is performing (see Box 7.2).

Box 7.2 Performance management for doctors and dentists

- Appraisal and revalidation
- Performance management for the service and staff
- Clinical audits
- Clinical targets
- Complaints register
- Patient satisfaction surveys
- Incident reporting system

Recognizing poor performance

- Appraisal and/or revalidation are not an appropriate way for concerns to be managed
- A distinction must be made between poor performance due to an inherent incapacity versus a wilful refusal to work to a satisfactory standard, as the management pathway will differ
- A disciplinary issue is behaviour that falls below the standard expected by the trust and profession, whereas a lack of capability is the inability to perform actions and work at the standard expected for their experience level. The trust's disciplinary and/or capability policies should be adhered to
- Underperforming staff who have the clinical capacity but lack motivation or drive should be approached differently to staff who have capability or capacity restraints
- Issues within employees' personal lives undeniably will have cross-over into their working lives at times; this can affect their ability to perform work tasks to their best standard or be fully engaged. It is now accepted that it is unrealistic to expect employees to 'leave their home life at the door' once entering work
- Employers are encouraged to take a more compassionate approach to external challenges which their employees may be facing; occupational health, counselling, or reasonable adjustments such as a temporary change or reduction in working hours, remote working should all be considered

- For employees with capability issues, every effort should be made to improve their performance and support them in their role and training (see conduct and capability below)
- Dentists and doctors in training roles will be under regular review and monitoring via competencies, work-based assessments, and portfolios with their respective deanery. Dentists in non-training roles also have a responsibility to achieve a satisfactory level of performance and behaviour and a failure to reach these standards requires investigation. Chapter 9 (Trainee management) outlines the process for trainees requiring additional support
- If there is any doubt that there may be complicating physical or mental health issues, a referral to occupational health to determine fitness to practice or disciplinary procedures should be arranged as a matter of urgency

Managing performance concerns

- The main consideration is patient safety and thus any concerns must be promptly raised (see Figure 7.4)
- For minor concerns that do not affect patient safety, issues should first be managed locally and informally. A meeting with the employee/trainee to discuss the concern and hear their insight should be arranged. Clear and documented objectives towards resolution or improvement should be set. Employees should be supported to achieve these goals, with training as required
- It may be necessary to limit the scope of clinical practice or instigate supervision, mentoring, or shadowing
- Concerns can be raised directly with the individual or with a more senior colleague. The line manager should also be notified
- Trainees have a designated clinical tutor and educational supervisor. They should be notified in the first instance. For ongoing or more grave concerns, further escalation is required including informing the postgraduate deanery or college/university
- If the concern relates to a consultant or senior staff member not in a training role, the clinical lead, head consultant, and/or medical directors should be involved
- If patient safety is at risk, an urgent review should be conducted. The medical director and team should be notified immediately
- If concerns are grave and are not being given adequate consideration or follow up, the trust's executives and chief executive should be involved. All serious concerns must be registered with the chief executive and a case manager appointed
- If concerns persist and have not been adequately managed, external steps must be taken by notifying the police
- Outcomes may be retraining, redeployment, being placed on alternative duties, dismissal, or if serious, external enquiries and criminal charges

Conduct and capability

- A case manager will be appointed; this may be the head of service, or a divisional manager. If the concern is about a director or consultant, the medical director will be the case manager

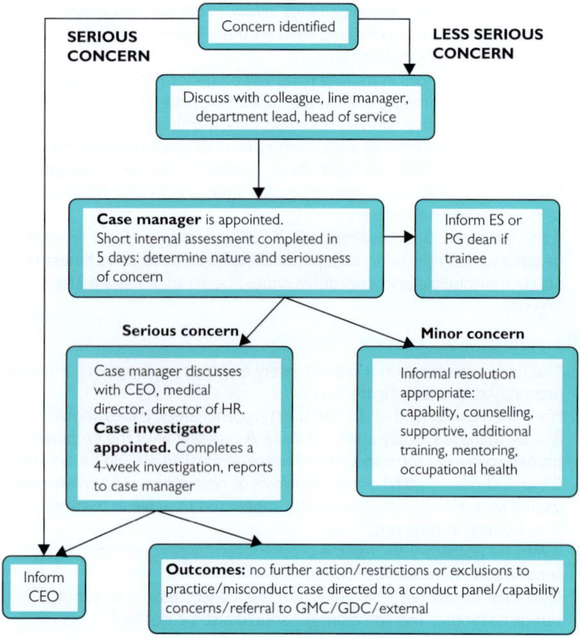

Figure 7.4 Flowchart for raising performance concerns

- The number of people involved and speed of escalation will depend on the gravity of the concern and potential risk to patient safety
- Capability issues can often be successfully managed with mentoring, additional training, and support, whereas conduct concerns may require management along the disciplinary pathway

Outcomes

- For issues that are not imminently putting patient safety at risk, the first-line management is often retraining, ongoing assessment, and support. The majority of issues do not require escalation to the next formal management steps
- Practitioner Performance Advice, or PPA (formerly National Clinical Assessment Service, NCAS) assists healthcare organizations to resolve concerns. This is a useful step before referring to a capability panel. PPA is a division of NHS Resolution. They can help direct the next steps forward, assist with restrictions and exclusions, clinical performance assessments, and generally provide support and advice for resolution of performance concerns in healthcare
- A case manager may determine that a disciplinary or capability hearing is required and thus the case is referred to a capability panel. The case is presented, the allegations or evidence discussed and the panel adjourns to deliberate. The employee is notified of the decision, often within 5 days (see Box 7.3)

Box 7.3 Outcomes from capability/disciplinary hearing

1. No action
2. Verbal agreement to increase performance within a timescale (confirmed in writing)
3. Written agreement to increase performance and steps, maintained on employee's file for one year
4. Final written warning
5. Termination of employment
   The employee may appeal the decision within approximately 25 days.

Challenges with performance management

- Appraisal and revalidation is criticised as being an ineffective way of monitoring doctors' and dentists' day-to-day productivity and performance. The processes involve limited use of objective data. Clinicians use reflective practice to identify learning objectives; this may not reflect actual performance
- Most trusts focus on performance management at a service or departmental level, rather than effectively evaluating individual clinician performance
- It can be difficult to obtain validated data on an individual's performance, especially for doctors and dentists not in training positions
- Medical and non-medical managers have expressed difficulty in challenging a doctor's performance, thus contributing to a lack of usable data (*Managing NHS hospital consultants*. London: National Audit Office, DoH, 2013)
- Poorly validated data can be detrimental to a clinician's career and the department, and the publication of such data could have negative consequences
- Hospital episode statistics (coding) data is often used to measure performance but is a poor reflection of an individual clinician's performance
- Empowering and enabling more successful performance evaluation and management strategies are preferable to a monitoring culture of measuring targets, as seen in non-healthcare sectors
- Bidirectional reviews are generally preferred to the more common 360 review. Colleague feedback is important but needs to be done within a context of improvements overall rather than personal criticism of one colleague
- More constructive is the 'continue start stop' approach: asking teams what colleagues should continue to do, start doing, and things that might not be effective and should be stopped
- Focusing on what clinicians like doing and how to facilitate more of that, ensuring that they feel supported in their progression
- Balancing professional accountability with performance growth and development. Using personal development plans to explore growth opportunities

Further reading

NHS Employers People Performance Management toolkit. Available at: ℞ https://www.nhsemploy ers.org/publications/people-performance-management-toolkit

Appraisal and revalidation

Doctors and dentists are required to carry out an annual appraisal. Revalidation, however, is only required for doctors, in order to maintain their GMC registration. Dentists are not required to undergo revalidation but instead must demonstrate that the required CPD, related to a personal development plan, has been carried out.

Revalidation

Revalidation is the process by which the General Medical Council (GMC) confirms the continuation of a doctor's licence to practise in the UK. It assures patients, the public, employers, and other healthcare professionals that licensed doctors are registered and fit to practise. GMC registrants must revalidate every five years. This is based on an annual appraisal to collate a portfolio of evidence. Doctors will have a connection to a responsible officer through their designated body (see Box 7.4). A recommendation is made to the GMC, who then decides if the doctor can retain their licence to practise.

Revalidation is not a requirement for registrants with the GDC, however dentists employed by an NHS trust are required to undertake this process as a contractual obligation. The Annual Review of Competency Progression (ARCP) is the equivalent for doctors and dentists in training.

Box 7.4 Revalidation definitions

Responsible officer (RO)

The responsible officer is usually a senior doctor in the trust (often medical director or a nominated representative). They are accountable for the quality assurance of the appraisal and clinical governance systems in their organization.

Designated body

For most doctors this is the organization in which they carry out most of their practice (such as NHS trust). They must appoint and resource the RO.

Medical appraisal

A medical appraisal is an annual meeting between a doctor and a colleague who is trained as an appraiser. It is a process of facilitated self-review supported by information gathered.

The medical appraisal enables doctors/dentists to:
- Reflect on their individual practice and performance
- Inform the RO's revalidation recommendation to the GMC
- Plan professional development and identify learning needs
- Demonstrate a doctor/dentist is up-to-date and fit to practise

There are three stages to the appraisal process (Figure 7.5):
1. Inputs into appraisal
2. Appraisal discussion
3. Outputs from appraisal

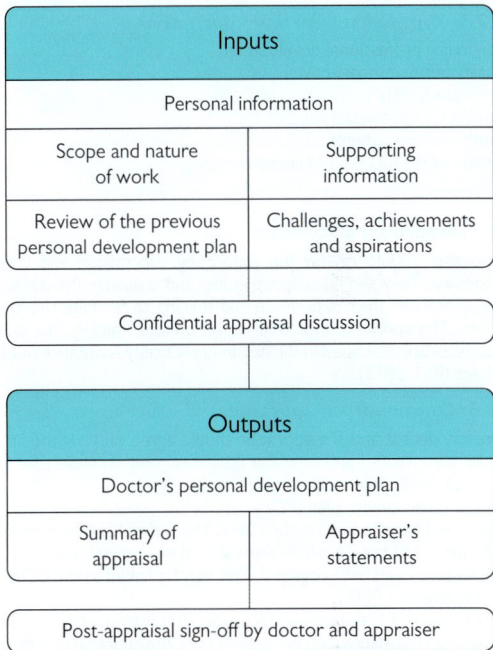

Figure 7.5 The appraisal process. Reproduced from Medical Appraisal Guide 2022, Academy of Medical Royal Colleges.

Stage 1: Inputs

The inputs should be submitted to the appraiser before the appraisal and must include:

- All roles and positions in which the dentist/doctor has clinical responsibilities
- Any other roles for which a licence to practise is required
- Work for voluntary organizations or private practice
- Managerial, educational, research, and academic roles
- Supporting information. This should relate to the *complete* scope of work (see Box 7.5)
- Review of the previous year's personal development plan
- Achievements, challenges, and aspirations
- Reflection is a key part of the appraisal inputs and process

> **Box 7.5 Types of supporting information**
> 1. Continuing professional development
> 2. Quality improvement activity
> 3. Significant events
> 4. Feedback from colleagues
> 5. Feedback from patients
> 6. Review of complaints and compliments

Stage 2: Appraisal discussion

The appraiser should review the supporting information and commentary provided. They should support, guide, and challenge the doctor constructively and use their experience and training to facilitate the appraisal discussion. The appraiser should have appropriate training. The skills and competencies are described in the document: Quality Assurance of Medical Appraisers (RST, 2013).

Stage 3: Outputs from appraisal

The doctor/dentist and the appraiser should agree on how the appraisal should be summarized and how the doctor is going to undertake further professional development. This must include:

- Personal development plan (PDP)
- An itemized list of personal objectives. There should be an indication of the period of time in which items should be completed and how completion should be recognized. This may be linked to the GDC requirement of a PDP
- The summary of the appraisal discussion. This is an overview of the supporting information and key elements of the appraisal discussion
- The appraiser's statements. These are statements to the RO which (where appropriate) inform the revalidation recommendation to the GMC

COVID-19

The appraisal process was paused in March 2020 to allow doctors to focus on the demands of the COVID-19 pandemic. Since then, the Medical Appraisal 2022 has been introduced as a new approach to appraisals. This has:

- A streamlined appraisal format
- Meets revalidation requirements
- Places more focus on well-being
- Reduces pre-appraisal paperwork requirements

Constituent nations

The GMC guidance on appraisal and revalidation is valid for the whole of the UK. There are variations in the management of the process:

- England—NHS England has published additional appraisal guidance
- Northern Ireland—DoH has published specific guidance
- Scotland—The Scottish Online Appraisal Resource (SOAR) is an administration tool for the completion and sharing of online forms and supporting documents and tracking appraisal history
- Wales—The Medical Appraisal and Revalidation System (MARS) is the online appraisal system used in Wales

Further reading

Academy of Medical Royal Colleges (2022). Medical Appraisal Guide. Available at: 🖰 https://www.aomrc.org.uk/wp-content/uploads/2023/07/Medical_Appraisal_Guide_2022_0622.pdf

BMA Appraisal and Revalidation. Available at: 🖰 https://www.bma.org.uk/advice-and-support/career-progression/appraisals/medical-appraisals

GMC (2013). Good Medical Practice Framework for Appraisal and Revalidation. Available at: 🖰 https://www.ombudsman.org.uk/sites/default/files/The_Good_medical_practice_framework_for_appraisal_and_revalidation___DC5707.pdf_56235089.pdf

GMC (2012). Supporting Information for Appraisal and Revalidation. Available at: 🖰 https://www.gmc-uk.org/registration-and-licensing/managing-your-registration/revalidation/guidance-on-supporting-information-for-revalidation

RST (2013). Quality Assurance of Medical Appraisers. Available at: 🖰 https://www.england.nhs.uk/revalidation/wp-content/uploads/sites/10/2014/02/rst-medical-app-guide-2013.pdf

Grievances and conflict resolution

Strong, cohesive teamwork is fundamental to the success of a department. Small disputes that are permitted to escalate unresolved have the chance of creating tension, poor interpersonal staff relations, and ultimately compromise patient care.

Having good basic principles to address and manage these issues in their early stages and as close as possible to the point of origin helps prevent escalation of minor issues into larger problems. Every trust will have its own grievance and disciplinary policy and it is worth being familiar with them when a dispute does arise.

Employees should be adequately supported when a dispute arises and it is important to have an unbiased view of the situation until a full investigation is completed (see Box 7.6). What may appear to be a disciplinary issue may in fact be a cry for help from an overwhelmed staff member or a trainee struggling with the programme and its responsibilities. Employees may be managing a challenging issue in their personal life which is encroaching on their work and a more lenient approach to support them during that time may be the better management strategy.

> **Box 7.6 When a conflict arises, consider**
> - Capability concern? Is the person struggling with the workload, do they require more training, are they not up-to-date with techniques/technology required, is there a personal/health issue that is impairing their ability to satisfactorily complete their work
> - Conduct concern? Is this a true conduct issue, is the employee being rude/offensive/exhibiting bullying or aggressive behaviour
> - Disciplinary pathway? Is the incident serious enough to warrant management along the trust's disciplinary pathway, which could ultimately lead to formal warnings or dismissal

Grievance

A grievance is an official complaint by an employee who feels they have been treated unfairly.

The employment grievance procedure is a formal way for an employee to raise a problem or complaint to their employer. It is usually best to try to raise a grievance informally in the first instance, unless the issue is so serious that it necessitates immediate formal escalation. Each trust will have its own grievance procedure, similar to Box 7.7. Acting promptly, effectively, and consistently, within the agreed policy and procedure will manage most issues at an early stage.

Mediation

Mediation can be used at any stage during conflict resolution. It involves the two sides working with an impartial person, to find a resolution. The mediator may be someone from within the department or trust or a paid external mediator service.

Bullying and harassment

The definitions of bullying, harassment and related terms are presented in Table 7.1. These are not limited to verbal behaviour but also include physical and written forms, including via text or email.

The trust, managers, and all individual staff are responsible for ensuring that the working environment is free from bullying, harassment, and victimization. The trust has a duty of care to its employees and is required

---

Box 7.7 Grievance procedure

Informal resolution
- Employee raises a grievance with their supervisor or line manager in writing
- Informal mediation meetings with HR to facilitate resolution
- Response in writing within 5 days of meeting
- If employee is dissatisfied with the response, proceed to formal resolution

Formal resolution:
- Formal meeting arranged with the manager, employee, and HR representative. Employee may be accompanied by a colleague or trade union representative
- An investigation may be planned, with a formal investigation report as the outcome
- Recommendations from the report will be considered as part of the final decision
- The employee may appeal the outcome

Table 7.1 Definitions of bullying and harassment (ACAS)

Bullying	Unwanted behaviour from a person or a group that is offensive, intimidating, malicious, insulting or an abuse or misuse of power that undermines, humiliates or causes physical or emotional harm to someone.
Harassment	Unwanted conduct related to a protected characteristic (Equality Act 2010) that violates people's dignity or creates an intimidating, hostile, degrading, humiliating or offensive environment.
Victimization	Someone is treated less favourably as a result of being involved with a discrimination or harassment complaint.
Violence	The use of physical force against another person or group that results in physical, sexual, or psychological harm.
Associative discrimination	Discrimination against someone because of their connection with someone/a group of people who have a protected characteristic.
Perceptive discrimination	Discrimination against someone because of a perceived protected characteristic.

by law to ensure that no employee is treated less favourably than any other. Individuals who experience bullying or harassment and those who are accused of being perpetrators often experience stress. Under health and safety legislation (Health and Safety at Work Act, 1974), the trust is responsible for the health, safety, and welfare at work of all employees. Harassment and bullying are harmful, cause distress, and can lead to accidents or illness, preventing employees from fulfilling their potential.

The key difference between bullying and harassment is that harassment relates to a protected characteristic set out in the Equality Act 2010 (Box 7.8), while bullying does not.

Box 7.8 Protected characteristics as per Equality Act 2010

It is against the law to discriminate against someone because of:
1. Age
2. Disability
3. Gender reassignment
4. Marriage and civil partnership
5. Pregnancy and maternity
6. Race
7. Religion or belief
8. Sex
9. Sexual orientation

Managing a bullying or harassment complaint

When managing a complaint, it is important to consider:
- The impact of the behaviour on the individual is the main consideration in determining the occurrence of bullying or harassment
- Both complainant and alleged perpetrator are entitled to a fair opportunity to give their version of events. Both parties have the right to be represented throughout the process. This may be by a trade union representative or a work colleague
- Resolution at an informal stage is preferred. If this is deemed inappropriate due to the gravity of the event or the informal process has failed, then the formal stage is entered
- If there is evidence of false or malicious allegations against another individual, it may be appropriate for an investigation to be conducted following the trust's disciplinary policy
- Each trust's policy document may vary slightly, with different time frames, etc., but they all will follow a similar outline from informal resolution to formal escalation to resolution, with the appeal process outlined (see Figure 7.6)
- The HR team will often be supported by and have recourse to the trust's legal team, due to the complexity of employment law, equity of outcome and the levels of compensation available, in particular for discrimination complaints

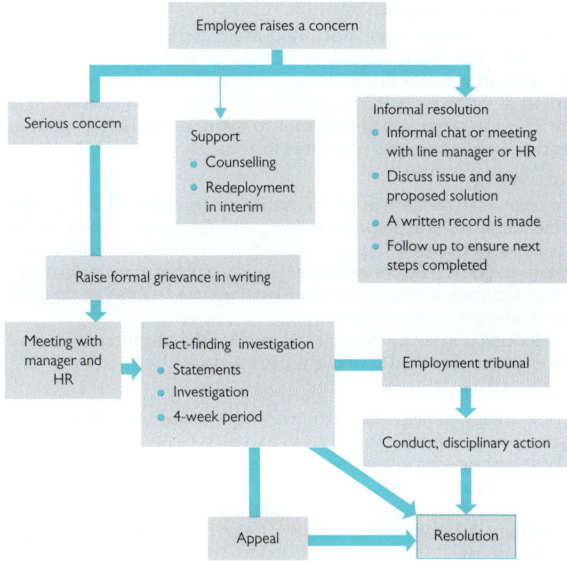

Figure 7.6 Flowchart for raising grievance.

Disciplinary issues

The line manager should aim to resolve any minor conduct issues informally and promptly by discussing the incident, setting expectations, and ensuring actions to rectify the issue. Incidents of gross misconduct may warrant summary dismissal; the immediate termination of the contract of employment without payment of statutory or contractual notice period.

- Misconduct is defined as an action falling below the standard of behaviour expected by trust policy or professional bodies (such as the GDC)
- Gross misconduct is any act or omission which causes irreparable damage to the relationship of trust and confidence between the employee and the trust. This includes actions such as theft, physical violence or gross insubordination

Managing disciplinary issues

Standard setting

A one-to-one meeting with the line manager and employee occurs, and underlying and contributory factors are discussed. This meeting may highlight supportive action required or training needs. The employee is reminded of the expected level of conduct and the trust's disciplinary policy, should further issues occur. A written summary of the meeting is sent to the employee.

Fact-finding and investigation

If there are repeated minor misconduct issues, the line manager may proceed to the fact-finding stage. They submit their findings to the case manager, who may decide that an investigation is required. The employee is notified of the terms of reference of the investigation. An investigating officer compiles a report and submits it to the case manager; an outcome decision is made or formally escalated to a hearing.

Formal hearing

The employee is notified in writing with five days notice. They can admit to the allegations as appropriate and forgo the full disciplinary hearing. The case manager chairs the hearing panel, which may decide that more investigation is required before making a decision. If there is a potential gross misconduct issue, a minimum of three members are required on the panel, one of whom is a HR representative.

A decision is made by the panel on whether the allegations are upheld. The employee is notified in writing within five days.

Disciplinary outcomes

- First written warning—for minor misconduct issues, remains on the employee's file for 12 months
- Final warning—for serious misconduct or multiple occurrences, remains on the employee's file for 18 months
- Dismissal—if severe misconduct or previous active final warning
- Summary dismissal—immediate termination of employment without notice or pay
- Alternatives such as demotion or transfer

ACAS codes of practice

The Advisory, Conciliation and Arbitration Service (ACAS) is an independent body whose role is to help foster good workplace relationships. They have developed codes of practice which help employers and employees navigate workplace conflicts, grievances, settlement agreements, etc. (Box 7.9). Although not legally binding, the codes of practice have been approved by Parliament and are used by employment tribunals as a benchmark for the minimum standards of fairness which workplaces should follow.

Relational intelligence in the workplace

Every trust has a grievance policy and procedures to resolve conflict. All employees know that conflict in the workplace is best avoided or managed at an early stage. But despite this, conflicts do arise and can persist unresolved, contributing to 'office politics' and tensions. Unease at work can lead to time off on grounds of stress and an increased workload burden on remaining colleagues, which can further increase tension.

There is a reason why simple algorithms for managing conflict in the workplace can be hard to follow. They ignore the human factors at play behind the majority of conflicts. Relational intelligence in the workplace has typically been overlooked; these are 'soft skills' that don't clear waiting lists or meet key performance indicators (KPIs) or revenue targets. The ability to get along well with other people in a department is not easily assessed at an interview. But there is a growing awareness of the importance of this in a happy, productive, conflict-free work environment.

Box 7.9 ACAS code of practice: discipline and grievance

- Employers and employees should raise concerns and resolve issues promptly
- Aim for informal resolution, wherever possible
- Employers should make every effort to listen to employees' grievances and make reasonable adjustments
- If informal resolution is ineffective, engage an independent third party mediator
- It is best practice for employers to have written policies in place for disciplinary and grievance procedures
- Employers are responsible for carrying out thorough and fair investigations to establish the facts of a case
- Employees must be given the opportunity to provide their side of the story before any decisions are made. They must be given the right to appeal any formal decision. They should be allowed to be accompanied during formal meetings
- If a party has not complied with an ACAS code of practice (with no justifiable reason), an employment tribunal can adjust financial compensation by up to 25%

The human factors underlying conflicts

When a conflict arises, it is important to consider both the issue at hand and also the people involved and what they bring to the situation. Most people have accumulated cognitive distortions throughout life and the person who enters the workplace doesn't leave all of that behind them. People hold different perspectives, beliefs, and thoughts, all of which are biased by their viewpoint and how they view the world. Colleagues may hold a completely different set of values and assumptions. These impact an individual's emotions, reactions, and ultimately on how they will handle a conflict.

What is happening in a conflict situation?

When we consider that 65% of start-ups fail due to conflict among cofounders (Noam Wasserman), the importance of relational intelligence at work becomes clear.

What is actually happening during a conflict though, is generally always more than just the issue at hand. The relational dynamics at play in any human interaction include a mix of power, rejection, fear, insecurity, trust, codependence… and many more. And this is all within a certain social, political, economic, and cultural context, all of which may be viewed differently by each of the parties.

Both parties involved in the conflict may have a degree of anger. There may be anger that the other person disagrees and can't see their perspective. Although they may not realise it, fear often plays a significant role. People are fearful that they are being attacked, taken advantage of, or misunderstood. There may be fear that they did something wrong and fear of retribution. This can make people feel vulnerable, insecure, ashamed, and this combination of emotions can lead to defensiveness. Defensiveness hinders problem-solving. The aim is to try not to defend anything—as each perspective is relevant and valid—and instead see the situation from the other side's point of view and what their fears may be.

How to resolve conflict

Look inwards first

- Look at yourself and try to understand your contribution to the situation. What cognitive or unconscious biases have led you to certain conclusions and assumptions?
- Self-awareness of your own character weaknesses; what past issues might you be bringing with you into work?
- Ability to accept and process feedback without defensiveness; are there areas of truth that you consider to modify your behaviour?
- Try not to take the issue personally. People do and say things that are more about themselves than the other person. One person might not have realized that something was hurtful or sensitive. Don't let your default assumption be that someone intentionally acted to cause hurt
- Draw on your empathy for others who have different cultures, ways of doing business, etc.

Change your perspective on the situation

- Stop trying to work out who is right and who is wrong. From varying perspectives, either could be argued as true for both sides since interpretations will vary
- Avoid trying to assign blame. Both parties are likely correct about some aspects and incorrect about others. Blame can lead to an impasse and defensiveness, it prevents the ability to determine what the contributing factors were and thus understanding how to mitigate these in the future
- Move away from blame and accusation towards a more neutral exploratory stance. Try to understand the other person's perspective, concerns, and reasons for their behaviour. Ask for clear information from them so that you can understand
- Once both parties feel heard and understood, it is easier to shift to a problem-solving mindset and to move forwards

Reaching solutions

- Show that you have insight into your role in the conflict and have taken responsibility for any negative contributions. This will encourage the other party to do similar and is a useful step in mediation and compromise
- As possible solutions to the conflict are discussed, continue to demonstrate that you understand the other party's concerns and motivations. Help them to understand your perspective
- Move away from either A or B are the only options in the situation. In reality, there are many different approaches and if neither party can agree on each other's, then find new options
- There may need to be multiple exchanges as the conflict resolution process evolves. Different options can be explored and then a meeting re-convened to express any further concerns

Benefits of a robust conflict resolution culture
- Quicker engagement with issues when they arise. This means issues won't linger in the department and become divisive among staff
- Employees will feel more confident to speak up to raise concerns, knowing that a fair resolution process is in place
- Employees will have a greater sense of satisfaction from engaging in effective communication and having their concerns addressed. This improves self-confidence, self-esteem, and ultimately happiness in the workplace

Unconscious bias

Unconscious (or implicit) bias is a term that describes the associations we hold, outside our conscious awareness and control. It can have a significant influence on our attitudes and behaviours, especially towards other people.
- Unconscious bias affects everyone
- It is caused by automatic, quick judgements and assessments
- They are influenced by our background, personal experiences, societal stereotypes, and cultural context
- This does not just relate to gender, ethnicity, or other visible diversity characteristics. Other factors such as height, body weight, names may also trigger unconscious bias
- It can influence key decisions in the workplace and can contribute to inequality

The following are some examples of unconscious bias:
- Affinity or similarity bias—Tendency to favour people who are like you in some way
- Confirmation bias—Once an opinion or decision is formed, the tendency to look for, and value, further information that confirms this. Incidents may be interpreted in a certain way, or other information that contradicts our confirmation bias is ignored. This can cause problems, if we fail to notice an issue or make misjudgments
- The halo effect—When one perceived positive feature or trait makes us view everything about a person in a positive way, giving them a 'halo'. This may lead us to ignore other aspects
- The 'horn effect'—The opposite of the halo effect, where focus is on one particularly negative feature

Reducing unconscious bias
- Being aware of unconscious bias. Increasing self-awareness allows individuals to mitigate it. It can be important to recognize and understand what biases you may hold
- Justify decisions by considering the evidence available and record the reasons for decisions
- Allow time to make decisions
- Keep a written record of why decisions are made
- Where appropriate, making decisions together as a team can help mitigate the biases of one individual
- Be open to conversations and challenges around decisions and potential biases
- Follow trust policies and guidelines

Reducing unconscious bias in recruitment
- Advertise a job vacancy in at least two different places to reach a wide range of people from different backgrounds
- Shortlist and interview based on the agreed essential criteria in the person specification. This allows objective evaluation, using numerical scores. This helps to treat each person as an individual, assessing them on their own merits against the criteria, rather than comparing candidates against each other
- Those involved in recruitment should agree to make each other aware if they notice stereotyping
- Blind sifting—Hold back some details such as the applicant's name or sex that could affect shortlisting opinions
- Consider having one interviewer conduct the interview by phone so they do not make decisions based on physical appearance
- Have multiple people involved in every stage of the job application procedures
- To reduce similarity bias, instead of considering whether an individual is a 'good fit' for the team, value diversity by asking 'what will this person add to our team?'

Further reading

ACAS Codes of Practice. Available at: ⬧ https://www.acas.org.uk/codes-of-practice
Wasserman N (2013). *The Founder's Dilemmas: Anticipating And Avoiding The Pitfalls That Can Sink a Startup.* Princeton, NJ: Princeton University Press. [Also see the Kauffman Foundation Series on Innovation and Entrepreneurship]

Scenario—Speciality trainee and nurse dispute

You are a dental consultant in the department. The restorative speciality trainee approaches you in frustration and says that she simply cannot work with a particular nurse anymore. She demands not to be rostered with that nurse again. How would you manage this situation?

Relevant policies
- Grievance and disciplinary
- Bullying and harassment
- Conduct, capability, and health

Immediate management
Attempt local resolution by finding out more information. This should be done in a confidential manner.

An informal discussion with the speciality trainee reveals her side of the story: the nurse arrives for the afternoon clinic exactly at 2pm (the session start time) and then proceeds to set up the equipment. The speciality trainee turns up early, to prepare for her afternoon session and so is ready to seat the patient in the dental chair exactly at 2pm, their appointment time. Because of the nurse's delay in setting up, the patient is often not seated until 2.15 pm or later. The nurse is unfamiliar with rotary endodontics and often passes the wrong files and the wrong sizes. When she has to leave the room to get another piece of equipment, the speciality trainee is kept waiting a long time and when she also leaves the room to check on the nurse, the speciality trainee finds her outside the clinic room, looking at her phone.

You could also discuss the situation with the lead nurse and see if there are any other ongoing issues within the department in general e.g., staff shortages or any personal issues affecting this nurse. Consider if the nursing staff are being given adequate lunch breaks and time to set up for clinics, to allow appointments to run on time.

On first impressions, this seems like a relatively straight-forward scenario to manage. The nurse requires additional training to support her in endodontic procedures and a reminder not to use her phone during active patient treatment and to arrive on time for clinics. You agree to roster a different nurse for the speciality trainee's next endodontic session. However, it would be inappropriate to arrange this for every session.

You arrange an informal meeting with the nurse, who gets upset and informs you: the speciality trainee is curt and rude. She demands equipment that is not usual for the scheduled procedure and rarely used. The nurse feels intimidated by the way the speciality trainee speaks to her in front of the patient. She uses the time outside the room to calm herself down. In addition, she is caring for her elderly mother at home and needs to check in frequently by phone. Finally, as the morning clinic session generally runs late, her lunch hour is already reduced, so she will not further reduce it by starting the afternoon session before 2pm.

Mediation

Continuing with informal resolution, you may choose to have another discussion with the speciality trainee now that you have more information. Alternatively, you may opt to bring both parties together for a discussion. Considerations:

- It is not feasible to have different staff members choosing not to work with each other as this could result in other staff requesting similar and disharmony in the department
- The speciality trainee does have an assertive communication style; this is not a negative trait but could be misinterpreted by others. Consider asking if other nurses have found this intimidating. Could this be a cultural difference or is there evidence of rudeness or bullying
- Is there staff capacity in the department to have a 'float nurse' with more flexible hours, to cover clinics that overrun and to set up for the subsequent ones. If not, is there a process for the nurses to log these reduced lunch breaks such that they get time in lieu? Or does the clinic schedule need to be changed e.g. with longer appointment times?
- Consider conduct and capability for each individual: Is there undue stress due to personal or professional reasons? Do either require training in endodontic procedures, are they aware of conduct at work policies and have insight into either of their failings? Do either of them need further performance management/support from more senior staff members?

If the situation is not resolved, it may be necessary to follow the grievance or disciplinary policy by escalating to formal management and appointing an investigating officer.

Leave and absence management

Absence is an expected occurrence in the workplace and employees are legally entitled to be absent on certain grounds. Authorized leave includes annual leave, bereavement, extended caring leave, maternity, and sickness and each trust will have its own policy regarding these.

Types of leave

Annual leave

Staff are entitled to annual leave and public holidays as per Table 7.2.

Table 7.2 Authorized absence periods

Role	Annual leave
Consultants	6 weeks
Associate specialist	6 weeks
Junior doctors (2016 contract): on appointment	27 days
Junior doctors (2016 contract): after five years	32 days
Other NHS Employees (including nurses)	
On appointment	27 days
After five years service	29 days
After ten years service	33 days

There is some variation in these allowances:
- Consultants on the 2003 contract for England or 2004 contract for Northern Ireland are entitled to an additional two days of leave, following seven years of consultant service
- Consultants in Wales are entitled to 6 weeks and 4 days annual leave per year

As consultants and junior doctors generally do not work a 9am-5pm regular working week but instead have variable working patterns, it can be difficult to define a working week. In addition, some consultants opt to complete their programmed activities (PAs) compressed within three days. Consultants may be able to agree a local solution to ensure that annual leave is taken equitably without them being away from the trust for a disproportionately longer time period than colleagues, owing to their compressed working hours.

Annual leave for part-time staff should be calculated on a pro-rata basis. If a consultant works half of a full-time commitment then their leave annual allowance should also be halved.

Maternity leave

All pregnant employees, regardless of their length of service in the NHS or hours of work, are entitled to a period of 52 weeks maternity leave. This comprises:

- 26 weeks of ordinary maternity leave (OML)
- 26 weeks of additional maternity leave

The level of pay during this time is dependent on:
- The length of employment with their current employer
- The length of employment with the NHS
- Whether they intend to return to the NHS
- Following maternity leave, flexible working arrangements can be requested

Paternity leave

A father-to-be or the pregnant employee's partner (including same sex partner) has the right to paternity leave and pay of 2 weeks to be taken within 8 weeks of the baby's birth.

Shared parental leave

Shared parental leave and pay allow eligible parents to share responsibility for a child in the first year of having a baby or adopting a child. Up to 50 weeks of leave and up to 37 weeks of pay can be shared.

Adoption and surrogacy

Adoption and surrogacy leave last for up to 52 weeks, as per maternity leave. A parental order or adoption order must be applied for within 6 months of the child's birth, for surrogacy rights, leave, and pay.

Parental leave

Parental leave is unpaid leave taken to look after a child's welfare, for example spending more time with children, helping children settle into a new school or childcare arrangements, etc. A parent is entitled to 18 weeks leave for each child and adopted child, up to the eighteenth birthday. A maximum of 4 weeks for each child in one year may be taken, and only as whole weeks, rather than days.

During maternity, paternity, shared parental, adoption, and surrogacy leave, employment rights are protected. This includes the right to:
- Pay rises
- Build up (accrue) holiday
- Return to work

Bereavement or compassionate leave

By law, there is a statutory entitlement to take time off on compassionate grounds (section 57 Employment Rights Act 1996) if a 'dependant' dies or their child is stillborn or dies under the age of 18 years. There is no statutory entitlement to be paid. The amount of time off is a 'reasonable' duration, specific to each situation. This is a 'day one' employment right; the employee does not have to be working at the company for a certain length of time first. ACAS have useful guidelines to detail the management of bereavement in the workplace.

Study leave

For all consultants, there is an entitlement to 30 days study and professional leave with pay and expenses within each 3-year period. This may be interpreted as 10 days per year by some trusts.
Study leave covers:
- Study (linked to a course or programme)
- Research

- Teaching
- Sitting examinations
- Attending professional conferences for educational benefit
- Rostered training events

Trainee dentists and doctors

Health Education England (HEE) oversees study leave and budgets and, from April 2018 implemented a new approach for study budgets (see page 347). This was in response to the Enhancing Junior Doctors' Working Lives review and wider contract negotiations within England. Local offices often provide course lists to assist trainees in finding the most appropriate courses for their needs. HEE continues to encourage attendance at courses or conferences if it benefits the curriculum or professional development of the trainee. UK-wide medical and dental recruitment has ensured that job specifications do not list named courses that are required.

In Wales, Health Education and Improvement (HEIW) has a policy document outlining the study leave policy for doctors and dentists in training. This is similar in Northern Ireland and Scotland.

Professional leave

Professional leave can be used for roles outside the employing organization that are still related to the completion of professional duties, for example, roles with the Royal Colleges, faculties, GMC/GDC. It should also be provided for interviews within the NHS, public health, or academic appointments.

Illness

Employees can self-certify that they are unable to work for up to 7 days. A GP or hospital doctor certificate is required if the period extends beyond seven calendar days (statement of fitness for work). Short-term sickness is absence that lasts less than 28 calendar days.

Staff must follow the absence reporting procedure in their trust; this is generally by phoning the line manager to inform them. Failing to do so may result in an assumption of unauthorized absence and ultimately, withheld pay and disciplinary proceedings.

The manager should consider providing assistance to the employee with the focus on the stay-at-work philosophy. This may include occupational health, counselling, rapid access services (i.e. faster access for NHS staff for certain treatments, provided it does not compromise the health needs of other patients e.g. physiotherapy, dermatology, mental health services).

Long-term sick leave

After 7 days of sick leave, employees need to provide a fit note. Long-term sick leave is more than 28 calendar days. The employee should be managed with the occupational health team and HR. When a member of staff is signed off work due to a chronic condition, occupational sick pay is provided. It is a maximum of six months of full pay, followed by six months of half pay, for those with more than five years of continuous service.

If after a prolonged period, it looks unlikely that the employee will be able to return to work in a reasonable timeframe, they will be invited to a formal interview. This will be actioned only after:

- Consideration of adjustments, phased return, and redeployment
- Discussion of ill health and early retirement
- The employee has been notified about the possibility of dismissal
- Advice has been sought from HR
- Following this meeting, a decision may be made to end the employment contract on grounds of capability

Return to work

A meeting should be conducted on the employee's first day back to see if any support or reasonable adjustments to the working arrangement are required. This ensures compliance with the Equality Act 2010; discrimination is prohibited where ill health, injury, or other impairment meet the relevant criteria under the Act. Engaging HR, occupational health, and carrying out a risk assessment is necessary when considering reasonable adjustments.

Occupational health (OH) (see also Chapter 7, page 267)

If an employee is on sick leave, the employer will refer them to OH to obtain advice on their condition and any adjustments to support them in the future. If the absence is due to a work-related reason, an immediate referral is warranted. Contact during sickness should not be avoided but should be performed sensitively.

Unauthorized leave

First consider if the employee may have come to any harm; contact with family, relatives, accommodation, or ultimately the police may be warranted. If they simply have just not turned up to work, then this is an unauthorized absence for which they may be dismissed or pay suspended on grounds of misconduct. The employee should be phoned and a voicemail left advising them to contact their employer as soon as possible. A recorded letter should be posted if phone contact has been unsuccessful.

Absence triggers are a way of managing attendance. For example, certain short-term or persistent attendance records may warrant further investigation, such as:

- Unusual timings or patterns (e.g. calling in sick every Monday or Friday)
- 8 or more days absence in a year
- 3 or more episodes of absence within 6 months

Bradford factor

The Bradford factor (BF) (see Box 7.10) is a means of measuring sickness absence within an organization. It assigns a numerical value to patterns of absence within a 12 months period, with a lower number being better. The

---

Box 7.10 Calculation of the Bradford factor

The formula is $S^2 \times D = B$

S is the total number of separate sickness absences an employee has had over a 52-week period

D is the total number of days absent

B is the Bradford factor score

- B = 150; may trigger a meeting with an employee's line manager
- B = 250–499; may result in a final written warning
- B = 450; dismissal may be warranted

BF puts more weight on individual absence episodes than the length of time of the absence, with the idea that multiple short-term absences are more disruptive from an employer's perspective than one longer period. However it doesn't consider the reasons for absence—which may be legitimate—nor measures that could help employees improve their attendance and some trusts are moving away from using the Bradford factor as a trigger. Open discussion is important when managing repeated absences.

Scenario—Absence management 1

You are a consultant in a teaching hospital. You have noticed that a staff nurse has been taking a lot of sick leave over the last 3 months, often on the same day of the week. How would you manage this situation?

Relevant policies
- Sickness and absence policy
- Flexible working policy

The head nurse is the line manager of the dental nurse and should be the primary individual to manage concerns regarding their attendance. Your concerns should be raised with them in the first instance, they may already be in the process of managing the situation or may not have realized there was a pattern of behaviour.

Accurate records of attendance should be maintained by the department for all staff to enable fact-based conversation about absence trends. The head nurse would review these and where there is a concern (a pattern of behaviour or if the Bradford factor score exceeds 150) an appropriate discussion should be arranged. Routinely, this is an informal discussion (and not a formal or disciplinary process) unless there have been previous concerns or if this is a serious concern. The informal discussion is still recorded and filed within the nurse's personal file.

The informal meeting should be supportive for the nurse and establish:
- The reasons for repeated sickness and if there is anything in particular leading to the nurse being off sick that specific day of the week
- Appropriate measures should be taken, such as directing them towards health and well-being, counselling, health screening, OH, physiotherapy, exercise classes, childcare, etc.
- Consider reasonable adjustments or a change in timetable
- Inform them that absence levels are reaching a trigger point for formal management
- Make a plan for sustained improvement, monitoring, and future management processes
- If a medical issue is affecting work, OH may become involved and carry out a risk assessment
- The details of the informal meeting should be documented
- Staff can request to work flexibly, but approval is at the discretion of the line manager and is dependent on:
  - Needs of the service
  - Service delivery
  - Health and safety legislative requirements
- HR would adjust their contract if flexible working is agreed
- The trust sickness leave policy should be used as a term of reference and advice may be sought from OH and HR

- For each meeting, the employee should be given 5 days' notice and a summary of the meeting sent to them within 5 days
- Where an employee fails to attend a meeting, it should proceed without them (with a summary of the discussion sent afterward)
- A period of monitoring should be agreed and established (usually three months)
- Informal meetings should be arranged within the monitoring period
- A meeting should be arranged at the end of the monitoring period. If there has been an improvement in attendance, a further (3-month) monitoring period may be agreed to ensure a sustained improvement
- Where there is no improvement in attendance, further discussion regarding adjustments, support, or an OH referral may be made and a further monitoring period agreed
- Following two periods of review (6 months), satisfactory improvement should lead to conclusion of the process. Any further absence exceeding the Bradford factor threshold established by the trust would lead to the process resuming where it was last concluded
- Where there has been further sickness and the manager is confident that all support and adjustments possible have been made, escalation, and a formal meeting should be arranged. At formal meetings, the employee has the right to be accompanied by a trade union representative or current work colleague from the trust. This meeting should be followed up with a written outcome and may result in a first written warning. If there is continued absence, a second formal stage is commenced
- If the absence continues, the final stage of the process may be initiated, which could result in dismissal. The employee may appeal this decision

Scenario—Absence management 2

You are a consultant and your speciality trainee has just emailed to say that his wife has been diagnosed with a critical condition and he will require long-term leave for caring purposes. How do you manage this situation?

Considerations:
- Trainee in difficulty
- Need to manage department and patients
- Special leave policy
- Deanery involvement

Immediate management
- Offer your support and show empathy; direct them to NHS staff counselling services, OH, and reassure them that their clinical workload will be redistributed
- Ask the speciality trainee what support they would like
- Meet the speciality trainee and ensure confidentiality
- You and/or their clinical supervisors should review their clinical diary for the immediate week or two. It is preferable to try not to cancel patients unless absolutely necessary. Other clinicians may be willing to work additional hours or consultants may offer to see patients during their SPA sessions, as an ad-hoc occurrence
- HR and the trainee's ES should be informed

- The trainee may want to take special leave (usually 5 days allowed, but at the discretion of their line manager)
- Advise the trainee to seek advice from their GP and OH

Medium-term management
- The line manager (as a trainee, this would routinely be the educational supervisor) should liaise with the clinical lead for the department. If service provision is expected to be affected for a long duration, then the divisional director should also be informed
- Review the compassionate/bereavement leave policy for the trust. There may be an entitlement for employees to be paid during time off
- Facilitate a meeting with HR and the speciality trainee to discuss their requirements—the projected amount of leave and if any reasonable adjustments could be made (compressed hours, flexible working, part-time training). It may be necessary to consider use of annual leave or unpaid leave if his absence from work is anticipated to be medium to long term. The trainee may apply for flexible working/training
- Consider the use of locum staff to fulfil clinical requirements. Postgraduate staff or clinical fellows may have capacity to help with clinics on a medium-term basis. If a therapist or dentist with a special interest (DWSI) is available, this could help increase clinical capacity, overseen by a consultant supervisor. It is unreasonable to expect all the other speciality trainees to increase their workload on a medium to long-term basis if they do not have capacity to do so and it could lead to resentment in the department if the remaining colleagues feel unsupported

Long term
- An extension to training may be required so it is necessary to liaise with the deanery via the educational supervisor and training programme director. If training time is suspended (the training clock stops), then the prospective end of training date will be reviewed at the ARCP. The decision to suspend training needs to be done in a formal manner with written agreement from the Postgraduate Dental Dean (see Chapter 9)
- An absence of 10 days or more in any 12-month period will trigger a review of the completion date at the next review of progression

Providing support

The line manager, head of department, and educational supervisor are all available to help guide employees and trainees. In the first instance, a helpful and supportive team culture can be fostered through:

- A culture of openness and engagement; clear goals and consistent support in achieving them
- Positive encouragement, developing resilience in staff and recognition of good service
- Focus on the importance of staff health and well-being, both mental and physical
- Providing regular opportunities for feedback from staff

Numerous initiatives are in place to help support employees by fostering optimal well-being in the workplace.

NHS health and well-being framework

This national programme was set up to support the well-being of NHS staff. It is a culture change initiative, rather than being one specific programme and can be adapted to suit individual organizations. The diagnostic tool helps the organization identify improvements it could make and strategies to better support the well-being of staff (see Box 7.11).

> **Box 7.11 The seven elements of the NHS health and well-being model**
>
> - Improving personal health and well-being
> - Relationships
> - Fulfilment at work
> - Managers and leaders
> - Environment
> - Data insights
> - Professional well-being and support

Growing Occupational Health and Well-Being (OHWB) Together

Growing OHWB Together is a 5-year strategy by NHS England to help improve the health and well-being of staff. It unites occupational health and well-being boards so that they can work synergistically. Growing OHWB Together is part of 2023/2024 NHS priorities and operational planning guidance, with ICSs mandated to act in this regard, thus emphasizing the increasing focus on employee well-being.

The Health, Safety and Well-being Partnership Group (HSWPG)

The HSWPG is the occupational health and safety subgroup of the NHS Staff Council. They have published a document 'workplace health and safety standards' to help organizations comply with health and safety legislation by combining good practice with legal requirements. The group aims to raise standards of OH and safety within healthcare settings by providing practice pointers. The HSWPG also publishes other guidance documents to help reduce the incidence of work-related injuries.

Well-being guardians and champions

A well-being guardian in the organization is often a non-executive director or clinical director. Their role is to hold the senior leadership and organization to account, advocating for optimal staff well-being by providing an assurance role at board level.

Well-being champions are individuals throughout the organization at all levels who promote health and well-being and help direct colleagues towards support in these areas as needed.

Health and safety at work

Health and safety in the NHS in England is regulated by the Health and Safety Executive (HSE) together with the Care Quality Commission (CQC). They share information, coordinate activities and liaise with other organizations such as the GDC/GMC. The OH team also helps to ensure compliance with health and safety regulations.

Employee assistance programme (EAP)

The NHS provides a 24/7 confidential, freephone, or online counselling service. Each trust may use a different independent body to provide its EAP, for example, the EAP at King's College Hospital NHS Foundation Trust is currently provided by Workplace Options. The EAP provides qualified advisors, who can then direct onwards to assistance in other areas as needed (e.g. legal, financial). An employee may contact the EAP directly or their manager may refer them.

A confidential text service also exists, which is available to all staff who need to access support and talk to someone; employees can text FRONTLINE to 85258.

Local support services in trusts

Most organizations will have a range of supportive measures to help their employees with both in-person and online assistance available (see Box 7.12)

Box 7.12 Supportive measures to improve health and well-being for employees

- Mental health support: mental health and well-being hubs, well-being apps, self-check tools, coaching services, counselling
- Physical health: organized walks and hospital exercise groups, digital weight management programme
- Support for specific groups of employees: armed forces, executive leaders, social care workers, workers affected by Long COVID, menopause, etc.
- Specific tailored support: financial well-being, staff accommodation, substance misuse, gambling, etc.

Practitioner Performance Advice

Practitioner Performance Advice (formerly the National Clinical Assessment Service, NCAS) was established in 2001 and is delivered by NHS Resolution. It aims to provide expertise and impartial advice to the NHS on resolving concerns regarding practitioners. PPA provides advice, assessment and intervention, training courses, and other expert services. Practitioners can contact them directly for general advice if they are concerned about some aspect of their clinical performance or health. They also provide information about other avenues of support that may be available.

Occupational health

The role of OH is to determine and maximize the health and fitness of individuals to perform operational roles. In this capacity, along with GPs or hospital therapeutic staff, they aim to coordinate the rehabilitation processes and enhance an individual's potential. Occupational health (OH) services help ensure that staff are fit for the work they do and that the work doesn't impact negatively on their health. This reduces sickness absence and improves staff retention. It is recognized that OH can provide the most support when it works collaboratively with other teams such as health and safety, HR, infection control, and line managers.

OH can provide advice and help manage:
- Pre-employment health assessments
- Sickness absence
- Return to work processes following absence
- Helping reduce and manage injuries sustained at work—slips, heavy lifting, falls, etc.
- Exposure to hazards—from contact dermatitis to repetitive strain
- Preventing infection in the workplace
- Employee assistance programmes (EAPs)
- Advising on employee capability concerns
- Advice on staff unable to work due to health problems
- Promotion of health and lifestyle, well-being services
- Rapid access for staff to specialist medical advice

Planning of referrals is essential early in the illness/injury period to ensure continued contact, consistency of treatment, and rehabilitation as well as constructing a feasible return to work plan. It is generally more effective to bring individuals back as soon as possible even if that means limited hours, to effectively reduce the total period of absence and isolation from colleagues. A phased return is not the panacea to recovery but it can reduce the barriers to making the transition back to employment as well as not overtaxing the member of staff.

The line manager should inform the employee of the reasons for the referral to OH and provide them with a copy of the referral letter. They should be reassured that OH is a supportive service rather than investigatory.

NHS Employers has provided guidance to support the implementation of OH services in the NHS, reinforcing the increasing role that OH plays in a happy, healthy workforce. Guidance is available to support commissioning teams and HR teams.

Areas of occupational concern within the dental profession

Dentists are exposed to blood borne viruses, dermatitis (often connected to allergies to glove material or frequent hand washing), musculoskeletal complaints (frequently related to the ergonomics of the operational role) and psychological pressures. Physical exposure to noise, radiation, and curing light requires careful evaluation and planned exposure reduction. Some OH departments will have in-house or direct access to professional counsellors and physiotherapists.

Exposure hazards are dealt with under the Control of Substances Hazardous to Health Regulations 2002 (COSHH), which covers both chemical and biological substance exposure. In addition to examining material data sheets, documented thorough risk assessments are mandatory. Careful consideration is required for those with a role within operating theatres with regard to anaesthetic gases and adhesives. Dental methyl methacrylate can compromise the protective nature of some gloves.

Although not specifically mentioned, OH provision is supported by the overarching legislation of the Health and Safety at Work Act 1974. In many trusts, more recently requests have escalated to OH for assistance in promoting the disciplines in the Management of Health and Safety at Work Regulations 1999 and the Equality Act (EA) 2010.

Stress at work

Stress is a physiological and psychological response to a perceived threat or challenge, leading to the release of stress hormones like cortisol and adrenaline. Not all stress is bad, and a little stress can be exhilarating and act as a driver to achievement. The Hungarian endocrinologist Hans Selye distinguished between positive and negative stress—eustress and distress. Distress can harm well-being; thus recognizing and managing it is important to maintain well-being and professional effectiveness. More than half (54.9%) of dentists have reported high job stress (British Dental Journal 2019).

Causes of stress in dentistry

Various causes of stress have been identified (see Figure 7.7). Cross and Dillon (2023) highlight the difference between stress, which is 'big, visible, and obvious' and microstress that is small, often invisible but 'pernicious because it is part of our everyday lives at a greater volume, intensity and pace than we have ever experienced before… increasing with technology and ubiquitous connectivity'. Microstress is a real threat in clinical practice because there are many moments of tension during a working day—they arise each time we carry out a clinical procedure for a patient. Perfectionism has been shown to be associated with greater anxiety and depression levels.

Consequences of unmanaged/chronic stress

- Physical health issues e.g. cardiovascular problems, heart disease
- Weakened immune system
- Digestive problems e.g. ulcers
- Anxiety and depression
- Insomnia and burnout
- Cognitive impairment
- Job dissatisfaction
- Reduced productivity
- Interpersonal relationship conflict and tension

Stress and burnout can lead to mental health issues and suicidal thoughts. One study in the UK (Collin 2019), found that 17.6% of respondents had seriously thought about committing suicide in the past. Dentists experience higher levels of suicidal thoughts than the general population. Methods to cope with stress are suggested in Box 7.13.

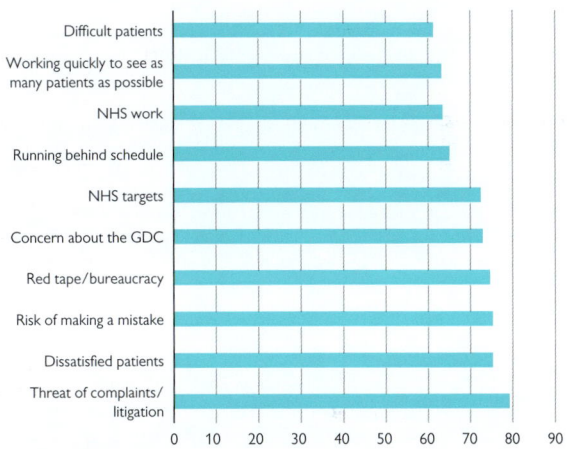

Figure 7.7 The most common stressors in UK dentistry. Data from Collin, V., Toon, M., O'Selmo, E. *et al.* A survey of stress, burnout and well-being in UK dentists. *Br Dent J* 226, 40–9 (2019).

Box 7.13 Stress management techniques

- Deep slow breathing
- Regular exercise to trigger endorphin release
- Progressive muscle relaxation (PMR)—tense and relax different muscle groups to release physical tension
- Balanced diet, adequate sleep, minimal alcohol, and caffeine
- Cognitive behavioural techniques (CBT) to reframe negative thoughts
- Meditation and yoga
- Prioritize tasks, set realistic goals, break larger tasks into smaller manageable steps to reduce feelings of being overwhelmed
- Share concerns with family, friends, colleagues to build a supportive network for emotional and practical assistance

Further reading

BDJ (2019) More than half of dentists say stress is affecting their practice. *Br Dent J*, 226:7.

Collin V, Toon M, O'Selmo E, *et al.* (2019). A survey of stress, burnout and well-being in UK dentists. *Br Dent J* 226:40–9.

Harvard Business Review (2023). The hidden toll of microstress. Available at: ℘ https://hbr.org/2023/02/the-hidden-toll-of-microstress

Fraud and bribery

Fraud, corruption, and bribery within the NHS are unacceptable and divert valuable resources away from patient care. NHS trusts should have robust controls, policies, and procedures in place to prevent and address this.

Terms of reference

While the principles are the same, there may be variations between NHS trusts on the exact process and values required for the declaration of interests and gifts. The following should be used as terms of reference for clinicians:

- The trust's 'Declarations of Interest and Gifts and Hospitality Policy'
- The trust's 'Fraud, bribery, and corruption policies'
- The NHS trust should follow:
  - Ministry of Justice
  - The Fraud Act, 2006
  - Guidance published by The NHS Counter Fraud Authority (NHS CFA)
  - The Bribery Act 2010

Definitions

Fraud is 'deception carried out for personal gain, usually for money. It can also involve the abuse of a position of trust'.

Bribery is the 'offering, giving, soliciting, or acceptance of an inducement or reward, which may influence a person to act against the interest of the organization'. Bribery does not have to involve cash or an actual payment exchanging hands and can take many forms such as a gift, lavish treatment during a business trip or tickets to an event.

Conflict of interest is 'a set of circumstances by which a reasonable person would consider that an individual's ability to apply judgement or act, in the context of delivering, commissioning, or assuring taxpayer funded health and care services is, or could be, impaired or influenced by another interest they hold'. These may lead an individual to benefit from the consequences of a decision they are involved in making.

A conflict of interest may be:

- Actual—there is a material conflict between one or more interests
- Potential—there is the possibility of a conflict arising in the future

Interests may be classified as:

- Financial interests
- Non-financial professional interests—e.g. increased professional reputation
- Non-financial personal interests
- Indirect interests—if an individual has a close association with someone who has a conflict of interest and could stand to benefit

Fraud

The NHS Counter Fraud Authority estimates the NHS is vulnerable to £1.264 billion of fraud each year. The Fraud Act 2006 gives a statutory definition of the criminal offence of fraud, defining it in three classes:

- Fraud by false representation
- Fraud by failing to disclose information
- Fraud by abuse of position

These offences occur when the act or omission is committed dishonestly and with intent to cause a gain or loss. The gain or loss does not have to succeed, so long as the intent is there

Local counter fraud specialist (LCFS)

- The LCFS embeds an anti-fraud culture to prevent and detect fraud, bribery, and corruption within the trust with preventative activity
- Decides whether internal/external referrals or matters raised through the whistleblowing process need to be investigated
- Investigates cases
- Assists with the recovery of funds fraudulently obtained where required
- Reports any case to the police where necessary, in consultation with the chief finance officer, the chief executive, and the NHS Counter Fraud Authority (NHS CFA)

Staff responsibilities

It is the responsibility of all staff to protect the assets of the trust and NHS. All staff should:

- Complete mandatory training
- Be aware of the provisions of the trust's countering fraud, bribery, and corruption policy
- Report any suspicions to the LCFS as soon as possible
- Unlike other concerns, fraud concerns should not be mentioned to anyone else or senior clinicians. Instead the LCFS should be notified as soon as possible, this is to prevent the individual from being alerted and giving them the opportunity to destroy any evidence (see Table 7.3)

NHS Counter Fraud Authority

The NHS Counter Fraud Authority is the special health authority charged with identifying, investigating, and preventing fraud and other economic crime within the NHS and the wider health group.

Types of fraud within the NHS

There are over 120 identified types of fraud in the NHS, the following are some examples:

Payroll fraud

- Working elsewhere while off sick
- Expenses or allowance fraud—false or inflated travel, expense claims
- Overtime or unsocial hours claims
- Timesheet fraud—claiming for hours that have not been worked

Employee/Identity fraud

- False identity/qualifications/professional registration
- Not having a legitimate right to work

Procurement and commissioning

- Accepting inducements from suppliers
- Ordering goods and services for personal use
- Collusion with suppliers to falsify deliveries
- False, intentionally inflated or duplicate invoices
- Payment diversion—organizations claiming to be an organization they are not

Overseas patient fraud
- People who are not resident in the UK and ineligible for NHS treatment

Help with health costs
- Purporting to be exempt from paying for prescription charges, dental treatment, or optical services

Contract, national tariff, and performance data manipulation
- Fraud in relation to national tariff and performance data, manipulation of data, and the payment by result (PbR) system
- Dental contractor fraud—submission of fraudulent claims to the NHS for a range of services provided to patients

NHS pension fraud
- Falsifying their circumstances or failing to notify the pension administration of a significant change in their circumstances

Fraud against NHS Resolution
- Fraudulent accident/insurance claims under the Liability to Third Parties Scheme (LTPS) or through clinical negligence

NHS bursary fraud
- False applications or the use of false documents to support a bursary application, other NHS funded training or financial support stream

What do you do if you suspect fraud?

Table 7.3 What you do if fraud or corruption are suspected

Do	Do not
Make an immediate note of your concerns	Do nothing
Report your suspicions confidentially to the LCFS or someone with the appropriate authority and experience	Be afraid to raise your concerns
Deal with the matter promptly if you feel your concerns are warranted	Approach or accuse individuals directly
Report to 24 hours NHS Fraud and Corruption reporting line on 0800 028 40 60 if you feel it cannot be done internally	Try to investigate the matter yourself
Alternatively, it is also possible to report fraud anonymously via the website ℘ https://cfa.nhs.uk/reportfraud	Convey your suspicions to anyone other than those with the proper authority

Sanctions
The LCFS will investigate any allegations of fraud and may impose one or more of the following sanctions against individuals:
- Criminal—the LCFS will work in partnership with the NHS CFA, the police, and/or the Crown Prosecution Service to bring a case to court against an alleged offender. The outcomes can range from a criminal conviction to fines and imprisonment

- Civil—Civil sanctions can be taken against those who commit fraud, bribery and corruption to recover money and/or assets which have been fraudulently obtained, including interest and costs
- Disciplinary—Disciplinary procedures through HR will be initiated where an employee is suspected of being involved in a fraudulent or illegal act. This may occur concurrently with civil or criminal court
- Professional body disciplinary—where appropriate, staff may be reported to their professional body as a result of a successful investigation or prosecution

Bribery

The Bribery Act 2010 makes it an offence to give, promise, or offer a bribe, and to request, agree to receive or accept a bribe. It is a corporate offence to fail to prevent bribery by an organization.

Examples of offences under the Bribery Act, include:

- The non-disclosure of personal interests with suppliers leading to the award of contracts to friends or relatives
- Staff receiving gifts and hospitality from suppliers or contractors in exchange for awarding contracts or orders for the supply of goods
- The acceptance of late tenders or where tender records are falsified or manipulated by trust staff in exchange for money or gifts

Declarations of interest and gifts and hospitality policy

All staff members with private or personal interests which might affect their role within the trust must declare:

- Any conflicts of interest when joining the organization
- Whenever the potential for conflict arises
- On an annual basis for decision making staff

This includes declarations such as private practice work, shareholdings, patents, loyalty interests, sponsorship from organizations. If an interest is declared but there is no risk of a conflict arising then no action is warranted.

Gifts

The trust maintains a policy and register of gifts, hospitality, and sponsorship. Staff should not accept gifts that may affect their professional judgement. Gifts from suppliers or contractors should be declined. An exception is made for low-cost branded promotional aids such as pens. All interests that might unduly influence an individual's judgement and objectivity should be declared. Modest gifts from patients do not need to be declared.

Staff responsibilities and principles

- Ensure that contracts are awarded solely on merit, taking into account the requirements of the trust
- No favouritism is shown to any company over its competitors
- Declare and record financial or personal interests in any organization with which they have to deal
- Be prepared to withdraw from those dealings if required, to ensure professional judgement is not influenced
- Refuse gifts, benefits, hospitality or sponsorship of any kind which might reasonably be seen to compromise personal judgement or integrity, or constitute an incentive or bribe

- Declare and register gifts, benefits, or sponsorship of any kind, within 28 days of receipt, (provided that they are worth more than £50), whether refused or accepted
- Ensure that donations of medical or IT equipment are subject to the appropriate approval by the biomedical engineering department or the ICT department and the procurement department

Nolan principles

These are a set of key guiding principles set out by the Committee on Standards of Public Life, set up by the government in 1994.

- Selflessness: Holders of public office should act solely in terms of the public interest. They should not do so in order to gain financial or other benefits for themselves, their family, or their friends
- Integrity: Holders of public office should not place themselves under any financial or other obligation to outside individuals or organizations that might seek to influence them in the performance of their official duties
- Objectivity: In carrying out public business, including making public appointments, awarding contracts, or recommending individuals for rewards and benefits, holders of public office should make choices on merit
- Accountability: Holders of public office are accountable for their decisions and actions to the public and must submit themselves to whatever scrutiny is appropriate to their office
- Openness: Holders of public office should be as open as possible about all the decisions and actions that they take. They should give reasons for their decisions and restrict information only when the wider public interest clearly demands
- Honesty: Holders of public office have a duty to declare any private interests relating to their public duties and to take steps to resolve any conflicts arising in a way that protects the public interest
- Leadership: Holders of public office should promote and support these principles by leadership and example

Whistleblowing

There is no universally accepted definition of a whistleblower but in general the term refers to:

1. The presence of work-related issues
2. An element of altruism or public concern
3. An ongoing risk to public well-being (illegal, immoral, illicit, unsafe, or fraudulent)
4. The reporting (disclosure) of these concerns to higher authorities; the 'protected disclosure'.

Historical cases

- Hospital medical care has historically experienced more whistleblowing cases than the dental field
- The first properly documented episode of NHS whistleblowing occurred in 1967 when psychotherapist Barbara Robb published her book 'Sans Everything. A case to answer'. This exposed the poor treatment of long-stay NHS psychiatric patients, triggering an NHS inquiry which was subsequently criticized for downplaying any issues and aiming to discredit the whistleblower
- The Bristol heart scandal was exposed by anaesthetist Steve Bolsin. It is estimated that 170 children died in the Bristol unit between 1986–1995, who would have survived in other NHS hospitals. Initially Bolsin was ignored but later the government report concluded that *'Bristol was a turning point in the history of the NHS. We are determined that some good can come from the tragedy that took place there'* (Kennedy, 2001)
- Over the next two decades however, other notable scandals occurred: Mid-Staffordshire, Morecambe Bay, Gosport, Shrewsbury and Telford and, more recently, the Lucy Letby scandal

The whistleblower

Whistleblowers can come from any culture or background with no defining characteristic that definitively marks out a potential whistleblower. However, Box 7.14 indicates some features that have been noted in whistleblowers. Most healthcare workplace issues should be dealt with internally or via regulators and should not become public knowledge. It is likely that many

---

Box 7.14 Features noted in whistleblowers (Travers, 2019)

- Slightly more likely to be male
- Have higher levels of education, higher salaries, and more tenure within the organization
- Typically more extrovert
- Score below average on the personality dimension of agreeableness and are more likely to have a domineering personality
- More likely to call out abrupt, unethical behaviour than unethical behaviour that increases gradually
- Usually take the side of fairness. (Whistleblowing represents a trade-off between the competing moral values of fairness and loyalty)
- Reflect the values of more individualistic cultures (Europe/USA) than collectivistic cultures (China, Japan, etc.)

scandals pass unreported, due to a reluctance to challenge poor behaviour (thereby risking unpopularity or retaliation) and the whistleblower may even be silenced (a gag or COT3 settlement). Whistleblowers may jeopardize their careers by speaking out, yet may equally be sanctioned and removed from their register for risking patient safety by not doing so.

The whistleblowing process

All hospitals will have their own whistleblowing policy, which should be consulted.

It is useful to have informal discussions with close colleagues. If the whistleblowing concerns are serious, there is safety in numbers and colleagues may have identified overlapping concerns. If no colleagues can be confided in or trusted, then discuss with a dental indemnity provider. Charities such as Protect UK and Whistleblowers UK can offer informal advice. A senior dental consultant in the department or service manager can be approached, if considered impartial and uninvolved. Otherwise approach the 'prescribed person'; in hospital practice this is the Freedom to Speak Up Guardian. The CQC and GDC (see Box 7.15) can also be approached. However, it is worth noting that such individuals, bodies and regulators have no power to intervene in the event of subsequent retaliation or detriment imposed by the employer. Nevertheless, if the employee is involved in litigation in the future, the fact that they declared their concerns to the correct prescribed person or regulator may act in their favour.

Legal protection

Employees have legal protection under the Employment Rights Act (ERA) 1996 and the Public Interest Disclosure Act (PIDA) 1998. This, in theory, provides full protection against being treated detrimentally by employers for raising a concern and protection against unfair dismissal if they report concerns pertaining to:

- A criminal offence or corporate lawbreaking
- A risk to someone's health and safety
- A risk or actual damage to the environment
- A miscarriage of justice
- The covering up of wrongdoing

What steps should the whistleblower take?

- Clearly identify the safeguarding issue. What is occurring and how do you know?
- Document the facts. Records should be meticulous and kept in a secure diary or notepad (time, date, place, etc.), separate from employer-accessible accounts. Protected disclosures to senior colleagues, managers, or a prescribed person should be noted as well
- Decide who needs to know
- Make a decision about confidentiality
- Make the call or submit your disclosure. Formally declare yourself as a whistleblower from early on in the process
- In the event of potentially hostile meetings, always take a trusted colleague as witness
- In the event of any 'pushback', make sure that a prescribed person or regulator is aware of your concerns early in the process, in order to establish your bona fides and formalize your protection under PIDA

Box 7.15 A summary of GDC guidance on whistleblowing

The GDC has expected standards of professional behaviour in the context of whistleblowing.

- You must raise any concern that patients might be at risk due to:
  1. A colleague's health, behaviour, or professional performance
  2. Any aspect of the treatment environment
  3. Someone asking you to do something that conflicts with your duty to put patients first and act to protect them
- Your duty to raise concerns overrides any personal or professional loyalties or concerns you may have
- You must act on concerns promptly. If in doubt, raise a concern
- You should not have to prove your concern for it to be investigated. If you fail to whistleblow by not raising a concern, your own registration could be at risk
- Where possible, you should raise concerns first with your employer or manager. If not appropriate or concerns are not acted on, then raise them with your local commissioner of health or CQC, Health Inspectorate of Wales, RQIA in Northern Ireland or Healthcare Improvement Scotland
- If the public/patients need to be protected from a GDC registered dental professional, then the issue must be raised to the GDC
- If a team member has raised a concern, the employer must:
  - Take the concern seriously
  - Maintain confidentiality, when appropriate
  - Investigate promptly
  - Make an unbiased assessment of the concern
  - Keep the staff member advised of progress, action taken, or reason for inaction
  - Monitor action taken to resolve the issue

Common challenges in whistleblowing

- It can induce conflict and retaliation within the department. Revenge whistleblowing and malicious reporting can occur
- Cognitive dissonance may occur within the whistleblower—if there is an internal clash between beliefs and actions this can induce psychological discomfort leading to an alteration in one or more of the whistleblower's attitudes, beliefs, or behaviours to reduce the discomfort and restore balance
- 'Normalization' of risk-taking can also be an issue. Most people will have little difficulty in registering and resisting dangerous behaviour when this happens suddenly. However, when the changes are slow and subtle, drawn out over a number of years, then 'normalization of deviance' and the acceptance of behaviour that is actually dangerous can become the new norm
- Whistleblowers can raise concerns anonymously, however it may be relatively easy to uncover their identity, especially in small departments. In addition, the GDC Fitness to Practise team will ask for consent to disclose identity as the informant for the majority of investigation cases

Outcomes following whistleblowing

Unfortunately and all too frequently, the whistleblower (perceived as a reputational risk to others in the organization), either loses their job or is 'managed' out of their position. This can take a number of forms. Sometimes, the whistleblower is simply dismissed, labelled as argumentative, disruptive and a 'non-team player'. Some Other Substantial Reason (SOSR), which falls outside the regular categories of fair dismissal is also frequently used.

Sometimes, the whistleblower is simply 'managed' out of their job. In essence, this simply means making life so impossible that the whistleblower resigns. Common tactics are pay cuts, demotions, hostile changes in terms and conditions, unjustified disciplinary action, and the removal of the whistleblower from their team and regular place of work, with isolation of the whistleblower in solitary and ill-equipped offices. Whistleblowers are frequently referred for psychiatric or psychological assessment, with all the stigma that is attached to such referrals. Whistleblowers are frequently referred vexatiously to their regulatory body and it is not unheard of for evidence against them to unexpectedly appear in the records, long after they have been forced out. Dental professional bodies have noted the increasing trend of 'blue-on-blue' referrals to the GDC by registrants who retaliate against fellow registrants for their own self-serving motives, such as attacking whistleblowers.

Support for the whistleblower

Unfortunately, whistleblowing can be an unpleasant and unsettling experience. It may also be a very emotional and character-testing process, where the whistleblower has to repeatedly defend their moral and ethical beliefs. In the first instance they should report this to the Freedom to Speak Up (FTSU) guardian. In the absence of support, report to the British Dental Association or Protect.uk (a whistleblowing charity) for free legal advice.

What are the options if the whistleblower loses their job as a result?
- Move on and seek employment elsewhere (although this can be difficult if they become known to be a whistleblower)
- Mediation through ACAS
- Career change
- Litigation

Litigation and employment tribunals

Litigation (brought through the PIDA 1998) while appearing superficially attractive, should be approached as a last resort. It is widely accepted that the large majority of employment tribunal cases for whistleblowing fail. A recent report suggests that of all those cases that go to a preliminary hearing, only 12% succeed (AAPG 2020). Some cases will have dropped out long before reaching this stage while others may have been settled out of court.

PIDA was introduced in 1998 but has recognized limitations:
- PIDA looks at violations of employment law, not risks to the public
- It offers only a small chance of redress once the detriment/dismissal has already occurred. It is therefore reactive rather than proactive
- For full compensation to be offered, the claimant (whistleblower) has to evidentially link the whistleblowing act with their subsequent dismissal or detriment. This can be difficult as the employer (the respondent) may claim some other reason for the detriment/dismissal

The future for whistleblowing

Better protections are needed for moral, diligent and committed staff who feel compelled to speak up and pressure is growing for a fundamental shift in the whistleblowing culture.

- NHS organizations need to appreciate the ability of frontline staff, including dental staff, to detect risk-taking and deviance from normal practice long before it becomes a scandal
- There is an increasing public sense that whistleblowers should be celebrated and congratulated, not demeaned and dismissed
- Regulators impose a duty of candour and safeguarding on front line staff and therefore also need to ensure whistleblowers' careers are protected, especially against potential malicious counter-reporting
- Review of the legal forum to ensure employers cannot discredit whistleblowers, close down safeguarding issues, and then escape responsibility; a more safety-orientated system of justice is needed

Further reading

All Party Parliamentary Group Whistleblowing. Making whistleblowing work for society. Available at: ℘ https://a02f9c2f-03a1-4206-859b-06ff2b21dd81.filesusr.com/ugd/88d04c_56b3ca80a07e4f5e8ace79e0488a24ef.pdf

Employment Rights Act (ERA) 1996. Available at: ℘ https://www.legislation.gov.uk/ukpga/1996/18/contents

GDC Standards. Available at: ℘ https://standards.gdc-uk.org/pages/principle8/principle8.aspx

Hilton C (2016). Whistle-blowing in the National Health Service since the 1960s. Available at: ℘ https://www.historyandpolicy.org/policy-papers/papers/whistle-blowing-in-the-national-health-service-since-the-1960s

Kennedy I (2001). *The report of the public inquiry into children's heart surgery at the Bristol Royal Infirmary 1984–1995. Learning from Bristol (Cm 5207 (II)).* London: HMSO.

Public Interest Disclosure Act (PIDA) 1998. Available at: ℘ https://www.legislation.gov.uk/ukpga/1998/23/contents

Robb B (1967). *Sans Everything: A Case to Answer.* London: Nelson.

Travers M (2019). What science tells us about the psychology of whistleblowers. Available at: ℘ https://www.forbes.com/sites/traversmark/2019/09/26/inside-the-mind-of-a-whistleblower/

Sellars S (2021). Speak up!. *Br Dent J,* 231:429.

General Dental Council

The GDC is the regulatory body in the UK for dentists and dental care professionals (DCPs). Its role is outlined in statute in the Dentists Act 1984. The main objectives of the GDC are:
- Protect, promote, and maintain the health, safety, and well-being of the public
- Promote and maintain public confidence in the dental professions
- Promote and maintain proper professional standards and conduct for members of the dental professions
- Promote high standards of education in all aspects of dentistry
- The GDC maintains a register of qualified dental professionals and investigates concerns about treatment or professional conduct

The GDC has different committees to fulfil these roles (see Box 7.16 and 7.18).

> **Box 7.16 GDC committees**
> - Professional Conduct Committee
> - Health Committee
> - Investigating Committee
> - Professional Performance Committee
> - Interim Orders Committee
> - Registration Appeals Committee

GDC standards and scope of practice

All dental registrants must practise in accordance with the GDC's published 'Standards for the Dental Team':
- Put patients' interests first
- Communicate effectively with patients
- Obtain valid consent
- Maintain and protect patients' information
- Have a clear and effective complaints procedure
- Work with colleagues in a way that is in patients' best interests
- Maintain, develop, and work within your professional knowledge and skills
- Raise a concern if patients are at risk
- Make sure your personal behaviour maintains patients' confidence in you and the dental profession

The GDC maintains a register for each of the seven dental care professionals in the UK: dentists, dental nurses, dental hygienists, dental therapists, orthodontic therapists, dental technicians, and clinical dental technicians. They publish a 'Scope of Practice' for each of these groups, outlining the practice skills for each group, which additional skills can be developed with training and those procedures which can be carried out under prescription.

Fitness to practise

Fitness to practise implies that the professional has the appropriate knowledge, skills, character, and health to carry out their dental profession to the standard expected. Concerns in this regard may be raised by a patient, member of the public, another organizational body (e.g. police) or a colleague. Fitness to practice concerns may also be raised if public confidence in the dental profession could be detrimentally affected, for example, a dental professional involved in criminal activity unrelated to dentistry.

The GDC will investigate if patients could be at risk or public confidence in dentistry could be damaged (see Box 7.17).

Box 7.17 Concerns that the GDC will investigate

- Serious or repeated mistakes in clinical care
- Failure to examine a patient properly, to secure informed consent before treatment, keep satisfactory records, respond reasonably to a patient's needs
- A practitioner working without professional indemnity insurance
- Cross infection issues
- Serious breaches of a patient's confidentiality
- Indications of a criminal offence including fraud, theft
- Poor health or a medical condition that could significantly affect a dental professional's ability to treat patients safely

---

There are a range of possible outcomes of a fitness to practise investigation:
- No action
- Issue a reprimand
- Place conditions on registration
- Suspend registration
- Remove an individual from the register

Illegal practice

The GDC will bring criminal prosecutions if it has evidence that individuals who are not registered are carrying out dental offences; practising dentistry, operating the business of dentistry or using protected titles.
- Section 38 of the Dentists Act indicates that it is a criminal offence for a person who is not registered as a dentist or a dental care professional to practise dentistry, hold themselves out as practising or as being prepared to practise dentistry
- Under sections 41 or 43 of the Dentists Act, the majority of the directors of a company carrying out the business of dentistry must be registered with the GDC
- Section 39 of the Dentists Act makes it an offence to use any of the dental professional titles, unless registered with the GDC

The GDC will instruct investigators to gather evidence. Their lawyers will assess if:
A. There is sufficient evidence for there to be a conviction
B. It is in the public interest to pursue the matter to prosecution

The lawyers may decide to take the case to the magistrates' court. A fine may be imposed if the case is successful.

Complaints to the GDC

Complaints to the GDC follow a four-stage process (see Figure 7.8). At each stage in the process, the parties involved are informed in writing about the progress of the case and decisions made.

Stage 1—Initial assessment team
The initial assessment team will assess the concern(s) to ascertain if the GDC is the most appropriate organization to deal with the concern.

Stage 2—Case worker
A case worker investigates the concern. The registrant is notified and relevant information is collected. This may include:
- In clinical cases, reviewing patient records and clinical advice
- In health cases, obtaining medical/psychological reports
- In criminal cases, obtaining certificates of conviction/police reports

A decision is made on whether the case necessitates referral onto stage 3, with summary allegations, for more detailed consideration by the case examiners. This decision is made within four months from the date that the concern is received.

Stage 3—Case examiners
The case examiners will consider the allegation and any comments from the dental professional and the person who raised the concern. They will decide whether to refer the allegation to a practice committee for a full inquiry. At this stage, all involved parties receive the paperwork pertaining to the case. Each case is considered by a pair of case examiners (one lay person and one dentist/dental care professional).
If the case examiners decide not to refer the registrant to the practice committee, the following outcomes may result:
- No further action
- A letter of advice or warning is sent to the registrant
- Agree a set of undertakings with the registrant

Stage 4
This stage involves a full public inquiry before a practice committee, which may be either of:
- Professional conduct committee (Box 7.18)
- Professional performance committee
- Health committee

These are the committees that investigate the allegations and conduct fact-finding; neither the investigating committing nor interim orders committees do this. A hearing will take place with full representation and presentation of the evidence. Expert reports will be used and a final decision made. The hearing may be held in private in the interest of parties, or to protect the registrant's private life, or if holding it in public would prejudice the interests of justice. The committee chair is an experienced panel member who ensures a fair hearing and helps to reach an outcome.

Box 7.18 GDC committees

Investigating committee (IC)

The IC considers allegations where a registrant's ability to practise may be affected and they decide if the allegations should be referred to a practice committee for a full inquiry. They can also decide to close an allegation or issue a warning. The IC considers cases that they may have previously adjourned or cases where the case examiners have failed to reach a decision. The IC meets in private and the committee is comprised of one registered dentist, one lay member, and a dental care professional if the case relates to one.

Interim orders committee (IOC)

The IOC considers if it is necessary to make an order impacting the clinician's registration, pending the outcome from a full hearing. This is in order to protect the public or in the interest of the individual concerned.

A case may be referred to the IOC at any stage and they may:
- Impose a suspension (up to 18 months, with six monthly reviews)
- Impose conditions (up to 18 months, with six monthly reviews)
- Decide that no order is necessary

Outcomes following a practice committee's consideration

1. No action needed. Registrant's fitness to practice is not impaired and the case is closed
2. Issue a reprimand
3. Impose conditions for up to 36 months
4. Suspend the registrant for up to 12 months
5. Erase the registrant from the register
6. Refer the case back to the case examiners, investigating committee, IOC, or any other practice committees

The GDC has come under some criticism due to the manner in which complaints were handled when requiring a practice committee hearing; in particular, the lengthy time period from when the complaint was raised to the final decision, which in many cases, resulted in 'no action needed'. This was causing protracted stress and anxiety for the dental registrants in question while they awaited an outcome. A favourable change was introduced in 2016 through the Section 60 Order which facilitated the introduction of case examiners, who could investigate complaints with increased transparency, without the need for a practice committee hearing.

Dental complaints service

The Dental Complaints Service (DCS) is a free and impartial service that helps resolve complaints in private dental practices. They will assist with complaints that are raised within 12 months of treatment or 12 months from becoming aware of an issue with the treatment. They will not assist with any complaints about NHS treatment.

If the DCS is unable to reach a local resolution, the issue is put before a panel, as the final stage. The panel always includes a dental professional, ensuring that professional expertise is considered in the final decision.

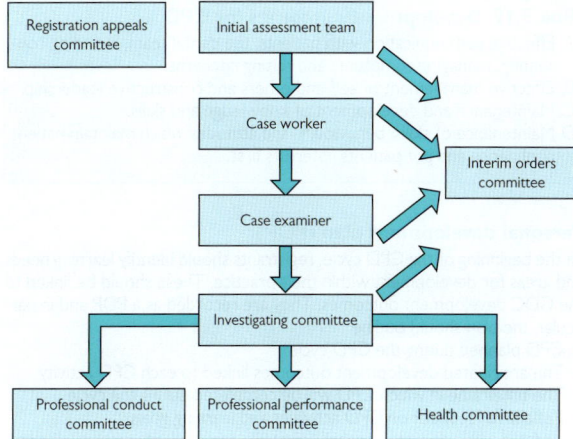

Figure 7.8 Stages of GDC complaint handling.

Dental continuing professional development (CPD)

CPD is a professional learning activity (lectures, courses, seminars, individual study) that is expected to advance dental professional development and is relevant to practise. It is compulsory for GDC registration.

Enhanced CPD scheme

In order to be compliant, registrants must:
- Complete the CPD hours for each 5-year cycle (see Table 7.4)
- Spread CPD hours evenly across the five-year cycle, completing a minimum of 10 hours every two-year period
- Make an annual CPD statement when renewing GDC registration
- Ensure that CPD is relevant to their field of practice
- Record CPD accurately, keep certificates, and link CPD to a development outcome (see Box 7.19)

Table 7.4. Minimum required hours of verifiable CPD

Dentist	100	Orthodontic therapist	75
Dental therapist	75	Dental technician	75
Dental hygienist	75	Dental Nurse	50
Temporary registrants (dentists)	20		

> **Box 7.19 Development outcomes for CPD**
> A. Effective communication with patients, the dental team, including con-senting, managing complaints and raising concerns.
> B. Effective management of self and others and constructive leadership.
> C. Maintenance and development of knowledge and skills.
> D. Maintenance of skills, behaviours, and attitudes which maintain patient confidence and put patients' interests first.

Personal development plan (PDP)

At the beginning of the CPD cycle, registrants should identify learning needs and areas for development within their practice. These should be linked to the GDC development outcomes. They are recorded as a PDP and in particular, the plan should outline:

- CPD planned during the CPD cycle
- The anticipated development outcomes linked to each CPD activity
- The timeframe in which CPD will be completed during the cycle
- Reflective feedback on CPD activities and learning goals

General Medical Council

The General Medical Council (GMC) is the independent regulator, registration and licensing body for all doctors working in the UK. It is a legal requirement to be registered with the GMC in order to practise as a doctor in the UK. The GMC outlines the duties of a doctor and the professional standards to maintain in order to continue active registration and enable provision of safe patient care.

History of the GMC

The GMC was first formed in 1858 as the General Council of Medical Education and Registration of the United Kingdom. Following the public inquiries of Bristol Royal Infirmary and the Harold Shipman case in the 1990s to early 2000s, significant reform occurred in the GMC. Self-regulation was replaced with professional regulation. Revalidation and clinical standards of good medical practice were introduced. The GMC began to set the standards and expected outcomes for medical training in the UK.

The role of the GMC

The GMC's role covers four main areas:
1. Registration and licensing of doctors
2. Setting professional standards of practice (see Box 7.20)
3. Medical education standards and quality assurance
4. Managing concerns-supporting patients and investigations

> **Box 7.20 Good medical practice standards**
> Domain 1—knowledge, skills, and performance
> Domain 2—safety and quality
> Domain 3—communication, partnership, and teamwork
> Domain 4—maintaining trust

Complaints to the GMC

Patients, the public, or colleagues may raise concerns to the GMC. The GMC will investigate only cases where the doctor poses a serious risk to patient safety or has significantly or repeatedly failed to meet the GMC professional standards. The GMC does not investigate issues such as minor clinical errors, disagreements over treatment plans or access to appointments.

Fitness to practise concerns

When a concern is raised, the GMC will assess:
- The seriousness of the concern
- The relevant context, including the culture of the organization the clinician is working in, the workload, etc.
- How the doctor has responded to the concern-their own insight, remedial steps, competency, etc.

Additional information may be collected during an investigation, such as witness statements, police reports, medical records, expert reports, or assessment of the doctor's performance or health.

It is important that the doctor is adequately supported during this period and there are bodies external to the GMC who can provide this support including indemnity organizations, personal support and counselling.

Outcomes

The evidence is considered by the GMC panel, which consists of both medical and non-medical advisors.

- No action taken and the case closed
- The doctor is issued with a warning—in cases where there is no ongoing risk to patients but they have departed from the expected professional standards
- Restriction of registration through agreed undertakings, conditions, or suspension—in situations that pose a risk to patients or the public
- Removal from the register and loss of practising licence

Cases with outcomes other than 'no action' are referred to the Medical Practitioners Tribunal Service (MPTS). A medical supervisor or responsible officer may be assigned to monitor any sanctions or restrictions imposed or the doctor may be required to undergo further assessments. A review hearing will be arranged for a later date to decide if the restrictions can be removed or changed. An early referral to the MPTS may be actioned if the doctor fails to comply with the conditions imposed or is deemed unsafe.

Further reading

DoH (2005). National Health Service (Appointment of Consultants) Regulation Good Practice Guidance. Available at: ℘ https://www.rcp.ac.uk/media/b3zn3oy0/nhs-appointment-of-cons ultants-good-practice-guidance-january-2005_0.pdf

GMC. Guidance for doctors: requirements for revalidation and maintaining your licence. Available at: ℘ https://www.gmc-uk.org/-/media/gmc-site/registration-and-licensing/guidance_for_ doctors_requirements_for_revalidation_and_maintaining_your_licence.pdf

GMC. Guidance on supporting information for appraisal and revalidation. Available at: ℘ https:// www.gmc-uk.org/registration-and-licensing/managing-your-registration/revalidation/guidance- on-supporting-information-for-revalidation

GMC (2013). Good medical practice. Available at: ℘ https://www.gmc-uk.org/professional-standa rds/the-professional-standards/good-medical-practice

NHS Appointment of Consultant Regulation 1996. Available at: ℘ https://www.legislation.gov.uk/ uksi/1996/701/contents/made

Professional indemnity

The General Dental Council (Indemnity Arrangements) (Dentists and Dental Care Professionals) Rules Order of Council 2015 introduced the requirement for registered dental professionals to confirm that they have appropriate indemnity or insurance in place for the work they undertake. This is a mandatory requirement, established in the Dentists Act 1984. It ensures that patients can claim and receive compensation.

The GDC recognizes individual indemnity arrangements or indemnity via employers provided by:
- Defence organizations
- Commercial insurers
- NHS/State indemnity arrangements

Indemnity and insurance options

Dental defence organization membership

Many dental professionals opt to join a dental defence organization. The three largest that operate in the UK as mutual, not-for-profit organizations are:
- Dental Protection (part of the Medical Protection Society)
- Dental Defence Union (DDU—part of the Medical Defence Union)
- Medical and Dental Defence Union of Scotland (MDDUS)

Traditionally, these organizations provide occurrence-based discretionary membership and do not have any financial limits on their products for individual members. In addition to indemnity for claims, membership also provides additional benefits including access to dentolegal advice, assistance with complaint handling, support in inquests and regulatory investigations (e.g. GDC Fitness to Practise).

Insurance policy

Registrants may choose an insurance policy from a commercial insurer. Insurance products may be arranged through a broker, insurance agent, or appointed representative. Insurers and their agents are regulated by the Financial Conduct Authority (FCA) and the terms of their products will be detailed in the insurance policy and schedule documents. These will confirm any financial limits, excesses and conditions/exclusions that apply. Insurance policies are often provided on a claims-made basis although occurrence-based options are also available. Insurance products can also include options for legal expenses cover and access to dentolegal advice and assistance.

Individual and group indemnity schemes

Individual protection

A dental professional may have indemnity or insurance in their own name which may be a requirement of their contract of employment. It is important to ensure that the product covers the full scope of work undertaken and meets any employer/contractual requirements e.g. with regard to meeting any financial limits.

Individual protection can be organized directly with the indemnity organization or insurer or may be accessed via membership of a professional organization e.g. via membership of the British Association of Dental Nurses (BADN).

Employer schemes

Employer indemnity schemes may be offered to employees such as dental nurses, as part of a practice-based package. It is important to consider what protection an employer scheme provides, as this is often limited to indemnity for clinical negligence claims and may not provide additional benefits.

NHS/State indemnity

Often referred to as 'crown indemnity', NHS indemnity provides cover for doctors, dentists and healthcare professionals working in NHS hospitals across the UK and for some NHS salaried dental services roles in primary care. Since April 2019, state indemnity also covers NHS GP medical work in England and Wales. The cover is limited to work undertaken on NHS patients in an NHS role and would not extend to include private work outside any NHS contract. This is indemnity which is paid for by the trust (and not by the crown) and is covered under the Clinical Negligence Scheme for Trusts (CNST).

NHS indemnity provides indemnity for claims but does not offer additional protection and support for the individual clinician who faces, for example, a regulatory investigation or an inquest or fatal accident inquiry.

Dental professionals with only employer or NHS indemnity arrangements should also consider additional individual protection to support them for clinical matters that fall outside the claims protection e.g. regulatory investigation.

Other indemnity considerations

Occurrence-based versus claims-made coverage

- Occurrence-based products provide the ability to request and receive assistance with incidents that occurred at any time the clinician was in membership or insured with an organization. This applies irrespective of when the assistance is requested which could be years after ceasing practice
- Claims-made assistance is dependent upon whether the policy in place covers both the date the incident occurred and when it is reported. It is usually a condition of the policy that any incident is notified to the insurer as soon as the insured clinician becomes aware of an event that might give rise to a claim. During any gap in practice or on retirement, 'extended reporting benefits' (often referred to as 'run-off cover') may need to be purchased to allow for any claims notified after a policy ends. If moving to another provider, 'retroactive cover' would need to be purchased to allow reporting of incidents and claims that come to light from previous years which were not known about at the point of changing provider

Excesses and financial limits

Excesses and financial limits are most commonly associated with insurance products.

An 'excess' is an amount that must be paid by the insured towards the overall cost of each claim under the policy. The amount can vary and may depend on the claims history of the applicant. When an excess exists, it is important to ensure that funds are set aside and available to cover the liability when a claim arises.

A financial limit is the maximum a policy will pay out and usually applies to each claim and claims in aggregate i.e. the total for all claims in a single policy period. Once the policy limit is reached, the insured would need to fund any additional payments. It is important to ensure that any limit is sufficient to meet any contractual obligations and provide adequate protection.

Vicarious liability and non-delegable duty of care

Patients may pursue claims alleging vicarious liability (VL) and/or non-delegable duty (NDDC) of care against a business owner.

VL focuses on the relationship between a practice owner/employer and the treating clinician, whereas NDDC claims focus on the business owner's relationship with a patient directly irrespective of who is providing the care.

Legal cases considering the position in dentistry highlight the complexities of these types of claims and liability is dependent upon the specific circumstances of each case. Although there is no obligation to have protection in place, business owners may consider purchasing additional products to provide indemnity if they face a claim.

The GDC issued guidance effective February 2024 which provides further information about what a registrant should consider regarding indemnity/insurance in order to meet their professional obligations.

Further reading

General Dental Council (2015). Indemnity Arrangements, Dentists and Dental Care Professionals. Rules Order of Council. Available at: ℅ https://www.legislation.gov.uk/uksi/2015/1758/contents/made

General Dental Council (2023). GDC publishes outcome report on its consultation to revise the Guidance on Indemnity and Insurance. Available at: ℅ https://www.gdc-uk.org/news-blogs/news/detail/2023/12/21/gdc-publishes-outcome-report-on-its-consultation-to-revise-the-guidance-on-indemnity-and-insurance

General Dental Council (2024). Guidance on professional indemnity and insurance cover. Available at: ℅ https://www.gdc-uk.org/docs/default-source/consultations-and-responses/guidance-on-professional-indemnity-and-insurance.pdf?sfvrsn=906330a6_7

Chapter 8

Information governance

Terminology

Information governance refers to the way in which organizations 'process' or handle information. It covers personal information relating to patients, service users and employees, as well as corporate information such as financial and accounting records.

Common terms used in the context of information governance are defined as:

Data controller

'The natural or legal person, public authority, agency or other body which, alone or jointly with others, determines the purposes and means of the processing of personal data'. Data Protection Act 2018 (DPA18).

In secondary/tertiary care, the NHS trust is the data controller.

Data processor

'Natural or legal person, public authority, agency or other body which processes personal data on behalf of the controller'. (DPA 2018)

This would include staff in an NHS trust or external organization working on behalf of the trust.

Data processing

Any action taken with data, e.g. collecting, recording, organizing, using, sharing, storing, erasing, disclosing, or destroying.

The movement of a healthcare record by a porter is considered transport of data and therefore a form of data processing.

Data subject

The subject is the person whose information has been collected. Any information relating to a person (a 'data subject') who can be identified, directly or indirectly, by reference to an identifier such as a name, an identification number, or location.

Personal data

If it is possible to identify an individual directly or indirectly (in combination with other information) from the data being processed, it is considered personal data.

Special category data

A subset of personal data that is afforded additional protection under the Data Protection Act 2018. This is information that reveals racial or ethnic origin, political opinions, religious or philosophical beliefs, or trade union membership, as well as genetic data, biometric data (processed) for the purpose of uniquely identifying a natural person, data concerning health or data concerning a natural person's sex life or sexual orientation.

Primary and secondary use of data

The primary use of data in a healthcare setting is clinical care. The law allows personal data to be shared between those providing care directly to patients, although this must be done securely.

Anything other than direct clinical care is a secondary use of data. This includes research, audit, commissioning, and public health planning.

Pseudonymization

This is the processing of personal data in a way that ensures it cannot be attributed to a specific data subject without the use of additional information, provided that additional information is kept separate.

Anonymized data

Anonymous information is data that does not relate to an identified or identifiable individual (i.e. data that is not personal data). Data protection law does not apply to truly anonymous information.

Corporate records

Information created or received and maintained by the trust in the transaction of its business or conduct of affairs and kept as evidence of such activity. Examples are:

- Corporate governance including agendas, meeting papers, minutes
- Staff records and occupational health
- Finance and procurement
- Estates
- Legal matters, complaints, and information rights

The legal and governance framework

The legal framework governing the use of personal confidential data in healthcare is complex. It includes the:

- NHS Act 2006
- Health and Social Care Act 2012
- Data Protection Act 2018
- Human Rights Act 1998 (Article 8)
- The Freedom of Information Act 2000
- Environmental Information Regulations 2004
- Access to Health Records Act 1990

Other codes of practice and guidelines of relevance for dentists in secondary care include:

- GDC Standards: Principle 4: Maintain and protect patients' information (see page 281)
- CQC's Outcomes Framework 'Outcome 21: Records', which outlines the controls against which dental providers can be audited
- NHS Code of Confidentiality
- The NHS Care Record Guarantee for England
- The Information Security NHS Code of Practice
- The Records Management NHS Code of Practice
- The common law duty of confidentiality

Duty of confidentiality

A duty of confidentiality means that when someone shares personal information in confidence it must not be disclosed without legal authority or justification. It is:

- A legal obligation derived from case law
- A requirement established within professional codes of conduct
- Included in all NHS staff members' contracts of employment

Examples of a legal basis for disclosing information include:

- The individual has capacity and has given valid informed consent
- Disclosure is in the overriding public interest
- There is a statutory basis or legal duty to disclose, e.g. by court order

NHS trusts will have a Confidentiality Code of Practice, often based on the NHS Code of Practice, published by the Department of Health and Social Care.

Data Protection Act 2018

The Data Protection Act 2018 (DPA18) governs the way organizations, including NHS trusts use, store, manage, and share personal information. It is the UK's implementation of The EU General Data Protection Regulation (GDPR).

It provides a framework for information governance and the application of the GDPR in the UK. It also sets out the Information Commissioner's functions and powers.

Principles of GDPR

The GDPR sets out seven key principles that 'embody the spirit' of the legislation. These are:

1. Lawfulness, fairness, and transparency

For the processing of personal data to be lawful, specific grounds for the processing should be identified. This is called the 'lawful basis' and there are six options defined in Article 6 of GDPR. The processing of special category data must fall into one of the conditions defined in Article 9 of GDPR. In dentistry this would routinely be one of:

(h) Health or social care (with a basis in law)

(i) Public health (with a basis in law)

(j) Archiving, research and statistics (with a basis in law)

2. Purpose limitation

Organizations must be clear and record the purpose of data processing. They must only use personal data for a new purpose if compatible with the original purpose.

3. Data minimization

Personal data being processed should be:

- Adequate—sufficient to properly fulfil the stated purpose
- Relevant—have a rational link to that purpose
- Limited to what is necessary

4. Accuracy

Personal data should be accurate and all reasonable steps taken to ensure it is not incorrect or misleading.

5. Storage limitation

Personal data should not be kept for longer than needed. Data retention policies in health are described in Table 8.5.

Data held should be periodically reviewed to erase or anonymize when no longer needed.

6. Integrity and confidentiality (security)

Appropriate security measures must be in place to protect the personal data held.

7. Accountability

Organizations must be able to demonstrate how they are complying with the other principles.

As a data controller of special category data, an NHS trust must demonstrate accountability by:

- Appointing a data protection officer (DPO)
- Adopting and implementing data protection policies
- Maintaining documentation of all processing undertaken in the trust
- Implementing appropriate security measures. This includes information security policies, access controls, security monitoring, and recovery plans
- Recording and, where necessary, reporting personal data breaches
- Adhering to relevant codes of conduct and signing up to certification
- Carrying out data protection impact assessments (DPIA)
- Taking a "Data protection by design" approach—Privacy and data protection issues should be considered at the design phase of any system, service or process and then continue that throughout the entire lifecycle

Rights for individuals

The GDPR provides the following rights for individuals:
- The right to be informed about the collection and use of their personal data
- The right of access to their personal data
- The right to rectification of inaccurate or incomplete information
- The right to erasure
- The right to restrict processing of their data
- The right to data portability so individuals can obtain and reuse their personal data for their own purposes across different services
- The right to object to the processing of personal data
- Rights in relation to automated decision-making and profiling

Exemptions and restrictions

There are exemptions and restrictions on the above that are relevant in the healthcare context, such as in instances to protect public health or if access is likely to cause serious harm to the physical or mental health of any individual.

Information Commissioner's Office

The Information Commissioner's Office (ICO) is the UK's independent body set up to uphold information rights.

The ICO is responsible for:
- Promoting good practice in handling personal data and giving advice and guidance on data protection
- Helping to resolve disputes by deciding whether it is likely or unlikely that an organization has complied with the GDPR when processing personal data
- Taking action to enforce compliance with GDPR, where appropriate
- Bring prosecutions for offences committed under GDPR, except in Scotland, where the Procurator Fiscal brings prosecutions
- The ICO may levy penalty fines which may be up to £8.7 million or 2% of the total annual worldwide turnover in the preceding financial year, whichever is higher

Registration

All data controllers must be registered with the ICO. In a secondary care environment this is the NHS trust. Individual clinicians do not routinely have to be registered. This may not be the case for the treatment of private patients in an NHS trust, or in dental practice. If the dentist is a data controller, they should register. If any doubt, contact should be made with the ICO.

Data breaches

A personal data breach is defined as a breach of security leading to the accidental or unlawful destruction, loss, alteration, unauthorized disclosure of, or access to, personal data. It includes:

- Any impact on the confidentiality, integrity, or availability of personal data
- Access by an unauthorized third party
- Deliberate or accidental action (or inaction) by a controller or processor
- Sending personal data to an incorrect recipient
- Computing devices containing personal data being lost or stolen
- Alteration of personal data without permission
- Loss of availability of personal data

The possible effects of a data breach for the individual and trust are summarized in Table 8.1.

Table 8.1 The possible effects of a data breach for the individual and trust

For the individual	For the trust
Loss of control over personal data	Loss of trust
Emotional distress	Reputational damage
Limitation of their rights	Litigation
Discrimination	Financial repercussions
Identity theft or fraud	
Financial loss	
Unauthorized reversal of pseudonymization	
Damage to reputation	
Loss of confidentiality of personal data	
Economic or social disadvantage	

Managing a data breach

In a dental department, a senior clinician (consultant) should manage a data breach in conjunction with the information governance team.

Figure 8.1 summarizes the steps taken when a data breach is identified.

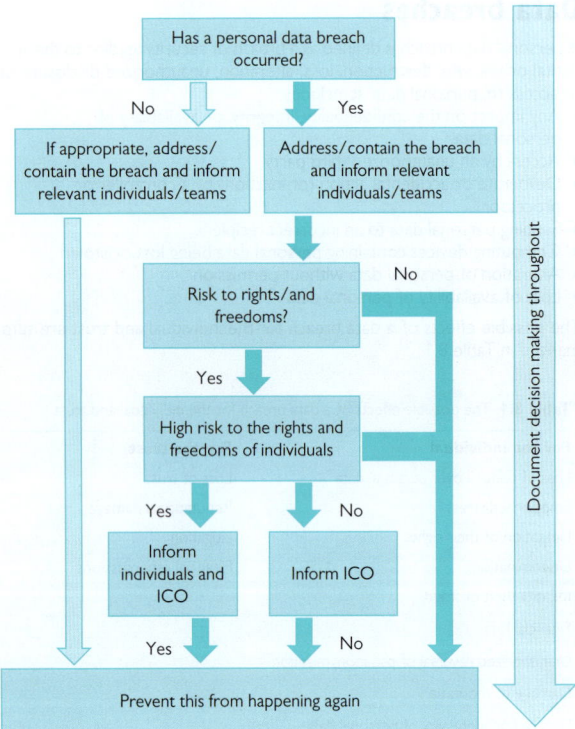

Figure 8.1 Managing a personal data breach.

Establish whether a personal data breach has occurred

Information should be gathered on:
- What has happened and why
- How many people were involved
- Timeline of when it all happened
- What actions have been taken so far

Data that has been anonymized is not considered personal data and therefore not considered a data breach. Although, it may be appropriate to investigate and respond to a breach to prevent the loss of personal data in the future.

Address or contain the breach and inform relevant individuals/teams

Immediate steps to contain a breach include:

- If information has been sent to someone by mistake, ask them to delete it, send it back securely, or have it ready for you to collect
- If a physical item has been lost, retrace your steps. Contact security and/or reception
- A stolen electronic device (laptop or phone) with appropriate systems installed may be wiped remotely. Inform the trust information and communications technology (ICT) team immediately
- A cyber incident may be contained by changing all passwords and ensuring other staff do the same

The appropriate teams and individuals within the trust should be informed. This may include the senior clinician (consultant), security, information governance team, DPO, ICT security. Completing an incident report (DATIX/ Ulysses) is a method of alerting the relevant trust teams.

Assess the risk to individuals (categorize the risk)
The risk of harm to the affected individuals (staff or patients) should be assessed. The DPO/risk management teams would undertake and/or advise on this. The level of risk is dependent on:
- Whether personal data was involved
- What personal data has been breached
- Who might have the data
- Number of people who will be affected
- Harm that may occur as a result of the breach

Examples of risk categorization relevant to the dental team are presented in the information governance scenarios (page 319).

Inform the ICO
The DPO will inform the ICO if the breach is 'reportable'. This is when:
- Personal data is involved
- If people's rights and freedoms are at risk
- If a risk is likely, the ICO must be informed, without undue delay and this must not be later than 72 hours of the trust becoming aware of the breach. If a breach isn't reported this should be justified and documented

Inform individuals
Where there is a high risk to the rights and freedoms of individuals, they must be informed directly and without undue delay.

This communication should be drafted and reviewed by the DPO, media team, legal team and senior clinician, with sign off by the directorate clinical lead and/or manager. This may be reviewed by a senior member of the trust management such as CEO or senior information risk owner (SIRO).

Document decision-making process
This process should be documented, particularly the reasoning for any decisions made. This would keep the trust in line with the requirements of the accountability principle.

Prevent the breach from happening again
Any breach should be investigated, and processes put in place to help prevent it from recurring.

Human error is the leading cause of reported data breaches (see Chapter 6, page 145).

The result of any investigation should be disseminated in the same way other patient safety incidents are:

- Reported in incident log
- Dental/department team meetings
- Risk action group (RAG) meeting
- Trust bulletins

Repercussions

The ICO may issue a monetary penalty for an infringement or issue a reprimand to the trust. Failure to notify the ICO of a breach can result in a standard maximum fine.

Where there has been misconduct, a data breach may result in disciplinary action, up to and including dismissal.

Information governance roles

There are numerous information governance roles at a national and local trust level. They are a source of advice, guidelines, and bodies to whom concerns may be raised.

NHS England and NHS digital

NHS England merged with NHS Digital in 2023, with responsibility for:
- Running critical national infrastructure for the NHS
- Collection, analysis, publication, and dissemination of data generated by health and social care services, to improve outcomes

NHS England had several cyber security responsibilities:
- Managing the security risks to NHS England data
- Enabling the wider NHS to reduce cyber risk
- Improving services and continuing to manage the overarching risks

National Data Guardian

The National Data Guardian (NDG) is the independent champion for patients and the public in matters relating to their confidential health and care information. They advise the health and care system to ensure that confidential information is safeguarded and used properly.

The Health and Social Care (National Data Guardian) Act 2018 gives the NDG a statutory role, including the issuing of official guidance about the processing of health and adult social care data in England, among other duties. The National Data Guardian owns and maintains the Caldicott Principles. The NDG is not a regulator and does not have investigatory or enforcement powers.

Data Security Standards

The National Data Guardian (NDG) has established ten Data Security Standards (DSS) (Table 8.2). They are intended to apply to every organization handling health and social care information.

The Data Security and Protection Toolkit

The Data Security and Protection Toolkit (DSPT) is an online self-assessment tool that allows organizations to measure their performance against the DSS. This is a mandatory annual assessment carried out by NHS England. All organizations that have access to NHS patient data and systems must complete this toolkit annually.

Accountable officer: chief executive

The chief executive is ultimately accountable for all information governance and security matters including compliance with the requirements of data protection law.

In relation to the Freedom of Information Act, they are the nominated 'qualified person' and therefore responsible for considering whether an exemption applies to any requested information (see Freedom of Information, p. 313).

Data protection officer

Organizations with more than 250 employees or firms which process more than 5,000 data subjects annually must appoint a dedicated DPO.

Table 8.2 NDG's data security standards (NDSSS)

Data security standard		Leadership obligation
1. Personal confidential data	All staff ensure that personal confidential data is handled, stored, and transmitted securely, whether in electronic or paper form	1. People: Ensure staff are equipped to handle information respectfully and safely, according to the Caldicott principles
2. Staff responsibilities	All staff understand their responsibilities under the NDGSS	
3. Staff training	All staff complete appropriate annual data security training and pass a mandatory test, provided through the revised Information Governance Toolkit	
4. Managing data access	Personal confidential data is only accessible to staff who need it for their current role and access is removed as soon as it is no longer required	2. Process: IT suppliers are held accountable via contracts for protecting the personal confidential data they process and meeting the NDG's Data Security Standards
5. Process reviews	Processes are reviewed at least annually to identify and improve processes which have caused breaches or near misses	
6. Responding to incidents	Cyber-attacks against services are identified and resisted and CareCERT security advice is responded to	
7. Continuity planning	A continuity plan is in place to respond to threats to data security, including significant data breaches or near misses, and it is tested once a year as a minimum	
8. Unsupported systems	No unsupported operating systems, software or internet browsers are used within the IT estate	3. Technology: Ensure technology is secure and up-to-date
9. IT protection	A strategy is in place for protecting IT systems from cyber threats which is based on a proven cyber security framework such as Cyber Essentials	
10. Accountable suppliers	IT suppliers are held accountable via contracts for protecting the personal confidential data they process and meeting the NDGSS	

The DPO:
- Monitors compliance with GDPR and organizational policies
- Informs and advises the trust and employees about their obligations
- Advises when a DPIA is required
- Acts as contact point for data subjects and the ICO
- In an NHS trust, the DPO will often oversee the process underlying subject access requests (SARs)

The DPO must:
- Be independent (although they can be a member of staff or contractor)
- Have expert knowledge of data protection law and practices
- They can perform another role in an organization but there should be no conflict of interest
- The DPO reports directly to the highest management level in an organization, i.e. the board/chief executive

Caldicott Guardian

The Caldicott Guardian role was established following the Review of Patient-Identifiable Information in 1997 by Dame Fiona Caldicott. There are eight established principles (Table 8.3).

A Caldicott Guardian:
- Is a senior person within a health or social care organization who makes sure that personal information is used legally, ethically and appropriately, and that confidentiality is maintained
- Provides leadership and informed guidance on complex matters such as breaches of confidentiality and information-sharing
- The role is advisory

All NHS organizations, local authorities that provide social services, and private or third-sector organizations that deliver publicly funded care must have a Caldicott Guardian. They must work at board or senior management level.

All four nations have chosen to have Caldicott Guardians, although there are differences in legislation and common law.

Senior information risk owner

The SIRO is one of two senior roles mandated by the NHS information governance framework, within each organization. The other being the Caldicott Guardian.

They are an executive director or member of the trust board. They:
- Have overall responsibility for the trust's information risk policy
- Are accountable for information governance
- Provide a focal point for managing information risks and incidents
- Are concerned with the management of all information assets—ensure that all care systems' information assets have an assigned information asset owner

Information governance steering group

The information governance steering group reports to the executive management team, through the senior information risk officer. It is responsible for overseeing day-to-day information governance issues and coordinating information governance in the trust through policies, standards, procedures, and guidance.

Table 8.3 The Caldicott principles

1. Justify the purpose(s)	Every proposed use or transfer of personal confidential data within or from an organization should be clearly defined, scrutinized, and documented, with continuing uses regularly reviewed, by an appropriate guardian.
2. Don't use personal confidential data unless it is absolutely necessary	The need for patients to be identified should be considered at each stage of satisfying the purpose(s).
3. Use the minimum necessary personal confidential data	Each individual item of data should be considered and justified for a given function to be carried out.
4. Access to personal confidential data should be on a strict need-to-know basis	This may mean introducing access controls or splitting data flows where one data flow is used for several purposes.
5. Everyone with access to personal confidential data should be aware of their responsibilities	Action should be taken to ensure that those handling personal confidential data — both clinical and non-clinical staff, are made fully aware of their responsibilities and obligations to respect patient confidentiality.
6. Comply with the law	Every use of personal confidential data must be lawful. Someone in each organization should be responsible for ensuring that the organization complies with legal requirements.
7. The duty to share information can be as important as the duty to protect patient confidentiality	Health and social care professionals should have the confidence to share information in the best interests of their patients within the framework set out by these principles. They should be supported by the policies of their employers, regulators, and professional bodies.
8: Inform patients and service users about how their confidential information is used	Patients and service users should be well-informed, have a clear idea about how and why their confidential information is used, and what choices they have about this. This should include providing accessible, relevant and appropriate information.

Information governance lead

The information governance lead is a source of information or advice in an NHS trust. They:
- Advise the SIRO and Caldicott Guardian on all aspects of compliance with information governance standards
- In conjunction with the DPO, investigate all serious information governance incidents and data breaches
- Are responsible for reporting and monitoring compliance with this policy

The patient safety team

This team is responsible for administering the trust's incident reporting system and risk registers including information incidents and risks.

They support managers to investigate serious information governance incidents within the trust including information governance and monitor delivery of the serious incident report.

The legal team

The legal team is responsible for processing all requests for information from the police, coroner, and solicitors, and in some instances requests for information from the local authority.

Director for cyber and information security

The director for cyber and information security ensures there are appropriate security measures in place to protect personal data. They:
- Inform, advise, and implement ICT security
- Review effectiveness of security controls
- Monitor compliance with or certification in legislation and standards, including:
  - Data Security and Protection Toolkit
  - Security elements of the UK GDPR and Data Protection Act 2018
  - Cyber essentials and cyber essentials plus
  - ISO 27001
  - Network and information systems (NIS) regulations
- Respond to and coordinate responses to security related incidents
- Cooperate with NHS Digital, the ICO and National Cyber Security Centre (NCSC)
- Champion and advocate for good information security practice in the organization
- Ensure the ICT Asset Register is regularly updated, maintained, and audited for accuracy and completeness

Information asset owners

Each clinical department will have an information asset owner (IAO) who is responsible for the information, information assets, and information flows within the department.

The individual varies by trust but they are always senior local operating managers (such as chief of service, clinical lead, or general manager).

The role of the IAO is to ensure that the information under their ownership is accurate, protected, and its value to the organization realized.

Information asset register

The information asset register (IAR) is a tool to record the information assets and their properties. An information asset is anything valuable to the trust that should be protected from unauthorized access, use, disclosure, modification, destruction, or compromise.

The following are examples of information assets in a dental department:
- Paper records
- Databases of data files, such as:
  - Laboratory work queues, patient laboratory box numbers
  - Patient waiting times

- Admission Lists
  - Patient data submitted to national registries (such as cleft outcome data)
- Audit data
- IT equipment
- Applications and system software
- Manuals and documentation
- Back-up and archive data
- Operations and support procedures
- Data encryption utilities
- Environmental services necessary for the safe operation of information assets (e.g. power and air conditioning)

Freedom of Information (FOI) team/coordinator

The Freedom of Information team/coordinator logs and responds to FOI/Environmental Information Request (EIR) requests. This may involve liaising with the trust's legal and communications teams.

Trust records manager

Responsible for the overall development and maintenance of health records management practices throughout the trust, in particular for drawing up guidance to promote best practice.

Dental department/senior clinicians

Senior clinicians in a dental department should take ownership of, and seek to improve, the quality of information within their services.

They are responsible for ensuring that the information governance policy, and related standards or guidance are built into local processes. These may be used to demonstrate accountability and as evidence to other regulatory bodies such as the CQC.

This can be done by:

- Implementing a culture of trust—dental staff should feel able to report incidents or near misses
- Regular review of:
  - Business continuity plan (BCP)
  - Information asset register
  - Data processes held by the trust
  - Trust policies to ensure that the department is compliant
- Obtain advice from the DPO/Caldecott Guardian/IG team prior to changing or establishing new processes or technology
- Complete DPIAs, as required
- Ensure security of the department when unattended
- Ensure staff have received appropriate and up-to-date training
- Establish clear guidelines, SOPs, and local policies
- Local induction and written manuals for new staff
- Regularly review and audit user access lists to ensure they are up-to-date. Remove staff no longer employed in the department
- Ensure encryptable/wipeable devices are available to staff
- Physical records should be kept in a designated area, which is secure but accessible 24 hours a day to authorized personnel
- Identify areas for storage of equipment when not in use

- Procure department cameras/equipment or establish an SOP for the trust's Medical Illustration department to obtain dental images
- Learn from incidents and near misses
  - Establish an incident log
  - Incidents and learning should be disseminated to the team
  - Attend RAG meetings
- Establish clinical audit or quality improvement programmes, particularly where a concern has been identified
- Take appropriate action and disciplinary measures where necessary

Dental team

All members of the team, clinical and non-clinical, are responsible for information governance. Some of the measures individual team members can take include:

- Maintain statutory and mandatory training
- Report near misses and incidents
- Work to the principle of 'check twice, send once'
- Appropriate disposal of records containing personal data:
  - Physical documents to be placed in confidential waste bins
  - Electronic items returned to ICT for data removal prior to disposal
- Do not allow others to access systems with their credentials
- Do not to share systems passwords
- Do not use personal phones to contact patients
- Do not use personal devices to share patient information
- Use trust/department devices (such as cameras)
- Non-encrypted drives to be wiped immediately
- Use password protected, limited access shared drives for storage
- Use the trust confirmed video conferencing (Zoom/Teams, etc.)
- Health records must not be removed from the department/ward from where the patient is located
- Report incidents when health records cannot be accessed
- Use trust or NHS email, only send emails within a domain name, etc., nhs.net to nhs.net
- Use secure filesharing or email encryption services to send emails outside of the trust established email system
- Ensure any data transfer containing identifiable information outside the trust is securely encrypted during transit
- Data should not be shared outside of the UK without the authority of the information governance team

Data protection impact assessments

Data protection impact assessments (DPIAs) are a key part of data protection by design approach and demonstrate the accountability principle for the trust and dental department.

Senior dental clinicians are likely to be required to complete a DPIA as part of any new process or technology being introduced to a department (see Figure 8.2). Examples include:

- Moving to 3D intraoral scanning and storage of 3D scans
- Creating a local database, e.g. physical study models
- New technologies that change how patient data is stored or processed
- Sending models/scans to a new (external) dental laboratory

A DPIA identifies and minimizes the data protection risks of new projects. It is a legal requirement before carrying out processing likely to result in high risks to individuals' interests. They should be completed prior to the processing of data.

Step 1: Identify the need for a DPIA

Inform the DPO (via the information governance team) of any new software, project, or process. They will advise if a project meets the criteria to undertake a DPIA.

Each NHS trust will have an established questionnaire template to complete. The DPIA is completed by the individual leading the project, usually

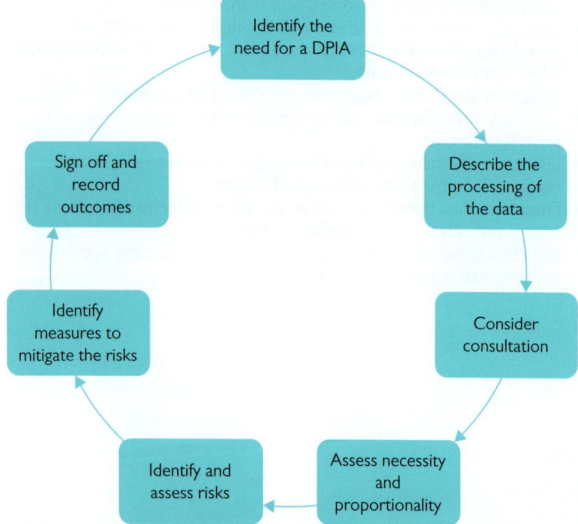

Figure 8.2 The process for completing a DPIA.

a clinician with the support of the information governance team providing guidance.

Step 2: Describe the processing
- Describe how and why the personal data will be used

Nature of the processing is what will be done with the personal data:
- How data will be collected, stored, and used
- Who has access to the data
- Who the data will be shared with
- Whether any processors will be used
- Retention periods
- Security measures
- Whether new technologies or novel types of processing are being used
- Which screening criteria are flagged as likely high risk
- Whether the information will be used for research

Scope of the processing is what the processing covers.
- Nature, volume, variety, and sensitivity of the personal data
- Extent, frequency, and duration of the processing
- Number of data subjects involved
- Geographical area covered

Context of the processing is the wider picture, including internal and external factors which might affect expectations or impact.
- Source of the data
- Nature of the relationship with the individuals
- How far individuals have control over their data
- Whether individuals include children or other vulnerable people
- Previous experience of this type of processing
- Relevant advances in technology or security
- Current issues of public concern
- Compliance with UK GDPR codes of conduct/certification schemes

Purpose of the processing is the reason why processing of personal data is required.
- Legitimate interests
- The intended outcome for individuals
- The expected benefits

Step 3: Consider consultation
This involves consulting individuals (patients) and other appropriate stakeholders such as ICT, legal team, estates and external software teams.

Step 4: Assess necessity and proportionality
Consider whether the plans help to achieve the stated purpose and if there is any other reasonable way to achieve the same result.
- The lawful basis for the processing
- How function creep will be prevented
- How data quality will be ensured
- How data minimization will be ensured
- How privacy information to individuals will be provided
- How individuals' rights will be supported
- Measures to ensure processors comply
- Safeguards for international transfers

Step 5: Identify and assess risks

A risk matrix (see Table 6.5, page 165) should be used. This should consider the potential impact on individuals and the trust (see section 'Data breaches,' page 299).

Step 6: Identify measures to mitigate the risks

For each identified risk, consider the options for reducing that risk. For example:

- Deciding not to collect certain types of data
- Reducing the scope of the processing
- Reducing retention periods
- Taking additional technological security measures
- Training staff to ensure risks are anticipated and managed
- Anonymizing or pseudonymizing data where possible
- Writing internal guidance or processes to avoid risks
- Using a different technology
- Making changes to privacy notices
- Data sharing agreement (DSA) established with external organizations
- Deletion of files from unencrypted memory sticks immediately after use (e.g. clinical camera)
- Limit sharing to established dental laboratories with whom a DSA exists

Step 7: Sign off and record outcomes

The DPIA should be reviewed by the relevant stakeholders, within a trust this would routinely include:

- The project lead
- Clinical lead
- IAO (usually the clinical chief of service/directorate)
- DPO
- ICT security and governance manager

Data transfers

A DPIA is likely required if a dental department is sending patient data to external organizations such as a dental laboratory. Increasingly these are based outside of the UK particularly for the development of surgical plans or guides. The transfer of personal data to receivers located outside the UK is termed 'restricted transfers'. Specific safeguards and precautions should be taken. The information governance team should be informed of any transfer outside the UK.

The following apply:

- The transfer of patient data to and from countries covered by adequacy regulations is permitted. These are countries or organizations the government has deemed provide an adequate level of data protection
- At the time of publication the UK has an adequacy decision with the EU Commission and transfers to/from the European Economic Area are therefore currently permitted
- Transfer to countries not covered by an adequacy agreement may take place subject to appropriate safeguards being in place
- The ICO's higher maximum penalty would be applicable where an appropriate restricted transfer has taken place

Records management

Records management is the process by which an organization manages all aspects of records whether internally or externally generated and in any format or media type, from creation, all the way through their lifecycle to appraisal and destruction.

For England, the Records Management Code of Practice for Health and Social Care, published by NHS England provides the framework for records management. It is based on established standards and has been reviewed by the ICO and NDG.

There is variation between the devolved nations:
- Scotland—SG HSC Scotland Records Management Code of Practice 2020
- Wales—HEIW records management policy 2020
- Northern Ireland (NI)—Good Management, Good Records disposal schedule

Data retention

The DPA18 states that personal data should be retained for no longer than is necessary.

Retention periods begin when the record ceases to be operational. This is at the point of discharge from care or the last entry (Table 8.4).

Varying retention regimes are in place for other care records such as mental health, maternity, cancer/oncology, patients with Creutzfeldt–Jakob disease (CJD) or long-term illness that may re-occur.

A log of destroyed records should be maintained.

At the time of writing there are two independent inquiries which have requested that large parts of the health and social care sector do not destroy any records that are, or may fall into the remit of the inquiry:
- The COVID-19 Inquiry
- The Infected Blood Inquiry

Electronic patient records

Electronic patient records should follow the same schedule if:
- There is the capacity to destroy records
- A 'metadata stub' can remain demonstrating that a record has been destroyed

Freedom of Information

The Freedom of Information Act 2000 (FOIA) gives members of the public the right to request recorded information held by a public authority, such as an NHS trust.

The Act came into effect on 1 January 2005 and covers non-personal information.

The trust has obligations under the FOIA:
- A duty to make information held in recorded form accessible to the public, unless it has an exemption (e.g. information about future publications, commercial interest data)
- Provide a publication scheme—specify the classes of information which a public authority (such as an NHS trust) publishes or intends to publish
- Respond to requests for information
- Provide access to and allow inspection of environmental information

Table 8.4 A summary of the retention schedules for the devolved nations

Record type	Children	Adults
England		
General dental services records	11 years or 25th birthday, whichever is longer	11 Years
Secondary care records	25th or 26th birthday*	15 years
Referrals (not accepted)	2 years	
Clinical audit	5 years, review and destroy if not required	
Operating theatre records	10 years	
Scotland	10 years or 25th/26th* birthday, whichever is longer	10 years
Wales community dental services	11 years or aged 25, whichever is longer, or eight years after death	11 years
Wales and NI hospital dental records	25th/26th birthday*, or eight years after death	8 years
Wales and NI general dental services and orthodontics	6 years	6 years
NI community dental service	25th/26th birthday*, or eight years after death	11 years

* Retain until 25th birthday, or 26th if the patient was 17 when treatment ended.

- It is a criminal offence to alter, deface, block, erase, destroy, or conceal any record held by the trust with the intention of preventing disclosure

Process
- To be valid, a request for information must:
  - Be made in writing, be legible and in a re-usable form (hardcopy or electronic format)
  - State the 'real' name of the freedom of information (FOI) applicant and an address for correspondence (postal address or electronic)
  - Include a description of the information requested
- The FOI must be forwarded to the FOI team immediately
- If received by letter, the date that the trust received the letter must be clearly marked

The FOI team, must:
- Respond to requests within 20 working days for FOIs or 40 working days for Environmental Information Regulations (EIR) to be compliant with ICO guidance
- The request timeline starts as soon as it is received by the trust, not by the FOI team
- Confirm or deny in writing if the requested information is held, unless doing so would reveal exempt information
- Provide the requested information, unless an exemption applies or the trust is technically unable to provide the information

- State what information cannot be provided and the reason for this (including specifying any exemptions and conditions which apply)

The clinical lead must:
- On receiving FOI requests from the FOI team, source the information requested and ensure that the response from their directorate/department is accurate. They are usually required to return this to the FOI team within 10 working days
- This constitutes 50% of the statutory timeframe of 20 working days, which allows for at least five working days before the FOI deadline

The executive team are notified when:
- Media-related or the information requested is deemed to be sensitive
- Potential for consequences to the trust's reputation
- Potentially prejudicial to the trust's commercial activities
- Information is requested that has previously been requested indicating a pattern

A fee may be charged under the Fees Regulations in the FOI.

Subject access request (SAR)

A SAR is a request to an organization (data controller) by an individual asking the organization for access to the personal information they hold on them.

The following legislation entitles the right to that access:
- Access to Health Records Act 1990
- DPA18

Who can place an SAR?

Individuals with capacity have the right to access their own health record. They may also authorize a third party such as a solicitor, member of parliament, or a family representative to do so on their behalf.

Process

- A request can be made verbally or in writing, including by social media. It can be directed to any part of the trust; it is not necessary to direct it to a specific person or contact point

A clinician who receives a request (in writing or verbally) should redirect it to the relevant team immediately, to prevent undue delay:
- The health records department is responsible for processing requests from a patient or person with parental responsibility
- The legal team is responsible for processing requests for information made by the police, solicitors, coroners, the GDC, or other regulatory bodies
- The human resources (HR) department is responsible for processing requests for information by previous employees and existing employees

The ICO requires all SARs to be processed within one month. Complex requests can be extended by two months.

In addition to the electronic and/or paper health record the following sources may also be searched:
- Information that has been archived
- Emails
- Complaints file
- Incident files (DATIX records and SI folder)

- Any other source of personal data (e.g. system or storage location) where there is evidence of personal data for the patient

A copy of the information must be provided free of charge (including postage costs) unless the request is identified as 'manifestly unfounded' or 'excessive'- in which case a 'reasonable' fee can be charged, or the trust can refuse to respond.

The national data opt-out

The national data opt-out (NDOO) was introduced to give patients a choice on how their confidential patient information is used for purposes beyond their individual care.

The opt-out applies where confidential patient information or personal data is used (i.e. data that is not in anonymized form):

- Is processed for research and/or planning
- Originates within the health and adult social care system located in England
- Relates to care that is funded or arranged by a public body

Research governance and GDPR

GDPR was not designed to impede research and allows research certain privileges.

Research can be exempt from some GDPR principles if the other data protection principles and safeguards are in place:

- Purpose limitation—existing personal data may be reused for research-related purposes
- Storage limitation—personal data may be kept indefinitely where the controller has set out legitimate justification

There is no specific lawful basis for research. Depending on the status and context, either 'legitimate interests' or 'public tasks' for this type of processing may be used. Research can be carried out on data which has been effectively anonymized as it is no longer considered personal data and data protection legislation does not apply.

Research retention

Research retention protocols vary from clinical records (see Table 8.5). The retention period begins at the end of the trial/research.

Table 8.5 Research retention guidelines

Record type	Retention period*
Advanced medical therapy research master file	20 years
Clinical trials—applications for ethical approval	5 years
Clinical trials master file	25 years
Research data sets	Not more than 20 years

Social media

Social media or social networking (see Table 8.6) are terms used to describe internet related tools which enable users to interact with the wider public.

Social media may benefit the dental profession and NHS trusts:

- An effective way of communicating on a personal and professional level
- A way for a trust to advertise services provided and encourage engagement with stakeholders and patients
- Collating opinions from within and outside the organization
- Keeping users/patients up-to-date with the latest developments
- A place to find advice about current practice

Principles of participating in online activities

The GDC standards for dental teams specifically mention social media: 'You must not post any information or comments about patients on social networking or blogging sites. If you use professional social media to discuss

Table 8.6 Main types of social media

Type	Use	Examples
Social networks	Used for advertising, persuading/influencing people using targeting metrics Cater to a wide and diverse audience	Facebook, X, Instagram, LinkedIn, TikTok
Discussion forums	Share ideas for market research by asking people what they think about brands and services	Reddit, Digg, Quora, Clubhouse, GDPUK
Image sharing networks	Share photos and related content	Instagram, Flickr, Photobucket
Blogging and publishing networks	Users publish thoughts on their jobs, current events, hobbies, and more	Medium, WordPress, Facebook, Tumblr
Consumer review networks	Display customer reviews of businesses	TripAdvisor, Yelp, OpenTable, Google My Business
Interest-based networks	Shared hobbies and interests	Strava, Peanut, Goodreads
Sharing economy networks	Access to resources by encouraging the sharing of goods and services	Lending Club, Couchsurfing, Eatwith
Social shopping networks	Sellers can reach customers who are looking for related products	Instagram, Poshmark, Etsy, Facebook
Video hosting platforms	Give individuals a platform to create videos for an audience	YouTube, TikTok, Snapchat, Vimeo, Instagram

anonymized cases for the purpose of discussing best practice you must be careful that the patient or patients cannot be identified'.

The following principles should be considered by those engaging with social media:

Maintaining standards

- The same standards are expected when communicating through social media as traditional media, including maintaining patient confidentiality and professional courtesy
- Compliance with GDC Standards and the trust's social media policy
- These apply even if you do not identify yourself as a dental professional (such as posting anonymously)
- You should not bring yourself or your organization into disrepute or damage public confidence in you as a dental professional
- Individuals are accountable for the sharing of offensive content, even if they did not create it
- Social media is not an appropriate way to raise concerns

NHS Organizations and social media

- All staff must be trained in information governance as part of their mandatory training
- Staff understanding of their organization's policy is key as they may use social media on a personal level and as a representative of the NHS organization they work for
- If a member of the public obtains a recording of an appointment, the rights to use this are independent of the NHS organization's policies
- Positive and negative reviews by the public on social media posts regarding an individual, service, or organization should not be managed personally. They must be reported to the appropriate team such as the trust media or ICT team
- Although image/video networks are not governed by copyright, it is important to understand the responsibility that an individual has prior to sharing content, as this content may be the property of the organization (and not the clinician)

Confidentiality

- Information posted online will be there permanently, even if deleted afterwards. Patients should be made aware of this
- Information which would identify a patient should not be published without their explicit consent. This includes specifying exactly what information will be published, what purpose, and where it will be available
- Although individual pieces of information may not breach a patient's confidentiality on their own, a number of pieces of patient information published online could be enough to identify them

Safeguarding

Safeguarding patients

Social media can pose a risk to patients:

- This includes online bullying, grooming, exploitation, or stalking, exposure to inappropriate comments or hateful language

- Concerns must be reported to the safeguarding lead within the organization in a timely manner
- If a child is known to be vulnerable, use of their image is not recommended, even if consent is obtained

Safeguarding yourself

- Privacy settings for each social media account should be reviewed regularly. The strictest privacy policy does not guarantee information will be kept secure
- A neutral profile image is recommended
- Do not engage in inappropriate conversations or content. Should you encounter such a situation, politely disengage, and seek advice from the media or ICT team
- Think carefully before accepting requests from patients

Social media and social networking are developing fast and therefore, it is important to check the intranet for updated policies as the recommendation is that these be updated at least every 6 months.

Scenario—Subject access request

You are a DCT2 in a restorative dentistry department in a dental hospital.

On your way into the department, an individual stops you and identifies themselves as the parent of a patient, AD. They would like to access records for their child, AD.

What do you do?

Advise the individual they will need to make a subject access request (SAR). Direct them to the trust website, or through Patient Advice and Liaison Service (PALS). They can also contact their child's lead or primary consultant for advice. There is sometimes a fee charged for acquiring copies of medical records If you are unsure what to do, you should ask your consultant for advice.

Do they need to provide a reason for the request?

No, an individual does not need to provide a reason for accessing their health records or the record of their child.

The individual states that due to 'Freedom of Information', they must be given the information immediately and do not have to apply for it.

Advise that access to personal sensitive information such as a health records requires that the request is verified, specifically proof of identity, and proof that they are entitled to the record for the child. This does not fall under FOI Act, but under the Data Protection Act 'right of access'.

FOI requests may be made by any means, with a statutory timeframe of 20 working days (and not immediately).

A subject access request timeframe of one month (set by the ICO) begins once the request has been received and verified.

The individual states their child is on a waiting list for treatment. They want to know how long the department waiting list is, how many people are on the waiting list and how many patients have been taken off the waiting list each month, for the preceding year.

This information would fall under the remit of an FOI request. You should offer to:

- Signpost to PALS or the trust website to obtain their contact details and information regarding the request
- If they do not want to do this, you should take their details (name and contact details, and the information they would like to request)
- You should inform a senior clinician of the FOI request. It may be more appropriate for a consultant to take these details and information from the outset
- Individual information regarding their child would not be provided
- The request should be sent in writing immediately to the FOI team
- Advise the individual, the information would routinely be provided within 20 working days

You are a consultant in the department. Your senior house officer (SHO) calls you to discuss with an individual at reception regarding an FOI request (the same request as above).
You are aware that a local newspaper has recently reported on long waiting lists in your department.

What should you do?

Advise the individual of the same information as above. You should forward the request to the FOI team immediately. Provide:

- All the details of the information requested
- The individual's contact details
- Highlight the media interest to the FOI team

You should also inform the trust media team and legal team about the request.

You should ensure that all staff are aware of the media/social media policy and ensure that any requests of information from the media should be sent to the media team.

- If the relevant information is your responsibility, you should begin obtaining it to ensure it is available within the 20-working day timeframe

You are aware of the child, and know they are likely to be booked for treatment in the next few weeks. What do you do?

You should not volunteer information regarding a patient, unless you are confident the individual has parental responsibility. If you cannot guarantee the date/timeframe, this information should not be given.

Three days later, you receive a subject access request for another child in the department. What do you do?

- Confirm that you are the most appropriate person to review the records i.e. the lead consultant for this patient
- If multiple specialities were involved in the patient's care, you should highlight to the health records department which speciality/individuals should also be approached
- The record should be reviewed as soon as possible (routinely within five working days), so that the trust adheres to the legal/trust requirement
- The patient records should be reviewed to ensure:
  - To the best of your knowledge whether disclosure might cause harm
  - To the best of your knowledge if the patient and/or parent (or anyone else) has requested that these records not be disclosed
  - Identify any missed records (such as dental study casts or images)

What information should be redacted?
- Other patient data
- 3rd party personal data e.g. information regarding other patients or details regarding family members that may be mentioned in the notes (unless they have agreed to their information being shared)
- Legally privileged information (e.g. solicitor letters, legal emails)
- Information that would cause harm if released
- Confidential information—if you are aware it is the patient's wish that this information should not be disclosed

You feel the comments may be upsetting for the patient, should this be redacted?
No, the 'serious harm test' should be applied. The ICO guidance states 'the exemption only applies to the extent that compliance with the right of access would be likely to cause serious harm to the physical or mental health of any individual'.

If you are unsure whether harm will be caused, who can you ask for help or a second opinion?
Where there is any doubt as to whether disclosure would cause serious harm, you should discuss the matter anonymously either with an experienced colleague, the DPO, the Caldicott Guardian, or the legal team.

You notice a mistake in the notes. Can you delete or correct it?
No, it is a criminal offence under the Data Protection Act 2018 to amend or delete records in response to a subject access request.

It is also against professional standards to amend the information. The most up-to-date information must be provided in response to a subject access request.

Amendments to records can be made, provided the amendments are made in a way which indicates why and when the alteration was made.

Scenario—Information governance breach

You are an SHO in a dental department. You lose your laptop on a train, it contains information for an audit that you are undertaking. You think the laptop was encrypted.

Considerations:
- Data Protection
- Confidentiality
- Consent
- Disciplinary issue
- Training Issue

What do you do?
- Immediately, if appropriate and feasible, you should try to recover the laptop
- If the laptop is recovered, you should still notify the:
  - ICT, to confirm that the device was encrypted and it is not possible for another individual to have accessed the data
  - DATIX the incident, inform the information governance team

- If the laptop is not recoverable, you should still inform ICT and complete a DATIX. You should ascertain whether ICT may be able to wipe the data remotely

You are informed by the IT department that the laptop was actually not encrypted. The details of 100 patients (date of birth, initials and diagnosis) were on the computer. Is this a concern?

- Yes it is a significant concern. The files were unsecured, so somebody could have accessed sensitive data
- As the laptop was not encrypted, there is no way for the you or the trust to determine whether the data had been accessed
- You cannot be certain that a risk to patients 'data subjects' did not occur
- The information was pseudonymized. It would be possible to determine the identity of individuals, and this is a data breach
- The information governance team, Caldicott Guardian, and consultant responsible for the audit should be informed. The DATIX should be updated
- While this would be managed by the appointed consultant/service manager you should immediately establish a list of the patients who are affected by this data breach
- The DPO would be informed, they would report the incident to the ICO
- The media/communications and legal team would draft a letter to potentially affected patients

Is the use of patient data in this manner lawful?

- The lawful basis for the processing of special category data (health data) under the GDPR or purposes of clinical audit falls under: 9(2)(h) ' … medical diagnosis, the provision of health or social care or treatment or the management of health or social care systems … '
- However, other principles of GDPR must be fulfilled including ensuring integrity and confidentiality, which may not have been fulfilled in this situation

Scenario—Lost memory card

You are a consultant in a department, a staff grade informs you that the memory card used for clinical photography went missing two days prior. They last used it to upload clinical photographs to their laptop for examination purposes.

What are the possible issues here?

- Loss of patient confidential data—data breach
- Professional conduct
- Failure to provide appropriate resources or processes
- Failure to foster an environment of trust—delay in reporting
- Loss of patient confidence
- Reputational and financial repercussions for the department/trust

What policies are of relevance and guide your response?
- Information governance policy
- Acceptable use of ICT
- Confidentiality policy

Who manages this situation
- As the responsible consultant you would manage the situation and ensure that appropriate action is taken now and preventative measures implemented to avoid future incidents
- The information governance response will be managed by the DPO and IG team including determining whether the situation is reportable to the ICO
- It may appropriate to discuss with the Caldicott Guardian if processes require reviewing
- The clinical lead and HR department would be involved if there is a concern regarding professional conduct. It is important to consider why was there a two-day delay before the issue was reported

What are your immediate concerns/actions?
The immediate goal is to minimize the risk to patient safety and determine what has happened. This will establish the gravity of the situation and appropriate response. Speak with the staff grade, establish:
- Is the memory card recoverable: Where did they last have it? Where and how it was lost? Can they retrace their steps?
- Confirm if it was a trust or personal device. A trust laptop may be encrypted and allow remote wiping of data
- If a personal device, was it encrypted or password protected?
- What data was involved. What the images comprised of (dental only, or face photos), the number of patients, the age of patients

If the card can be wiped remotely, does this still present a data breach?
- If the data is not backed up and is unrecoverable, this is still considered a data breach

Short-term action
The relevant teams should be informed. This includes the information governance team, who will:
- Investigate and keep a log of the incident
- Under the DPO, they will determine if the breach is reportable to the ICO (within 72 hours). Information will be passed to the CQC
- Determine whether it is necessary to inform patients, i.e. if there is a risk to their rights and freedoms. If so, a list of patient names should be established
- Involve the media/communications and legal teams, based on the number of patients involved and the type of images. They will review the communication prior to it being sent to patients. This will include:
  - What happened including what data was lost and where
  - What measures the trust and department are undertaking to prevent this occurring in the future
  - The complaints process

- Report the incident using the Department of Social Policy and Intervention (DSPI) reporting tool
- Incident form (DATIX) should be completed. This will also alert the relevant teams, including:
  - Complaints team
  - Risk management team
  - It will also be placed for allocation and discussion on the RAG, to ensure appropriate follow-up has been undertaken

Take action to prevent the situation from recurring, for example an agreement that:
- Clinical photographs are only taken by medical illustration
- An email to all staff, advising them that clinical photos should be immediately uploaded and deleted

You should ascertain why this situation arose and why there was delay in reporting the incident. This will be through speaking with the staff grade and other members of the clinical team. Contributing factors may be:
- A failure to follow an established protocol
- A lack of awareness or insight into the importance of information governance—a failure of induction and/or training
- A deficiency in the process of taking clinical photographs—such as lack of clear standard operating procedure (SOP) or lack of departmental resources (clinical camera or encryptable drives)
- This is likely a difficult/stressful situation for the staff grade. Regardless of conduct, you should offer support from the outset. Any conversations with them should not be accusatory, instead aim to establish what has happened and how this will be prevented in the future. You may signpost occupational health and/or advise them to speak with their indemnity provider for additional advice

Medium-term action

The incident should be disseminated to the rest of the department:
- Logged in the department incident book
- Raised at a departmental team meeting
- If there was a failure to follow established protocol, leading to a data breach, the trust disciplinary process should be followed (see Chapter 7, Staff management)

In instances where there was a lack of knowledge:
- Review statutory and mandatory training records for each member of staff
- Additional training for the department as a whole
- The induction policy should be reviewed

In instances where there is an inappropriate or deficient workflow. It would routinely be the 'owner' of the incident, appointed by the local RAG who leads on finding a solution. This would usually be a member of the consultant body or service manager. This may be:
- Service level agreement and/or training of medical illustration
- Procurement of hardware
- Establish a clear protocol for clearing of non-encryptable hard-drives
- Establish a secure location for non-encrypted memory card/drives
- If the delay in reporting reflects a poor working environment, this should be investigated, and measures taken to improve this. This would

be established by speaking with the staff grade, other members of the junior dental team and nursing/support team
- The annual trust staff survey or a review of other patient safety incidents may provide further insight

Additional limited information governance scenarios

The following are examples drawn from the ICO on risk categorization:
For each, regardless of actual harm or near miss, the standard principles of obtaining further information, escalation, risk management, and dissemination as described in the previous examples should be taken.

A consultant copies a clinic letter to a child's birth parents; it contains the name and address of foster parents.
- This presents a high risk to the child and foster parents' safety
- The foster parents, safeguarding team, and local authority should be informed as soon as this becomes apparent, allowing steps to minimize the risk to be taken—such as moving the child and perhaps foster parents into alternative accommodation or putting additional safeguarding measures in place
- This is a reportable incident to the ICO and warrants an investigation and possible steps to prevent recurrence

An urgent '2-week' referral is sent to the orthopaedic department instead of the oral and maxillofacial department.
- The referral should be redirected immediately to the correct department
- Despite the data being special category—both the sender and recipient work for the trust with the same data security measures, and should have completed training on working with vulnerable people
- It is very unlikely that there would be any risk of harm or detriment
- The breach does not need to be reported to the individual or the ICO
- The process to direct referrals should be reviewed
- This may warrant additional staff training, given the clinical risk

An administrative member of dental team accidentally deletes the study leave records of the dental team. The details are later re-created from a back-up.
- This is unlikely to result in a high risk to the rights and freedoms of those individuals
- The individuals or ICO do not need to be informed about the breach
- The regularity of data back-up for these and other records should be reviewed

A member of the administrative team accidentally sends incorrect health records to another member of the administrative team. They inform the sender immediately and delete the information securely.
- This is unlikely to result in a risk to the rights and freedoms of the individual
- The individual or ICO does not need to be informed about the breach

A dental nurse opens an email and inadvertently enters their login credentials into a website. The following day they notice they are no longer receiving emails.

The ICT and information governance teams are informed, and they establish that a third party responded to several emails using a spoofed email account, requesting funds from patients for treatment undertaken.

- Regardless of whether payments are made, this incident poses a high risk to patients' rights and freedoms
- The ICO and affected patients should be notified about the breach

Further reading

CQC (2018). Information Governance Policies. Available at: ℘ https://www.cqc.org.uk/sites/defa ult/files/20190228%20CQC%20Information%20Governance%20Policies.pdf

GDC (2024). Guidance on using social media. Available at: ℘ https://www.gdc-uk.org/docs/defa ult-source/guidance-documents/guidance-on-using-social-media.pdf?sfvrsn=de158345_2

General Medical Council. Confidentiality guidance: Sharing information with a patient's partner, carers, relatives or friends. Available at: ℘ https://www.gmc-uk.org/professional-standards/ the-professional-standards/confidentiality/disclosing-patients-personal-information-a-framew ork#:~:text=In%20such%20cases%2C%20you%20should,deciding%20to%20disclose%20 the%20information

Gov.uk. Data protection. Available at: ℘ https://www.gov.uk/data-protection/find-out-what-data- an-organisation-has-about-you

Gov.uk (2003). Confidentiality: NHS Code of Practice: Department of Health guidance on con- fidentiality. Available at: ℘ https://www.gov.uk/government/publications/confidentiality-nhs- code-of-practice

Gov.uk (2010). Confidentiality: NHS Code of Practice Supplementary Guidance—Public Interest Disclosures: Department of Health guidance on when you can share information for the good of the public. Available at: ℘ https://www.gov.uk/government/publications/confidentiality-nhs- code-of-practice-supplementary-guidance-public-interest-disclosures

ICO. For organisations. Available at: ℘ https://ico.org.uk/for-organisations/

ICO. UK GDPR guidance and resources. Available at: ℘ https://ico.org.uk/for-organisations/uk- gdpr-guidance-and-resources/

ICO (2019). Data protection if there's no Brexit deal. Available at: ℘ https://ico.org.uk/for-organi sations/data-protection-and-brexit/data-protection-if-theres-no-brexit-deal/the-gdpr/intern ational-data-transfers/

ICO (2019). Guide to data protection. Available at: ℘ https://ico.org.uk/media/for-organisations/ guide-to-data-protection-1-1.pdf

Information Governance Alliance. The General Data Protection Regulation—What's new. Available at: ℘ https://www.lanarkshirelmc.org.uk/wp-content/uploads/2018/04/IGA_-_GDPR_What s_new_guidance_V1_FINAL.pdf

Information Governance Alliance. The General Data Protection Regulation—Guidance on Consent. Available at: ℘ https://www.lanarkshirelmc.org.uk/wp-content/uploads/2018/04/IGAGDPR Consent.pdf

NHS England (2021). Records Management Code of Practice 2021. Available at: ℘ https://transf orm.england.nhs.uk/media/documents/NHSX_Records_Management_CoP_V7.pdf

NHS England. Transformation Directorate: Information governance. Available at: ℘ https://transf orm.england.nhs.uk/information-governance/

NHS England. NHS England launches new universal information governance templates. Available at: ℘ https://www.dsptoolkit.nhs.uk/News/templates

NHS England. About information governance. Available at: ℘ https://www.england.nhs.uk/ig/ about/

NHS England (updated 2024). Social media. Available at: ℘ https://www.england.nhs.uk/long- read/social-media/

Nuffield Trust (2011). Information governance in health. Available at: ℘ https://www.nuffieldtrust. org.uk/research/information-governance-in-health

Royal College of Psychiatrists. Carers and confidentiality in mental health: issues involved in information-sharing: guidance on sharing information on a patient's mental health with their carer. Available at: ℘ https://www.rcpsych.ac.uk/docs/default-source/improving-care/better-mh-pol icy/college-reports/college-report-cr209.pdf?sfvrsn=23858153_2

Schlegel DR, Ficheur G (2017). Secondary use of patient data: review of the literature published in 2016. *Yearb Med Inform*, 26(1):68–71.

UK Council of Caldicott Guardians guidance (2017). Caldicott Guardian Manual. Available at: ✄ https://www.ukcgc.uk/caldicott-guardians-manual

Your Europe. Data protection under GDPR. Available at: ✄ https://europa.eu/youreurope/business/dealing-with-customers/data-protection/data-protection-gdpr/index_en.htm#shortcut-6

Chapter 9

Trainee management

Regulators and training bodies

High-quality dental postgraduate training is the responsibility of multiple training organizations and professional bodies (see Box 9.1).

Embedded within these organizations are individuals and training committees that share the responsibility of ensuring excellent training is delivered and patient safety is prioritized.

General Dental Council

- Protects patient safety
- Registers all qualified dental professionals and investigates concerns of fitness to practise
- Sets standards of conduct, performance, and ethics for dental teams
- Sets standards for UK providers of dental education and training
- Quality assures speciality training (with exception of post-Certificate of Completion of Speciality Training (CCST))
- Approves speciality curricula
- Monitors continuing professional development of all registrants

Joint Committee for Postgraduate Training in Dentistry

- Develops speciality curricula
- Makes recommendations to the GDC on speciality training
- Develops assessments and examinations for speciality training
- Advises the GDC on applications for specialist listing based on claimed equivalence
- Makes recommendations to the GDC on recognition of previous training towards speciality training

---

> ### Box 9.1 Key organizations and professional bodies involved in postgraduate dental training
>
> - General Dental Council (GDC)
> - NHS England, Workforce, Training, and Education Directorate NHSE (WT&E)
> - Health Education and Improvement Wales (HEIW)
> - NHS Education for Scotland (NES)
> - Northern Ireland Medical and Dental Training Agency (NIMDTA)
> - Committee of Postgraduate Dental Deans (COPDEND) working through Dental Foundation Advisory Group (DFTAG), Dental Core Training Advisory Group (DCTAG) and Dental Speciality Training Advisory Group (DSTAG)
> - The Joint Committee for Postgraduate Training in Dentistry (JCPTD) working though the Royal College Specialist Advisory Committees (SACs)
> - Employers; NHS trusts, universities, lead education providers (LEP), NHS practices, NHS boards, health boards

---

Postgraduate dental deans

- Quality management of all dental postgraduate training

- COPDEND develops and approves curricula for dental foundation and dental core training
- Approval of training programmes and posts
- Appointment of trainees and trainers for Foundation and Vocational training, Training Programme Directors (TPD) and Speciality Training Committee (STC) Chairs
- STCs operate on behalf of Postgraduate Dental Deans (PGDD) to implement policy, standards, and regulations for speciality training and ensure the curriculum is delivered
- Review of trainee progress (see review of progress, page 340)
- Recommends speciality trainees to the GDC for the award of a CCST (see completion of training, page 344)

Employers

- Provide a supportive training environment for both the educator and the trainee and to ensure patient safety
- Ensure all those with supervisory responsibility are appropriately trained and have sufficient time dedicated to support their role as an educator
- Provide appropriate facilities and equipment to support the delivery of training
- Ensure access to suitable patients for training requirements

The training pathway

A new model for postgraduate dental training is under development and is being designed, following graduation, to incorporate exposure to primary and secondary care settings. The intention is to enable a broader experience of managing complex care and development of transferable skills which will facilitate career progression. The current dental training pathways in England, are illustrated in Figure 9.1. The Academic training pathway is detailed in a later section (see academic training pathway, page 346).

Dental foundation/vocational training

- The majority of graduates from dental schools in the UK undertake dental foundation training (DFT) or the Scotland equivalent, dental vocational training (DVT)
- This is an established means for newly qualified dentists to practice, improve their skills, and acquire necessary competences to work independently in NHS general dental practice
- All training is mapped to a curriculum approved by COPDEND
- The assessment system is approved by COPDEND for DFT and NHS Education for Scotland (NES) for DVT
- Trainees gain knowledge of clinical governance and practice management as well as gain more experience in clinical skills
- 12 months or equivalent spent in a practice setting with study days

Dental core training

- Varies in length from one to three years
- Posts may be longitudinal, offering two years of dental core training (DCT) or a combined two-year programme of joint dental foundation core training (JDFTC)
- It is not a statutory requirement but an opportunity to undertake further training
- The curriculum and assessment system is approved by COPDEND
- Training takes place in practice, community, and hospital settings
- Exposure to a wide range of dental disciplines and educators, offers a valuable opportunity to acquire further knowledge and skills and enables clarification of career intentions
- Undertaking three years of DCT can equip an individual with the necessary skillset to progress to provision of enhanced care or entry to speciality training

Dental speciality training

A dentist in the UK is not restricted from undertaking any treatment provided they have the capability and are appropriately indemnified. However, any dentist must be registered on the specialist list if they are to refer to themselves as a specialist. The GDC recognizes and approves the curricula for 13 dental specialities (see Table 9.1). The majority of entrants onto a specialist list follow the Certificate of Completion of Speciality Training (CCST) pathway, which requires:

- GDC registration as a dentist
- Have successfully completed an approved programme (with National Training Number (NTN)) including all entry, training, and assessment criteria

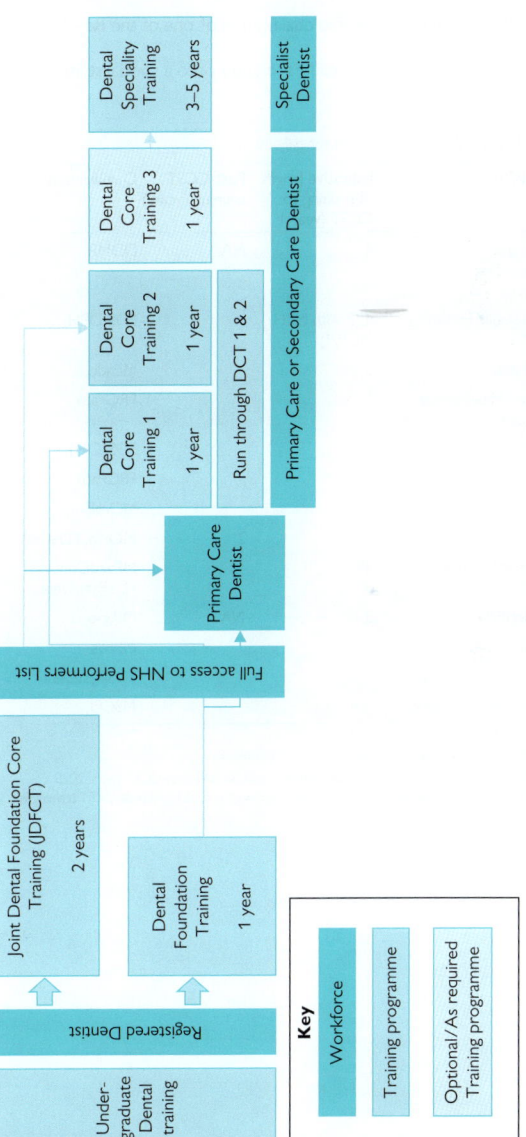

Figure 9.1 Current dental training pathways in England. Reproduced from NHS England, Workforce, Training and Education Directorate.

- Hold the relevant membership qualification of one of the Royal Colleges
- The GDC offers alternative routes to entry onto a specialist list

Table 9.1 GDC-approved dental specialities

Speciality	Indicative length of training to CCST (years)[a]	Post-CCST training (years)	Qualification
Dental and Maxillofacial Radiology	4	NA	DDMR
Dental Public Health	4 (3 with MPH/MDPH)		FDS(DPH)
Endodontics	3		MEndo
Oral and Maxillofacial Pathology	5		FRCPath
Oral Medicine	5		FDS(OM)
Oral Microbiology	5		FRCPath
Oral Surgery	3-4		MOralSurg
Orthodontics	3[b]	2	MOrth, FDSOrth
Paediatric Dentistry	4[b]		MPaedDent, FDSPaedDent
Periodontics	3	NA	MPerio
Prosthodontics	3		MPros
Restorative Dentistry	5		FDSRestDent
Special Care Dentistry	3-4		MSCD

[a] Length of training may be reduced in specific circumstances.

[b] Run-through training posts are available, combining CCST, and post-CCST years. 2025 Paediatric dentistry have introduced a four year pathway to CCST and post-CCST training will be phased out.

Training management

Since 2009, considerable efforts have been made to provide guidance for trainees and their trainers, to outline the regulations and assessment processes for all training pathways. There have been various editions and iterations of these documents but they have most recently been distilled into key references.

Key framework documents

- A Reference Guide for Postgraduate Dental Foundation Training in England, Wales, and Northern Ireland, The Dental Blue Guide. 2nd edition 2022
- The Dental Gold Guide: A Reference Guide for Postgraduate Dental Core and Speciality Training in the UK. DGG 4th edition September 2023
- Guidance on DVT Assessment. NHS Education for Scotland 2023–2024

Curricular requirements, assessment modalities, and the length of training differ considerably across the training pathways and specialities but guidance is provided within these documents on key themes.

In addition to the roles of the wider organizations (see Regulators and Training Bodies) and other training committees, there are a number of individuals with specific roles and responsibilities relating to the management of postgraduate training and reviewing the progress of each trainee.

Associate Postgraduate Dean or equivalent
- Supports the management of training programme
- Provides guidance and support for all educators
- Available to support progress reviews
- Assists PGDD with those trainees requiring additional support

Training programme director
- Participates in local arrangements for managing training programmes
- Supports national and local recruitment processes
- Plans programmes to account for the collective needs of the trainees and ensures curriculum delivery
- Provides guidance and support for all supervisors and trainers
- Chairs the STC (regional variations may exist)
- Contributes to all progress reviews (often chairs panel)
- Assists with those trainees requiring additional support including the necessary escalation of concerns to the PGDD

Educational supervisor
- Overall responsibility for supervision and management of a trainee's progress
- Appropriately trained to deliver their responsibilities including knowledge of the relevant curricula, educational theory, and practical educational techniques
- Provides regular assessment opportunities (DFT and DVT)
- Provides opportunities to regularly feedback to the trainee and revise learning plans

- Contributes to the review of progress through completion of a formal report
- Provision of career guidance
- Understands the processes in place for escalation of concerns

Clinical supervisor
- Appropriately trained to teach, undertake assessments, and provide regular opportunities for feedback in the clinical setting
- Provides a level of supervision commensurate with the trainee's capability and learning needs and consistent with maintaining patient safety at all times
- Contributes to the formal review of progress through clinical supervisor reports
- Understands the processes in place for escalation of concerns and liaises closely with the educational supervisor (ES)

Academic supervisor
- Responsible for overseeing academic progress of a specified trainee
- Appropriately trained to provide regular opportunities for feedback in the research setting
- Contributes to the review of progress through completion of a formal report

In different pathways an educator may take on more than one supervisory role. In DFT the ES will also be the clinical supervisor (CS) for the majority of the week. In DCT and dental speciality training (DST) there are likely to be multiple CSs in a particular placement and this may or may not include the ES.

Recruitment

The recruitment of dental postgraduate trainees is predominantly via a national recruitment process overseen by a National Recruitment Working Group. In England this is the only process for recruitment of DFT, DCT, DST, and post-CSST posts. In Scotland, NES runs a centralized recruitment process for DVT. The PGDDs of NES, HEIW, and NIMDTA can elect to hold a local recruitment for dental core, speciality, or post-CCST training. Oriel is the UK-wide portal for recruitment to postgraduate dental training. Applicants use Oriel for all stages of recruitment.

Key stages of recruitment

All recruitments should follow the principles of values-based recruitment which includes:
- Fair to all candidates
- Openly competitive and designed to identify and rank candidates most likely to successfully complete the training programme
- Compliant with employment law and best practice in recruitment and selection

The specific details of the recruitment process will vary from programme to programme and may change annually but the key steps usually include:
- Online application process through Oriel. All applicants must carefully review the person specification, eligibility criteria, and job description before applying
- Selection process which may include any of the following:

- Situational judgement test
- Self-assessment
- Assessment centre (online) with a multistation format
- Ranking of candidates
- Preferencing of schemes or posts by candidates
- Offering of posts and acceptance

On occasion, where posts have not been recruited to via a national process, there may be an opportunity for local recruitment. These posts may be for a specified time period and while competencies may be gained while in post it will not necessarily count towards a future training pathway.

Academic recruitment

Applicants for academic posts must apply through a local or national academic selection process and unless already in a speciality training post with a NTN, must be benchmarked at the relevant national DCT or DST recruitment process. Benchmarking is only valid until the next round of recruitment (see also: academic training pathway, page 346).

National Certificate of Dental Core Equivalence (NCDCE)

Applicants wishing to apply for speciality training are required to demonstrate they have achieved the requisite competences consistent with completion of UK DCT year 1 at the time of interview and of UK DCT year 2 at the time of post commencement. The NCDCE was developed to facilitate entry into speciality training for those who have not followed the standard UK training route. Applications for NCDCE occur annually. This process can also be used by applicants for DCT3 posts if they have not already undertaken a DCT2 post.

Undertaking a training programme

Performer list numbers

- All DFTs (England and Wales only) must have a performer list number by time of appointment
- Inclusion in the NHS performers list in England and Wales (or equivalent in Northern Ireland) is a legal requirement for a dentist to work in NHS primary care dental services
- Application for a performer list number should commence well in advance of the start date of the training programme. For most this will be on receipt of a graduation certificate
- Graduates from non-UK dental schools, and graduates from dental schools with more than 12 months of experience working as a dentist may apply to join the Performers List by other routes
- Training will end in the following circumstances and only in certain situations can the trainee appeal the decision:
  - Successful completion of training
  - Trainee voluntarily resigns from training prior to completion
  - PGDD decides trainee is not suitable to continue in training
  - The trainee does not hold GDC registration, has had their name erased or suspended from the register or placed under restrictions which are incompatible with continued training
  - Unable to gain entry, erased, or suspended from the NHS performers list or equivalent

National training numbers
- National training numbers (NTNs) are reserved for those trainees who have been recruited through open competition for a place on a speciality or post-CCST training programme
- NTNs may only be issued by the PGDD
- The number is unique to the trainee and is speciality and location specific. This enables the PGDD to have oversight of the location and progress of trainees
- The numbers provide valuable workforce information and assist with planning education delivery and future recruitment
- A trainee holds the NTN until training is completed (including a period of grace), they resign, or the NTN is withdrawn
- Withdrawal of the NTN occurs under the same circumstances as training ending (see above)
- When the PGDD decides to withdraw the NTN, the employer must be informed. This normally leads to termination of the employer contract
- DCTs are not allocated NTNs

Defence primary healthcare
- The Defence Postgraduate Medical Deanery (DPMD) works with the relevant PGDD to identify an appropriate training placement in practice to allow for the training of foundation dentists to meet the needs of the armed forces
- Dentists selected by the defence dental services suitable for undertaking speciality training must be benchmarked at the relevant national recruitment process
- The DPMD will identify an appropriate training programme in discussion with the PGDD
- Review of progress follows the same process as for other postgraduate dental trainees but with the inclusion of a representative from the DPMD on the panel at least annually

Less than full-time training
All trainees, at the time of appointment are eligible to apply for less than full-time training (LTFT). In a bid to provide more flexibility in training opportunities, retain the workforce, and offer better work-life balance, applications for LTFT are carefully considered and, where possible, approved but they are not guaranteed. Training programme capacity and service needs must also be considered with LTFT applications therefore decisions are made jointly between the education provider and the employer.
- Applications may be submitted at the time of appointment or at any point during training and will usually take three months to process
- Training is ordinarily no less than 50% of the full-time equivalent
- Any changes in working hours, once LTFT has commenced requires further approval from the PGDD
- Training reflects the same balance of work as those in full-time posts
- Any additional work undertaken outside of the training programme is declared on Form R
- All LTFT trainees should have a review of progression at least annually

Breaks in training

The most frequent requests for a break in training are for statutory reasons such as maternity/paternity/adoption or sick leave. However, to promote more flexible training pathways, retain the workforce and career enhancement other Out of Programme (OOP) opportunities exist for speciality trainees but require PGDD approval: career break (OOPC), clinical experience (OOPE), research (OOPR), and training (OOPT).

- OOPE, OOPT, and OOPC are usually approved for one year but can be extended to maximum of two years at discretion of the PGDD
- OOPR is normally approved for no longer than three years but exceptional approval may be granted by the PGDD up to a maximum of four years
- Any Time out of Training (TOOT) has the potential to impact on a trainee achieving the competences required of their programme. An absence of 10 days or more in any 12-month period will trigger a review of the completion date at the next review of progression
- A break in training, particularly one longer than three months, requires careful planning of the return with the training programme director (TPD) and educational supervisor (ES). Patient safety is always the priority

Inter-deanery transfers

- An inter-deanery transfer (IDT) is available to those DCT (certain posts only) and DST trainees who have experienced a significant change in circumstance since commencement of their training programme. Requests are not usually considered until a trainee has been in post for a minimum of 12 months
- Eligibility criteria are in place but there is no right to a transfer
- A nationally agreed process exists for reviewing IDTs and requires approval from the PGDD in both regions affected
- The acceptance of an IDT into certain regions outside of National Health Service England (NHSE) will also be dependent on the trainee's review of competency progression (RCP) outcome

Form R

Form R, a 'registration for postgraduate training form' is a self-declaration form completed by postgraduate dentists for the purposes of registration and monitoring. This form is obtained from and should be returned to the postgraduate dental dean.

The form:
- Initiates the issuing of an NTN
- Ensures the trainee is registered on NHSE, HEIW, NES, and NIMDTA database
- Initiates the review of competence progression (RCP) system through which trainee progress is monitored
- Allows the postgraduate dental dean to inform the relevant SAC of the appointment
- Enables the postgraduate dental dean to inform the trainee's employer of the trainee's starter information and the NTN
- Records the date of entry into the programme and likely CCST date

The form is completed annually as part of the annual review of competency progression (ARCP) process, and includes:

- Dentist's whole scope of practice, including work outside of training programmes
- Declaration of good clinical practice
- Declaration of significant events

Review of progress

A review of competency progression (RCP) is a mandatory requirement for those in postgraduate dental training. It is a formal process and all pathways have at least one review in any 12-month period. Assessment requirements for DVT in Scotland are determined by NES.

Review of competency progression panels

Table 9.2 details the type of review, timing, and panel construction.

- Review of competency progression (RCP)
- Annual review of competency progression (ARCP)
- Final review of competency progression (FRCP)

External representatives are a key component of the quality management procedure. At DFT and DCT level this is usually provided by a TPD or associate dean (AD) from another scheme or region. In addition, a lay representative reviews the process and panel conduct, and provides assurance of consistency and fairness. Speciality reviews require the presence of a SAC representative who also reviews a proportion of portfolios and may offer advice to the panel. The external representatives provide a formal report on completion of the process.

Table 9.2 Review timing and panel construction

	Review	Timing (months)	Panel construction (minimum requirements)
Dental foundation/ vocational	RCP	6	AD or equivalent
			TPD or equivalent from another scheme in region
	FRCP	10	AD and AD from another region, or TPD from another programme in or out of region
			Lay representative
Longitudinal	RCP	6, 10, & 18	As above for RCP
	FRCP	22	As above for FRCP
Dental core	RCP	6	PGDD or nominated deputy TPD and/or ES or CS
	FRCP	11–12	Academic member[a]
			AD from a different region
			Lay representative
Dental speciality and post-CCST	RCP	6[b]	As above for DCT but external member from the relevant SAC rather than AD from a different region
	ARCP	10–14	

[a] if academic trainee is being reviewed

[b] a mid-point review is usually only undertaken for those in year one of speciality or post-CCST training

At each review the following is expected:
- Careful assessment of all evidence of a trainee's progress and performance; the ES report is central to this
- Trainee's ES is not involved in the outcome decision
- Outcome decisions are based purely on the evidence contained within the e-portfolio as all reviews are *in absentia*
- Assess the impact of any time out of training that has occurred
- A judgement as to whether sufficient progress will allow continuation of training or recommendation for completion of training

Portfolios

Each curriculum will clearly state, often in the form of a checklist, what the requirements are to achieve a satisfactory outcome at the time of each review. The use of checklists and decision aids for trainees and their educators when preparing for reviews, provides clarity as to what is expected and assists with standardisation and consistency across the UK. Electronic portfolios (e-portfolios) have replaced paper-based versions and different platforms are used across the training pathways and organizations (see Table 9.3). A trainee will need to provide evidence of any assessments and other evidence may be included (see Box 9.2).

Assessments

Assessment is used to inform learning, provide feedback, and inform decisions regarding progress. Formative assessments are designed to assess learning with a focus on current strengths and weaknesses and provide feedback to create new learning plans and set goals. Summative assessments are assessments of learning and provide a gate-keeping function. One of the consequences of our education system, from school to higher education, is learners are conditioned to be more focused on summative assessments. Each training pathway has its own assessment system but the key to the success of any programmatic assessment is:
- Training of assessors
- Timing of assessment—spread throughout the programme
- Richness of the feedback from multiple assessors

All aspects of the curricula are assessed using one or more components of the assessment system. However, one of the defining characteristics of

---

Box 9.2 Additional information in portfolio
- Personal development plan
- Curriculum vitae
- Progress or completion of an audit or quality improvement project
- Progress or completion of a research project
- Progress or completion of speciality specific project work
- Clinical activity logbook
- Study day and/or CPD log
- Self-declaration of time out of training, involvement in any complaints or significant events
- Reflective log
- Publications

Table 9.3 Portfolios used in postgraduate dental education

e-Portfolio	Training pathway/speciality
Dental e-portfolio	Dental foundation training (except Scotland)
	Dental core training (except Scotland)
Turas	Dental vocational training (Scotland)
	Dental core training (Scotland)
Intercollegiate speciality curriculum portfolio (ISCP)	Endodontics
	Oral Medicine
	Oral Surgery
	Paediatric Dentistry
	Orthodontics
	Periodontics
	Prosthodontics
	Restorative Dentistry
	Special Care Dentistry
Royal College of Pathology Learning Environment for Pathology Trainees	Oral and Maxillofacial Pathology
	Oral Microbiology
Royal College of Radiologists Kaizen	Dental and Maxillofacial Radiology
NHS e-portfolio	Dental Public Health

DST is the requirement to pass professional exams prior to completion. Workplace Based Assessment (WBA) and Supervised Learning Event (SLE) are used interchangeably and refer to a range of assessments (see Table 9.4).

Following implementation of the revised specialty curricula in 2024, the assessment system will also undergo change. Validity and reliability of assessment methods are considered two of the most important characteristics of a well-designed assessment process. The validity of WBAs may be high if multiple assessments and assessors are involved. It is problematic, however, when detailed and effective feedback is not provided. Dentistry is likely to bring about changes that will reflect a more outcome-based assessment system with greater reliance on narrative feedback from senior clinicians and educators and less focus on the number of assessments.

RCP and ARCP outcomes

All trainees are issued an outcome during and on completion of training (see Table 9.5) Trainees should receive detailed formative feedback to help plan their development in their next phase of training. Appropriate preparation and educational meetings prior to the review ensure that a trainee receives an outcome that is expected.

At speciality level an outcome 2 or 3, also described as a developmental outcome, will usually necessitate an additional review of progress to be planned within six months. This ensures clear, time-limited objectives are

Table 9.4 Examples of assessments in postgraduate dental training

Formative	Summative
A dental evaluation of performance tool (ADEPT)[a]	Educational supervisor report
Longitudinal evaluation of performance (LEP)[b]	Trainer and adviser statement[b]
Direct observation of procedural skills (DOPS)	Review of competency progression (RCP)
Case-based discussion (CBD)	Annual review of competency progression (ARCP)[d]
Clinical evaluation exercise (CEX)	Final review of competency progression (FRCP)
Multisource feedback (MSF)	Professional exams[d]
Patient satisfaction questionnaire (PSQ)	
Assessment of audit (AoA)[c]	
Assessment of teaching (AoT)[c]	
Project-based assessment (PBA)[d]	

[a] Dental foundation training only

[b] Dental vocational training only

[c] Dental core and speciality training

[d] Speciality training only

set out to support the trainee in achieving the required competencies to progress to the next stage or complete training.

Any outcome 3 or 4 requires ratification by the PGDD. A panel will make a recommendation for the length of any extension in the event of an outcome 3 (maximum of 12 months (DFT and DCT) or 24 months (DST)). Adequate trainee engagement with the training programme is required to grant an extension.

Reviews and appeals of outcomes

Although a trainee should not be surprised by any outcome issued, they do have the right to request a review (outcome 2) or an appeal (outcome 3 or 4).

- Request for a review or an appeal must be in writing, stating the reasons, and within 10 days of the RCP outcome being issued
- A review requires the original panel to review the outcome, including any relevant information or additional evidence submitted by the trainee
- An appeal request ordinarily commences with the review process as described above. If a review panel decides the original outcome should stand the PGDD will confirm with the trainee their wish to proceed to an appeal panel. The appeal hearing requires a new panel to be convened that does not include original panel members. The decision of the appeal panel is final
- An appeal would normally be refused in situations where the GDC have erased a dentist from the register or a trainee has not completed training due to exhausting the number of attempts at an exam sitting

Table 9.5 Review of competency progression outcomes

Outcome		Definition
1		Satisfactory progress—achieving progress and the development of competences/capabilities at the expected rate.
2		Development of specific competences/capabilities required—additional training time not required (applicable for DCT).
3		Inadequate progress—additional training time required.
4	W	Released from training programme—with or without specified competences/capabilities.
	VR	Trainee voluntarily resigns from the programme.
5		Incomplete evidence presented—this is a holding outcome to allow for evidence to be uploaded, the panel must agree conversion to a final outcome.
6		Recommendation for completion of training—all required competences and capabilities have been achieved.
7		Applicable only to those in post-CCST training
	7.1	Satisfactory progress in or completion of training.
	7.2	Development of specific competences/capabilities required—additional training time not required.
	7.3	Trainee has not made adequate progress for this period of training.
	7.4	Released or resigned from training programme—with or without specified competences/capabilities.
	7.5	Incomplete evidence presented—this is a holding outcome, following a specified period of time, to allow for evidence to be uploaded, the panel must agree conversion to a final outcome.
8		Out of programme for clinical experience, research or a career break (OOPE, OOPR, OOPC). This is not applicable to DFT/DVT or DCT.
N		No outcome is issued when a trainee is out of training for statutory reasons.

Completion of training

Dental foundation and vocational training

Since 2004, satisfactory completion of DVT has conferred eligibility for a VT number and, in turn, an NHS performer number which allows a dentist to practice as an associate or principal within the NHS or as a salaried dentist in the Public Dental Service (PDS).

On satisfactory completion of DFT a trainee will be recommended, by the PGDD, for the award of Certificate of Satisfactory Completion of Dental Foundation Training (CSCDFT). This confers eligibility for the dentist to have their conditional inclusion in the NHS performers list changed to unconditional inclusion.

Dental core training

On completion of a DCT post, a trainee will receive a certificate to indicate they have undertaken training in an approved programme. The certificate will detail the outcome received at the FRCP.

Evidence of the skills and knowledge learnt during DCT may allow a trainee to successfully progress to speciality training.

Specialist listing

On receipt of an outcome 6 at a final RCP the PGDD will recommend the trainee for inclusion on the relevant GDC specialist list.

Acting up as consultant/specialist

Trainees may act up as a consultant/specialist within six months of their CCST date. 'Acting up' provides trainees with the experience of navigating the transition from a junior to a more senior position, while maintaining the supervision associated with being a trainee.

Opportunities to act up are not available to all trainees and are only possible if an employing or host local education provider/trust extends an invitation. Acting up must not be confused with undertaking a locum post, the trainee is moving into an established, substantive, approved post. (e.g. if a consultant is on extended leave).

The trainee must:
- Have the PGDD's and employer's approval
- Have passed the relevant examination
- Satisfactorily completed training to date
- Be deemed by the ES to be competent to undertake the role
- Must have appropriate named supervision arrangements in place at all times and continue to have an educational supervisor
- CCST holders in Orthodontics and Paediatric Dentistry must have completed 18 months (pro-rata) in a post-CCST appointment before acting up
- LTFT trainees can act up but on a pro-rata basis. Trainees can act up for individual sessions or longer periods of time (until end of training)
- Trainees acting up can credit time towards training if this has been prospectively approved by the PGDD. Such appointments do not affect the CCST date or grace period. The trainee maintains their National Training Number throughout the acting up opportunity

Academic training

The traditional funded route into dental academic training in the UK commences with an application for a National Institute of Health and Care Research (NIHR) Academic Clinical Fellowship (ACF). NIHR funded clinical academic training programmes allow dentists who have academic/research interests to have dedicated research time and support to prepare a PhD proposal. Their training programme time is split as follows: 75% clinical and 25% research. The complete eligibility criteria for the NIHR ACF can be found in the ACF guidance document on the NIHR website.

Academic training pathway

There is a two-stage process for securing an ACF post.
- Applicants submit an application, are shortlisted, and deemed appointable at the initial academic interview stage. The highest ranked applicant receives a conditional offer
- Candidates progress to the second stage of clinical benchmarking to ensure minimum clinical competencies. Candidates successful at this stage receive unconditional offers for ACF posts
- Each dental school is allocated two speciality ACF posts each year from the 12 dental specialities
- There is only one recruitment round each year if a successful applicant is identified
- These three-year fixed term posts are therefore competitively sought after due to their limited availability
- Candidates are expected to demonstrate an academic portfolio, ideally comprising of peer-reviewed publications, presentations, awards, research projects, etc. Many candidates opt to complete the HEE leadership fellowship and the NHS clinical senate leadership fellowship. For teaching experience, qualifications such as the Postgraduate Certificate in Dental Education are advantageous

Completion of PhD project

The principal challenge of the academic pathway is that during the ACF training, the academic needs to secure external funding for a PhD, which entails formulating a fundable project which is strengthened by preliminary research findings obtained during the 3-year funded ACF post.

Obtaining funding for a PhD remains extremely competitive, necessitating exploration of multiple funding sources, such as research councils, charitable organizations, and industry partnerships. One such example includes the NIHR doctoral fellowship, which fully funds the PhD, including part-clinical work and salary. They have dedicated advisors to provide guidance and support.

Following completion of the PhD, the applicant can apply for a HEE funded NIHR clinical lecturer post. Similar to ACF posts, these are competitive and subject to national recruitment and clinical benchmarking to be appointable. If successful, the progression from here relies on applying for an advertised university-appointed senior clinical lecturer post.

Study leave and courses

Generally, all dentists in postgraduate training have access to up to 30 days of study leave each year. The manner in which this allocation is used in each training programme will vary considerably but the purpose of all study leave and associated courses is to support curricula delivery.

- In DFT and DVT the full 30 days are committed to a mandatory study programme
- In DCT and DST a proportion of the study leave allowance may be allocated to mandatory and/or didactic teaching
- There is greater flexibility in the use of study leave during DCT and DST with a focus on curricula delivery and personal development
- Approval processes and funding for DCT and DST study leave will vary across specialities and regions
- All trainees must follow local employer processes for study leave applications

Trainees requiring additional support

Trainees may face all manner of challenges throughout their training pathway and may require additional support. Labels such as 'trainee in difficulty' are to be avoided as the stigma of this type of terminology has been a factor in learners being reluctant to seek out appropriate help and support. Formal guidance and protocols in place in the employing organization and at deanery/local education provider (LEP) level must be followed and should provide a systematic approach for both learners and their educators; the primary goal is to ensure that patient safety is not compromised and secondly, to facilitate continued training.

Key principles

- The training environment is supportive for both the educator and the trainee
- Trainees are confident in the skills of their educators to deliver their roles and responsibilities
- Effective and appropriate communication between educators and trainees is established early
- Early identification of problems and implementation of interventions
- Access to specialist educational and professional support services is available for trainees and their supervisors
- Remediation is proportionate and relevant based on clear criteria with the trainee taking personal responsibility in finding solutions and seeking appropriate support
- Concerns, discussions, and learning plans must be documented within an e-portfolio and/or trainee file and shared with the trainee. Reports must be written in a factual manner avoiding opinion and in language that is appropriate to be shared with those that need or request access
- Individuals (e.g. trainee, educator, training programme director, (TPD), postgraduate dental dean (PGDD)) and organizations (e.g. trust, LEP, health education institute (HEI), health board, National Health Service England (NHSE)) must have a clear understanding of their roles and collective responsibilities in ensuring patient safety and providing support to the trainee. This includes awareness of referral mechanisms to those who can provide additional support

The resources and support available for learners requiring additional support, and advice for educators, are plentiful and should be explored and used.

Roles and responsibilities

Personal and professional misconduct issues are in a minority and the vast majority of issues are quickly and effectively resolved with close working between the trainee and their supervisors.

Trainee

- Trainees are employees and subject to formal management guidelines and protocols within their organization
- Trainees need to take personal responsibility for their training including full engagement with the educational process and an active role in

highlighting any difficulties, finding solutions, and seeking the appropriate support
- Inform their TPD of any involvement in a serious incident, formal complaint or referral to the GDC (at the time of an ARCP this is now required to be declared on Form R)

Employer
- Responsible for performance management and disciplinary procedures
- Ensures employment laws are upheld and robust processes in place to identify, manage, and support any dentist in training where their performance, health or conduct has been a cause for concern, including advice from human resources (HR) and referral to occupational health
- Ensures clinical and educational supervisors are appropriately trained and that their job plans support the delivery of their educational responsibilities
- In Trusts/LEPs it is often the role of the Director of Medical Education (DME) to confirm how allegations or concerns are investigated in accordance with local HR policy
- Facilitates collaborative working between the DME, ES, and TPD to put in place appropriate support
- Guardian of Safe Working monitors hours of work

NHSE/health board/deanery
- Overarching responsibility for quality management of postgraduate dental education
- Provision of a TPD-led educational framework to respond to any dentist in training requiring additional support
- Planned programme of support for those returning to training following a prolonged absence
- Facilitates access to specialized support e.g. via Professional Support Unit
- There is a national system in place for the appropriate transfer of information from undergraduate to postgraduate training (Education Transition Document) and across postgraduate training organizations to allow for implementation of any necessary additional training support

GDC
- Must be made aware if a dentist in training is, for whatever reason, not deemed fit to practice and patient safety is at risk
- Referral to the GDC may be based on evidence of the following:
  - Serious and repeated mistakes in diagnosis or treatment
  - Fraud or theft
  - Treatment of patients without consent
  - Inappropriate behaviour towards a patient
  - Serious criminal offence or conviction
  - Failure to safeguard children or vulnerable adults

Identifying issues

Early warning signs for trainees facing difficulties may be noticed by any member of the team and shared with the clinical and educational supervisors. It is well recognized that periods of transition, such as changing jobs, moving regions, or commencing a new training programme may trigger a change in behaviour and increased vigilance is recommended. This of course can be problematic in itself. Training programmes where trainees are in one place for a longer period of time rather than rotating every six months can afford a better opportunity to observe any changes in behaviour. Knowledge of a trainee also helps to distinguish between one-off events or repeated patterns of behaviour. Paice and Orton (2004), described seven early warning signs, however, the list of possible signs is not exhaustive (see Box 9.3).

Exploring the underlying causes

An early conversation between the supervisor and the trainee, to establish and clarify the facts, usually allows for prompt identification of the cause, classification of the problem, and development of a specific learning plan, with effective interventions. The reasons for a trainee requiring additional help are wide-ranging but categorizing the cause may help:

Clinical capability
- Knowledge, skills, communication
- Limited experience in a specific clinical area
- Exam failure
- Complaints and serious incident involvement
- Colleague reports

Health and home
- Known or new medical condition, substance abuse
- Personal/family stress, isolation, or lack of integration
- Career frustrations
- Financial issues

Personality and behaviour
- Risky behaviours
- Professional/personal conduct issues
- Motivation
- Self-awareness and impaired insight
- Religious or cultural issues

Box 9.3 Early signs of trainees facing difficulty
- The disappearing act—lateness, absenteeism, unreliable
- Rigidity in thinking—inability to compromise or cope with ambiguity
- Low work rate—slow at completing tasks, poor documentation, arrives early, and leaves late without demonstrable productivity
- Lack of engagement in educational process—last-minute organization of assessments and appraisals, poor completion of e-portfolio
- Inappropriate emotional outbursts or rude and dismissive with colleagues
- Bypass syndrome—other team members avoid engaging with them
- Poor self-awareness—failure to respond to constructive criticism, defensiveness, counterchallenge
- Career problems—uncertainty over career pathway, exam failure, recruitment rejection, failure to learn and change
- Unkempt appearance, tiredness

Organizational issues
- Workload including workforce issues and lack of support
- Poor workplace culture, including bullying and harassment
- Service re-design

Planning remediation

Establishing the most effective interventions requires careful joint planning between the trainee and supervisor. Reports and feedback, from a variety of sources such as WBAs, clinical observations and MSF can provide the necessary 'diagnostic data' to identify the support and learning experiences required to address the underlying cause (see Table 9.6).

It is essential that remediation plans are bespoke to the individual, specific and time defined. Allowing the trainee to identify underdeveloped areas in their learning and create a specific learning plan, with guidance from their supervisor, encourages them to take a lead in the process. The learning goals are regularly reviewed to monitor progress and success.

Table 9.6 Identification of the cause and planning interventions

	Identify	Intervention
Practical skills	Assess or observed practice (DOPs) Feedback from colleagues	Specific feedback and guidance Observation of those highly skilled in procedure Simulation training Repeated opportunities to practice with 1:1 supervision
Clinical reasoning	CBD Clinical teaching Over-reliance on investigations Diagnostic errors	Develop subject knowledge Data interpretation Role modelling Increased clinical exposure, use of CBD with focus on decision making
Communication skills	CEX, DOP MSF Patient feedback	Specific feedback and guidance Video recording with self-review Formal training
Insight into performance	MSF with self-ratings Capacity to self-evaluate	Frequent opportunities to compare self Professional coaching and mentoring
Health concerns	Self-reported Sickness record and observation Feedback from colleagues	Immediate advice from OH and HR in matters of patient and personal safety Adjustments to work, short and long-term Break in training
Deficiencies in educational environment	Trainee feedback Serious incident report Workforce survey Exam failure	Local adjustments Quality intervention Suspension of training

Classifying concerns and escalation

- Organizations and education providers may classify concerns in different ways, e.g. level 1, 2, 3; low, intermediate, high. The level at which a concern is categorized will influence escalation processes and access to available support
- Most situations where a trainee requires additional support are resolved locally within the service or training programme with close collaboration between the clinical and educational supervisors
- Health concerns need particularly careful management especially in relation to sharing of confidential information. HR and OH may advise referral to other professional services
- The impact of any remediation plans on progression of training should be made clear within the e-portfolio. This then allows any future RCP or ARCP to consider the evidence when making outcome decisions including the need to delay progression or extend training
- Serious incident involvement needs to be declared by any dentist in training within their e-portfolio on Form R. The TPD and Associate Dean should also be informed. While the employer is responsible for undertaking an investigation, and ensuring there is learning from any serious incidents, it is important that pastoral support is also in place for the trainee
- In the rare event of serious professional or personal conduct issues the employer undertakes a formal disciplinary investigation and the PGDD must be informed, particularly if referral to the GDC is recommended. Poor performance of this magnitude is usually complex and often relates to interpersonal and personality difficulties. Educators must also be supported and fully understand their supervisory boundaries

Pedagogical theories

Ensuring that trainees are supported throughout their training pathway also extends to the use of the appropriate teaching styles. Many departments and academic programmes will use blended teaching methods, as there is a move away from didactic lecture-style teaching only and an increased awareness of varying learning theories and individual styles.

Psychology of learning

There are various general schemas which underpin the psychology involved in an individual's ability to learn. The two main concepts are:

Behaviourism

Underpinning concept: Learning is a behaviour; the learner becomes conditioned through stimulus and response.

- Learning occurs through repetition, which reinforces neural pathways and reduces the time between stimulus and response
- The response to the stimulus then becomes a reflex
- This is useful in clinical situations such as managing medical emergencies, however wider application in healthcare and education is limited

Activities associated with a behaviourist approach:

- Reading, reviewing, and analysis of provided text and materials
- Individual work submitted directly to the teacher for correcting
- Structured assignments directly linked to learning objectives
- Little or no cohort discussion

Constructivism

Underpinning concept: Learning is actively constructed by the student, not the educator. Individuals analyse and evaluate information and learn through processing the information and their responses.

- The main types are cognitive and social constructivism
- Cognitive constructivism refers to learning through making sense of an individual's own experiences; constructing meaning from them
- Dialogue enables the learner to reflect, contribute and share their understanding of concepts, and develop deeper learning as a result
- Social constructivism uses the zone of proximal development; the individual's current understanding is just exceeded, promoting learning
- Limitations of constructivism: learners are responsible for intelligent behaviour, success measured in terms of speed of learning and length of recall

Activities associated with a constructivist approach:

- Application of principles—case studies and projects
- Open-ended assignments linked to changing learning objectives
- Assignments reflect 'real world' conditions and requirements

Learning styles

Learning styles identify the preferred approach of the individual learner. There are a multitude of learning styles in educational research, with Honey and Mumford's 1992 index being the most commonly used. No single learning style has been identified as superior to others.

Activist

Underpinning concept: Active experimentation results in the best learning.
- Keen to try new ideas
- Activists learn best:
  - The learning is exciting especially if a new experience
  - Rapidly changing environment
  - They lead the teaching
  - They are set challenges yet given freedom in exploring them
- Activists learn least:
  - No social engagement, reading or writing on their own
  - Long explanations with passive listening or reading
  - Following specific instructions

Reflector

Underpinning concept: Experiential learning followed by reflection results in the best learning.
- Reflectors learn best:
  - Observe prior to starting the task
  - Given time to consider and reflect before starting
  - Having the opportunity to review and reflect after the task
  - Working towards a deadline
- Reflectors learn least:
  - Starting a task without preparation
  - Forced into leadership of a group
  - Rushed by a deadline

Theorist

Underpinning concept: Theoretical learning followed by trying out in practice results in the best learning.
- Theorists learn best:
  - A task is structured and reinforced with concepts and ideas
  - Opportunity to question
  - A task which requires complex understanding
- Theorists learn least:
  - Unstructured tasks
  - Tasks which involve a significant emotional factor
  - A task without knowing the principles involved

Pragmatist

Underpinning concept: Practical learning where an example or theory can be copied results in the best learning.
- Pragmatists learn best:
  - The task is demonstrated with clear and practical aspects
  - Feedback is received from the educator
  - The task can be replicated or emulated by the learner
- Pragmatists learn least:
  - There are no or unclear guidelines
  - Purely theoretical task, with no practical aspects
  - There is no immediate practical benefit

In reality, the preference for a particular learning style can change, depending on the task and also factors which are both intrinsic and extrinsic to the learner.

Philosophies in learning and teaching

There are various types of learning practice and a well-rounded trainee will ideally have experience of all types.

Experiential learning

Underpinning concept: Knowledge is created through transformation of experience (Kolb 1984).

- Experience is combined with reflection, to form abstract ideas, which are tested in a new situation. This is thinking critically about the learning experience encountered
- Each action leads to a paradigm shift, the subsequent cycle starts at a different initial point
- Does not account for learning indirectly through 'second-hand' experiences

Reflective practice

Underpinning concept: Learning occurs through observing real life situations (Schön, 1987)

- Students learn from listening, watching, doing, and coaching from the educator to perform the task
- Reflective process: Knowledge in action (observe)—reflection in action (during the task)—reflection on action (after the task)
- A limitation is that some tasks cannot be observed

Problem-based learning

Underpinning concept: Effective learning occurs through enquiry (Carl Rogers 1969.)

- Learning objectives are changed into a problem, where successful solutions are considered by the learner
- Group discussions analyse successful solutions, and formulate new questions / problems as new learning objectives
- The process: Problem (learning objective)—solution (with explanation)—discussion (small group discussion)—questions (unanswered questions are new learning objectives)
- Learners can deviate from the topic however and without a moderator there is a risk of significant variation of learning outcomes

Scenario—Repeatedly late trainee

You are a consultant in a Dental Hospital, you notice the new senior speciality trainee repeatedly attends late and often switches their clinic with another trainee.

Who manages this situation?

- As the responsible consultant for the clinic, it is your responsibility to ensure that the clinic runs safely and that patient care is not compromised. Initially you should investigate the situation
- If the situation is not resolved locally, concerns should be raised with the ES, who is responsible for the trainee
- Even if the situation is resolved locally the ES should still be informed. They will assess if this reflects a pattern of behaviour, if the situation requires additional investigation or if the trainee requires additional support

Can a trainee switch a clinic with colleagues?

- There are situations where a clinic switch is acceptable. However prior permission from the consultant responsible for the clinic should be sought
- Where a trainee is involved, this should be confirmed by the educational supervisor of both trainees. Trainees have requirements to meet to reach a level of clinical competency, thus they cannot choose clinics to change/omit at their own discretion

What do you do?

Speak to the trainee

- Establish if there are any difficulties with attending the clinic on time
- There may be an established change to the trainee's timetable (e.g. due to childcare) agreed with their educational supervisor, of which you are unaware
- Establish why they have switched clinics
- If this reflects an unfortunate coincidence, the situation may be resolved locally. The trainee should be reminded of their obligations to patient care and their own learning
- The educational supervisor should be informed. Depending on the trainee's insight and response, no further action may be required

You are the educational supervisor. A clinical supervisor reports the trainee is consistently late for clinics. What do you do?

- Gather more information. You need to establish if this affects this individual clinic or is a more generalized issue. Speak to other clinical supervisors and/or support members of the team such as nurses (if appropriate)
- Speak to the speciality trainee. Establish if there is insight into their behaviour and if it reflects a lack of professionalism. There may be a specific reason for being late and the trainee should be given the opportunity to highlight any personal or professional issues they may have. Examples include:
  - Personal commitments (e.g. childcare)
  - Workload/timetable

You establish that the trainee finds it difficult to manage their workload. They are late to afternoon clinics because they run late from the morning clinic.

Establish whether the trainee has an unfair workload, or if the workload is appropriate and they require additional educational or clinical support. Benchmark the trainee against their expected development. To assess this:

- Review the trainee's clinic session—the number of patients seen and length of time allocated for each patient, based on complexity
- Review their portfolio, specifically previous experience and logbook of current patients
- Review clinical supervisor comments
- Review with the TPD, the expected number of patients per session
- Check that the clinical environment is conducive to the workload (adequate nursing support, functioning equipment available)

The workload is excessive:

- If the workload is excessive or the clinical environment not conducive, this should be rectified. The clinical supervisor of these sessions should be involved in conversations to ensure that patient safety/care is not compromised. Patients may be transferred to other clinicians or concerns raised with the nurse manager if appropriate. The trainee should be adequately supported to reach their training objectives and the work environment should not be detrimental to this. This should be reviewed with the trainee and changes reviewed after an established time period (e.g. 3 months)

The workload is appropriate:

The trainee should be supported to improve their clinical skills. Initially 'diagnose' the areas that require improvement which may be clinic preparation, clinical decision-making, or practical skill. This may be established by:

- Speaking to the trainee (who may or may not have insight into where they require support)
- Review their portfolio and experience
- Review WBAs, CS comments
- Review record of training courses attended

Arrange regular developmental conversations to create an open, trusting relationship for the trainee to offer advice and guidance on how to keep up with the workload:

- Set SMART goals for improvement e.g. manage a specified number of patients during a clinic session within six months
- Temporarily reduce the number of patients seen on clinics
- Arrange observational shadowing of senior clinicians
- Arrange simulated training or courses e.g. typodont or surgical
- 1-to-1 supervision
- Check whether the trainee has a regular dedicated study session and whether this is used effectively
- Clinical supervisors should be made aware of the additional support the trainee requires and given advice on how they may facilitate this
- Complete WBAs to provide direct, tailored feedback to the trainee on how they can improve

Ensure retention of accurate dated and signed records of feedback, supervision, and appraisal sessions of the trainee. These will highlight the trainee's progression and also manage and support the trainee.

Ensure all information is included for the trainee's ARCP so that an independent assessment may be made of the trainee's progress. This may lead to:

- Outcome 1—Satisfactory progress—the trainee is now developing competencies/capabilities at the expected rate
- Outcome 2—Further development of specific competences/capabilities required but additional training time is not required
- Outcome 3- Inadequate progress—additional training time required, the training period may be extended

There is little measurable improvement in the trainee, they are also late for morning clinical sessions consistently.

- The trainee's lack of progress will be reflected in the portfolio of evidence at their ARCP
- The reason for lateness should be reviewed with the trainee

- Where reasonable adjustments are appropriate (see chapter 7: Staff management) these should be implemented
- Where there is a concern regarding professionalism, the trainee should be managed as a trust employee through informal and formal disciplinary processes (see chapter 7: Staff management)
- The ES/ TPD should be involved in this process and would likely lead on the information gathering process for the trainee and be present for informal/formal meetings

Scenario—Consultant cover

You are a senior paediatric speciality trainee (ST4) in a dental hospital. You are asked by your supervising consultant to cover a clinic with complex patients as they will be on annual leave.

What do you do?
- If you are competent to cover this clinic, then this is acceptable
- It is the responsibility of the consultant to ensure appropriate cover, this may be another consultant or a speciality trainee/staff grade. If there is any uncertainty, they should review the clinic notes in advance to ensure they are within your competency
- If you are unsure, you should check with the consultant in the first instance and/or review the patient notes to ensure you are comfortable seeing these patients. You should also establish if there is another consultant available for advice on the day or if the responsible consultant is available/willing to be contacted
- If there are patients beyond your competency, you should highlight this to the consultant. These patients may be reappointed or seen by a more appropriate colleague; it may be possible to run a reduced clinic list
- Your ES should be informed whenever there is a change in your timetable, even temporary
- This should be reflected in your timetable, i.e. your own clinic cancelled or time given in lieu
- If there are areas of your knowledge/skills that require development to allow you to cover this clinic, these could be added to your portfolio or discussed with your clinical supervisor/educational supervisor to establish ways to develop these
- Additional experiences such as this should be recorded in your portfolio

The consultant repeatedly asks you to cover clinics. What do you do?

This should be raised with the consultant. If you feel unable to, you should speak with your ES.

Service provision may require a permanent change in timetable. This should consider several factors:
- You should not be expected to see patients beyond your competency and there should be appropriate supervision arranged
- A change should not be detrimental to your development
- Your timetable should adhere to the recommended number of treatment, clinic and SPA/admin sessions
- Any timetable change should be uploaded to your portfolio for review at your ARCP

They are your educational supervisor. What do you do?

If you feel comfortable to do so, speak with the consultant. If not, speak to either your training programme director, the clinical lead of the department or another consultant in the department.

Scenario—Obtaining a new trainee

You are a consultant in a district general hospital. You have no speciality trainees in your department and have an interest in teaching.

How is a trainee funded?

Trainees are funded by NHS England (previously Health Education England) with the department reimbursed up to 100% of their salary plus related employer costs. You therefore may not need to undertake a business case specifically to obtain funding for such a position.

Additional costs of a trainee (such as nursing costs or equipment) are not funded. Additional activity generated by the trainee (if under PbR contract) would contribute to the department budget.

What are the terms of reference for setting up a training post?

There are several documents that explain the requirements and standards of trainers and the training process:

- The Dental Gold Guide
- The relevant speciality curriculum
- The GDC Standards for speciality education. This includes standards on protecting patients, quality evaluation and review, and trainee assessment
- COPDEND Standards for dental educators. This has standards over five domains: teaching and learning; assessing the learner; guidance for personal and professional development; quality assurance; and management

What resources are required to support a training post?

Clinical/academic resources

- The consultant team must be able to deliver the curriculum both clinically and academically. This will likely be in association with a teaching hospital
- An appropriate case mix and volume of patients for teaching is required
- Appropriate colleagues should be available to facilitate training and cross-cover if appropriate
- Non-clinical training opportunities—particularly for speciality trainees for whom managerial/leadership projects are required
- Consultant time—an additional 0.25PAs per week should be allocated to the educational supervisor for each trainee. This requires incorporation into job plans
- Clinical supervision—every clinical session must have a named clinical supervisor with the required skills and experience
- Potential education and clinical supervisors should have appropriate training. This may include postgraduate certificates or qualifications in dental/medical education or 'train the trainer' courses

Support services
- Additional clinical capacity including clinic chair, nurse, and equipment
- Adequate lab capacity and administrative support to facilitate the increase in patients seen
- Non-clinical space—access for the trainee to office space, computer and printing facilities to support clinical and academic needs
- Access to library facilities

Who would you speak to regarding your plans?

Internal to the trust
- Consultant colleagues
- Nursing and administration support to assess capacity
- Clinical director—changes to job plan will be required
- Service manager—particularly if a business case is required to increase capacity
- Identifying the resources required—nurse manager, administration lead

External to the trust
- The local PGDD and TPD. They would confirm if an NTN and therefore funding is available, often through discussions with the SAC
- Royal College Specialist Advisory Committee Chair for advice (but not for permission)
- Commissioners—to ensure that commissioning aligns with an increased service delivery
- Consultant in DPH may assess service provision in the local area
- Dental Hospital—if affiliated with a dental hospital for to provide training and courses
- University—if the post will likely be linked with a university or Master's programme

Who would approve a new training post?

The PGDD would approve a training post. They will consider:
- The needs analysis locally and or nationally
- Training capacity
- Compliance with curriculum and knowledge of assessment framework
- Knowledge of the potential trainer's ability to train/completion of appropriate courses

Further reading

Dental Blue Guide. A Reference Guide for Postgraduate Dental Foundation Training in England, Wales, and Northern Ireland. 2022. Available at: https://www.copdend.org/wp-content/uploads/2022/09/Dental-Blue-Guide-September-2022.pdf

Dental Gold Guide 4th Edition.DGG4. A Reference Guide for General Dental Council. Specialist List Application Pack. Management of Health and Safety at Work Regulations 1999 (Statutory Instrument 1999/3242). Available at: https://www.gdc-uk.org/registration/your-registration/specialist-lists/specialist-list-application-pack

National Certificate of Dental Core Equivalence (NCDCE)—COPDEND. Available at: https://www.copdend.org/postgraduate-training/header-dental-core-training/dct2-equivalence-process/#:~:text=If%20a%20dentist%20has%20not%20undergone%20UK%20Dental,DCT2%2C%20they%20can%20apply%20to%20have%20this%20confirmed.

Paice E, Orton V (2004). Early signs of the trainee in difficulty. *Hosp Med*, 65(4):238–40.

Postgraduate Dental Core and Speciality Training in the UK 2023 Available at: https://www.copdend.org/wp-content/uploads/2023/11/DGG4-v10-2023.pdf

Chapter 10

Research governance

Research governance

Research governance is the framework of principles, regulations, and processes guiding research activities. It is essential for the safe and ethical management and conduct of research studies within the UK. It ensures:

- Research is conducted ethically with oversight by ethics committees
- Methodologies are transparent
- Conflicts of interest are managed
- Participant welfare is safeguarded
- Reliable and trustworthy outcomes are obtained
- Legal compliance
- Data integrity

Research governance safeguards the credibility of research, fosters public trust, and promotes responsible and accountable research.

It is the researcher's responsibility to ensure that they are aware of their responsibilities and the approvals that are needed before they start their research project. They must follow established guidelines, obtain informed consent, and ensure that data is reliable and valid.

Dentists working in secondary care environments are likely to be involved in research as investigators or to encounter patients who are enrolled in research studies. Dental consultants should be aware of these principles given that their patients and/or junior doctors/dentists within their team may be involved in research projects.

Declaration of Helsinki

The Declaration of Helsinki is a statement of ethical principles developed by the World Medical Association (WMA) for medical research involving human subjects, including research on identifiable human material and data.

It has been periodically amended, most recently in 2013 and its principles are divided into:

- General principles
- Risks, burdens, and benefits
- Vulnerable groups and individuals
- Scientific requirements and research protocols
- Research ethics committees
- Privacy and confidentiality
- Informed consent
- Use of placebo
- Post-trial provisions
- Research registration, publication and dissemination of results
- Unproven interventions in clinical practice

Good clinical practice

Good clinical practice (GCP) is a code of international standards concerning the design, conduct, performance, monitoring, auditing, recording, analysis, and reporting of clinical trials.

It is consistent with the Declaration of Helsinki and provides assurance that a study's results are credible and accurate and that the rights and confidentiality of the study subjects are protected.

GCP training
- All investigators must have an up-to-date GCP certificate
- This may be obtained through online learning on the National Institute of Health and Care Research (NIHR) website
- Refresher courses are recommended every 2–3 years to keep up to date with best practice
- Separate courses on informed consent and paediatric consent may also be required

Research ethical considerations

Ethics is a crucial aspect of research governance, ensuring that research is conducted in a manner that is respectful of participants' rights and interests.

Researchers must consider the ethical implications of their research which includes:

- Informed consent from participants
- Maintaining confidentiality
- Managing conflicts of interest
- Seeking ethical approval from appropriate regulatory bodies
- Ensuring that all risks identified have mitigation plans in place

Informed consent

Informed consent must be obtained before any research-related procedures are undertaken. This requires that participants have a clear understanding of the research's aims, procedures, risks, and benefits before consenting to participate. Informed consent forms a key role in good clinical practice (GCP).

If researchers are not intending to obtain patient consent, they may need to apply for Confidentiality Advisory Group (CAG) approval to use participants' data without consent.

Participants should be informed of any updates or changes during the life cycle of the study that may affect their continuing participation such as updated safety information or if other treatments become available.

The person taking consent must be:

- GCP trained
- Suitably qualified and experienced
- Have been delegated this duty by the chief investigator or principal investigator on the delegation log

Each participant has the right to withdraw from the study at any time.

Confidentiality

All researchers must ensure that participants' personal and medical data is protected and kept confidential in compliance with data protection laws such as the General Data Protection Regulation (GDPR) as well as the NHS Code of Confidentiality. See Chapter 8, Information governance.

Managing conflicts of interest

Researchers must declare any potential conflicts of interest (COI) and take steps to manage them appropriately. This is particularly relevant if researchers have a financial or professional interest in the outcome of the research. All NHS trusts and higher education institutions maintain conflict of interest registries and staff are required to update these when COIs arise.

Seeking ethical approval

The ethical approval process is a legal requirement for conducting research within the NHS. Researchers must seek approval from the appropriate regulatory bodies before conducting any research involving human participants. This may include the:

- Health research authority (HRA)
- Research ethics committee (REC)
- University ethics committee
- Medicines and healthcare products regulatory agency (MHRA)
- Approval from the HRA and REC may be obtained by completing the integrated research application system (IRAS) form

Identifying and mitigating risks

All potential risks and burdens associated with the research should be considered and documentation made of the actions taken to mitigate these risks. A risk assessment may be required (see Chapter 6, Risk management).

The IRAS form requires researchers to identify all potential risks and burdens to the participant. This should:

- Include any potential for distress, discomfort, and/or inconvenience
- Consider the likelihood and consequences of potential harm
- Explain why the intervention is necessary and steps taken to minimize the effects
- Describe and compare the risks and benefits
- Consider the risks associated with any breach of confidentiality or failure to maintain data security

Typical risks that need to be considered include:

- Physical risks—discomfort, pain, injury, illness, or disease
- Psychological risks—anxiety, depression, guilt, loss of self-esteem, and altered behaviour
- Social risks—disclosures that could affect a participant's standing in the community, in their family, or their job
- Legal risks—activities that could result in a criminal offence or might lead to a participant disclosing criminal activity
- Economic harm—this includes the opportunity cost of the time taken to undertake the study such as loss of earnings

It may be appropriate to involve the patients, carers, service users, or members of the public to help identify risks.

Potential risks and burdens should be described in the participant information sheet in such a way that potential participants can clearly understand what is involved if they consent to participate.

The potential risks to researchers, other service users and the organization/sponsor (such as the NHS trust) should also be considered. This includes reputational, legal, and/or economic risks.

Research sponsors should have systems in place to monitor and respond to developments as the research proceeds, particularly those which put the safety of individuals at risk, and to ensure the design and conduct of the research is modified accordingly.

Adverse events

All adverse events (AEs) should be recorded in the medical notes of the participant and an adverse event log in the investigator site file.

If anyone other than the principal investigator (PI) will be evaluating AEs, they must be named on the study delegation log.

It is good practice for the chief investigator (CI) to review serious adverse events (SAEs) with the PI at defined intervals.

In research, an SAE is defined as an untoward occurrence that:
- Results in death
- Is life-threatening
- Requires hospitalization or prolongation of existing hospitalization
- Results in persistent or significant disability or incapacity
- Results in a congenital abnormality or birth defect
- Is otherwise considered medically significant by the investigator

All serious adverse effects, other than those defined in the protocol as not requiring reporting, must be reported to:
- The sponsor/CI within 24 hours of the PI becoming aware
- The research ethics committee (REC)
- An adverse event may require an amendment to the study (see page 375)

Regulatory framework

The regulatory framework governing research in the UK is complex, with several organizations overseeing different aspects of governance.

Health research authority

The health research authority (HRA) aims to protect and promote the interests of patients and the public in health and social care research:

- It provides guidance on research ethics and governance
- Reviews research proposals to ensure that they meet ethical and regulatory requirements
- Coordinates and standardizes research regulatory practice
- Provides independent recommendations on the processing of identifiable patient information where it is not practical to obtain consent

Research ethics committees

Research ethics committees (REC) are independent committees that review research proposals to ensure that they meet ethical and regulatory requirements. They play a vital role in:

- Protecting the rights and welfare of research participants
- Ensuring that research is conducted in an ethical and safe manner
- Participants are fully informed and consent to the proposed research

Ethical approval from a REC or confirmation that approval is not required, must be sought before conducting any research involving human participants in the UK.

Medicines and Healthcare products Regulatory Agency (MHRA)

The MHRA is part of the UK's Department of Health and Social Care. The Agency is responsible for regulating medicines, medical devices, and blood donations for transfusions within the UK.

If a new drug (investigational medicinal product) or device is used, permission from the MHRA is required. If a device is used within its intended purpose as per its UKAS marking (United Kingdom Accreditation Service) or CE marking, then approval may not be required.

Sponsorship

The Medicines for Human Use (Clinical Trials) Regulations and the UK Policy Framework for Health and Social Care Research stipulate that all clinical trials of investigational medicinal products in the UK and/or any research carried out in the NHS or social care must have an identified sponsor.

The sponsor is the organization legally responsible for a project's administration and management. They:

- Maintain oversight and provide advice during the research study
- Confirm whether a project is research or may be better classed as an audit or quality improvement programme
- Advise on the documents that are required before submission to regulatory bodies such as the REC, HRA, and MHRA
- Check and approve these documents prior to submission

- The sponsor may have additional templates and documents that require completion before submission is approved, such as:
  - Insurance certificates for non-NHS Sponsors
  - Nationally agreed Model Agreements
  - Costing documents depending on sponsor type (such as commercial or non-commercial sponsor)
- The sponsor may delegate some of their responsibilities to the CI or a clinical research organization. They would maintain appropriate oversight of all delegated duties and continue to provide advice

The 'sponsor' is not the same as the 'funder'. The funder may only provide the financial resources, without taking legal responsibility for the project. However, a funder may also take on the role of sponsor.

Student research

If the researcher is undertaking a research study for an educational qualification (including both MSc and PhD level students), the Higher Education Institute is expected to act as the sponsor, unless there is a compelling reason for a trust to do so, such as:

- The study continues after the student has finished their degree
- The educational qualification element is a small part of the study

Chief investigator and principal investigator

The chief investigator (CI) takes on the overall responsibility of running the study and is accountable to the study sponsor. Within a dental department this is usually a dental consultant.

It is a requirement the CI has a permanent or honorary contract with the NHS trust or university within which the research is being undertaken.

For clinical trials of investigational medicinal products, a PhD student does not qualify as the chief investigator.

A principal investigator takes on the responsibility for the study at their site, but not the overall responsibility for the entire study.

Research approval process

Decision tools

There are two decision tools which can be used to determine whether a study is classified as research and whether NHS ethical approval is required (see Box 10.1).

Sponsor approval

The researcher should consult with their proposed sponsor before starting the project. They will:
- Confirm whether the study is research
- Confirm the approvals and permissions that are required
- Check and approve the documents before submission to the REC, HRA, and MHRA (if applicable)
- Provide sponsor templates as required. This would include using the sponsor's approved protocol, participant information sheet, and consent form templates

HRA approval

While officially named HRA and Health and Care Research Wales Approval (HRA/HCRW Approval), this process is more commonly known as HRA approval.

This must be sought when an NHS organization has a duty of care to participants such as patients, service users, or NHS staff or volunteers. It also applies to participants whose NHS data or tissue is involved in a research project.

HRA approval brings together the:
- Assessment of governance and legal compliance, undertaken by dedicated HRA staff
- Independent ethical opinion by a research ethics committee (REC)

Box 10.1 Determining if a study is research

1. Is my study research?

This tool is based on the table published by the Health Research Authority (HRA) summarized on page 114. It confirms whether a project is research, clinical audit, or service evaluation. https://www.hra-decisiontools.org.uk/research

2. Does the study require NHS ethics approval?

Also published by the HRA, this decision tool confirms whether REC review is required.

https://www.hra-decisiontools.org.uk/ethics/

Even if NHS ethics approval is not needed, HRA approval may still be required. This is the case when studies involve NHS staff only or the use of previously collected routine clinical data for research purposes by a member of the normal care team.

Researchers only have to submit a single application using the Integrated Research Application System (IRAS) form. Health and Social Care Northern Ireland and NHS Research Scotland are responsible for the approval process in their respective countries. However, the IRAS submission process is similar for each of the four UK nations, regardless of where the study is led from.

Figure 10.1 gives an overview of the process for simple studies. More complex studies may require additional organizations.

Documentation

The documentation required varies based on study design. All documents submitted for review must be dated and version controlled. Required documents for submission include, but are not limited to:

IRAS form

The IRAS form is a single system which contains all the necessary forms for applying for permission/approvals for health and social care and/or community care research in the UK. A series of initial questions about the study design filter the form to ensure that only questions relevant to the study appear.

Protocol

This is a full description of the study. It is used as a reference by the research team to ensure that they are following the study requirements.

Participant (or Patient) Information Sheet—PIS

This document is given to potential participants and contains a full description of the tests/assessments that will be conducted. The content will vary depending on the study, but includes:

- Why the potential participant is being approached
- Risks and benefits (if any) of taking part
- Contact details if there is a problem or complaint
- Details about the sponsor and funder
- Potential sample requirements
- What will happen to their data
- Indemnity arrangements

Consent form

A short document with clauses for the participant to initial, showing they consent to taking part in the study.

Curriculum vitae (CV)

A short CV of the chief investigator. The CI is also likely to be required to provide evidence of good clinical practice (GCP) training.

Trial registration

If the study is interventional, the study should be registered on a publicly accessible database. This is a requirement if there is an intention to publish the study. The International Committee of Medical Journal Editors have made it a requirement to be registered on a database before the first patient is enrolled into the study. There are several databases that meet their criteria including clinicaltrials.gov and International Standard Randomized Controlled Trial Number (ISRCTN).

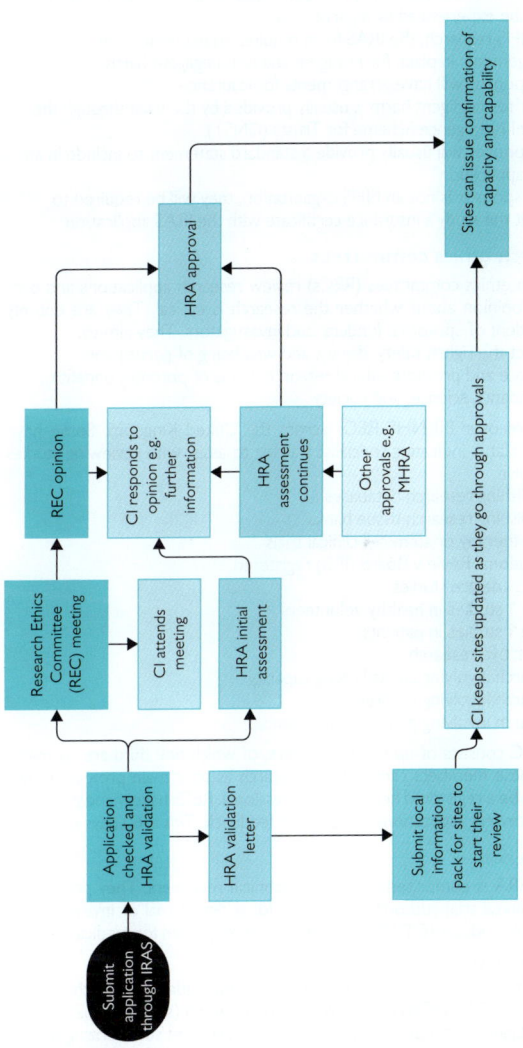

Figure 10.1 HRA and ethical approval process flow diagram.

Insurance
- Insurance is required to provide cover against harmful events which could be experienced by a participant
- For NHS research, the IRAS form requires an explanation of arrangements in place for negligent and non-negligent harm
- The sponsor will have arrangements for insurance
- Cover for negligent harm is usually provided by the trust through the Clinical Negligence Scheme for Trusts (CNST)
- The sponsor will usually provide a standard statement to include in an IRAS application
- If the sponsor is not an NHS organization, they will be required to submit the study's insurance certificate with the IRAS application

Research ethics committees

Research ethics committees (RECs) review research applications and provide an opinion about whether the research is ethical. They are entirely independent of sponsors, funders, and investigators. They aim to:
- Protect the rights, safety, dignity, and well-being of participants
- Facilitate and promote ethical research that is of potential benefit to participants, science, and society

There are over 80 NHS RECs across the United Kingdom. Some have 'flagged' status indicating specialist training to assist with reviewing studies that involve:
- Establishing research databases
- Establishing research tissue banks
- Gene therapy or stem cell clinical trials
- Institutional Review Board (IRB) registered
- Medical device studies
- Phase 1 studies in healthy volunteers
- Phase 1 studies in patients
- Qualitative research
- Research involving adults lacking capacity
- Research involving children
- Research involving prisoners or prisons

Each REC consists of up to 15 members, of which one third are lay members. These members cannot have research as their main profession, nor can they be a registered healthcare professional. RECs have mandated timelines to review applications and provide feedback. This is 60 days currently.

MHRA review

The MHRA is comprised of expert technical reviewers. They provide either a clinical trial authorization (CTA) for a clinical trial of investigational medicinal products (CTIMPs) or notice of no objection for medical devices.

Documentation
Based on the study design and type, documents additional to those submitted for HRA/ HCRW approval may be required (see Box 10.2):
- Investigator brochure—This is a detailed document summarizing the information about the investigational medicinal product or device

> **Box 10.2 Applying for MHRA review**
>
> ***Device-only studies***
> These studies are submitted through IRAS, but each body (REC and MHRA Devices) reviews them independently and hence questions may come from both bodies separately.
>
> ***Combined review***
> Clinical trials of investigational medicinal products (CTIMPs) and combined medicine and device trials, go through the combined review process.
>
> Researchers submit a single application on the IRAS website. This goes in tandem to the MHRA, a REC, and study wide review such as HRA/HCRW Approval.
>
> The reviews by both MHRA and the REC are done in parallel and any requests for further information (RFIs) are raised jointly. The investigator sends a single response to these requests which will result in a single decision from both reviewers.

- Labels—A mock-up of the label to be used for the investigational medicinal product or device under investigation
- Investigational Medicinal Product Dossier (IMPD)—data on the quality and production of the IMP under investigation

Other committees

Permissions from additional committees may be required. Common examples include:

- Confidentiality Advisory Group (CAG)—Approval is required if confidential patient information is being used without consent, outside the direct care team. This is done through IRAS
- Public Benefit and Privacy Panel (Scotland only)—Approval is required where health data without consent is used in a study involving more than one NHS board in Scotland. Applications are made to Research Data Scotland (RDS)
- Administration of Radioactive Substances Advisory Committee (ARSAC)—A licence is required for the use of radioactive substances

Imaging in research

Many dental studies use imaging modalities. The Ionising Radiation (Medical Exposure) Regulations, (IR(ME)R) cover the following:

- General radiography, interventional imaging, CT scans, DEXA scans, mammography, and dental radiography
- Radiotherapy
- Administration of radioactive substances (e.g. nuclear medicine, PET)

If studies use any of the procedures covered under IR(ME)R, even if the procedures are considered standard care, the imaging section on the IRAS form must be completed. This requires:

- Lead medical physics expert (MPE), who performs a radiation dose/risk assessment for all the radiation exposures proposed
- Lead clinical radiation expert (CRE), who assesses all radiation exposures at any site in the study and advises the CI and the REC on the suitability and clinical justification for additional exposures

Only the imaging detailed in the IRAS is approved by the site. If researchers need further imaging, an amendment is required.

For studies which include the administration of radioactive substances:
- The site must hold a licence
- Each ARSAC practitioner must hold their own licence
- The sponsor of the study is responsible for obtaining ARSAC approval for the study

Confirmation of capacity and capability (CC&C)

Confirmation of capacity and capability (CC&C) is the confirmation from each trust that it has the resources to conduct the study after reviewing the study documentation.

To initiate the CC&C process, researchers submit all the documents listed on the HRA validation letter. This is known as the local information pack (LIP). The LIP should be submitted to each trust's R&D department that will take part in the study.

There are three elements to CC&C: assessing, arranging and confirming.

Assessing

The NHS trust reviews the proposed study and confirms whether it has the capacity and capability to undertake the study.

Arranging

The NHS trust puts in place practical arrangements to deliver the study. This includes identifying the staff needed to manage the study such as research nurses, doctors, allied health professionals, and clinical trial practitioners (CTPs).

The R&D office at each trust confirms with each relevant service support department that they have the resources to undertake required activities.

Complex studies that require many service support departments may take longer to approve and this should be factored into study timelines.

Examples of service support departments that may be approached to confirm that they have the ability to conduct the study include:
- Research costings and contracts team. They ensure the proposed budget covers the cost of the study and check any legal agreements
- Imaging modalities such as radiology or medical illustration
- Pathology/labs/histopathology
- Information governance—any data flows are identified and anonymization/pseudonymization processes are confirmed
- Clinical trial pharmacy—full review of the IMP and any production requirements identified and storage conditions/reconstitution

Confirming

Once all reviews are complete, the R&D office confirms that they have the capacity and capability to deliver the study and are committed to its delivery.

Amendments

Amendments are changes made to a research project after approval from a review body has been given.

The process to apply for an amendment depends on whether it is considered to be substantial, non-substantial, or an urgent safety measure.

Types of amendments

Substantial

These are changes to the protocol or any other supporting documents that are likely to affect the safety of the participants, the scientific value of the study or the conduct/management of the study.

These require submission to REC/HRA and MHRA (CTIMPs) for review. Examples of substantial amendments include:

- Changes to the procedures undertaken by participants
- Significant changes to study documentation such as participant information sheets, consent forms, questionnaires, etc.
- Change of sponsor(s) or sponsor's legal representative
- Appointment of a new chief investigator
- Change to the insurance or indemnity arrangements for the study
- CTIMP or regulated investigation of a medical device adding a new non-NHS/health and social care site
- Temporary halt of a study to protect participants from harm, and the planned restart of a study following a temporary halt
- Change to the definition of the end of the study

Non-substantial

These are changes to the conduct of the clinical trial that do not have a significant impact on the safety of the participants or the scientific value of the study.

Non-substantial amendments do not require submission to the REC or MHRA. Examples of non-substantial amendments include:

- Minor changes to the protocol or other study documentation, e.g. correcting errors, updating contact details, minor clarifications
- Updates to the investigator's brochure (unless there is a change to the risk/benefit assessment for the trial)
- Changes to the chief investigator's research team
- Changes in funding arrangements
- Changes in the documentation used for recording study data
- Changes in the logistical arrangements for storing or transporting samples
- Changes to the research team at trial sites
- Inclusion of new sites and investigators
- Change to the study end date

Changes to contact details for the sponsor, chief investigator, or other study staff are minor amendments but should be notified to the REC that approved the original application.

Urgent safety measures

An urgent safety measure is taken by the sponsor or investigator to protect the participants of a clinical trial against any immediate hazard to their health or safety. These can be implemented immediately without prior authorization from a regulatory body. However, they should be notified as soon as possible.

Amendment process

Amendments cannot be submitted without prior authorization from the sponsor. An amendment is submitted through the completion of the IRAS amendment tool. This:
- Categorizes the amendment
- Advises whether an update to the original IRAS form is required
- Lists the organizations to be notified of the proposed amendment

If no review by HRA/REC is required, changes may be implemented. If REC/HRA approval is needed, an amendment pack can be sent to each site to review the changes during the review process. Once approval is given, the site will issue trust approval for the amendment.

Amendment categories

The amendment tool will state the amendment category (A, B, or C) once completed. This is distinct from whether it is substantial or non-substantial. The categorization confirms whether the amendment has delivery implications for all, some, or none of the participating organizations. It indicates whether any action is required to implement the amendment. Amendments in category A have implications for all participating organizations and require REC/HRA review, category B has implications for specific participants, while category C are minor changes.

Amendment implementation

Unless the proposed amendment is an urgent safety measure or a category C, researchers must wait until they receive trust approval at each site before changes are implemented. Amendments may be implemented after 35 days if the trust does not object.

Data management

Research data should be managed in compliance with the relevant legislation including data protection regulations (see Chapter 8).

Measures to ensure compliance include:

All study and source documents should be stored securely and only accessible by study staff and authorized personnel:

- Physical data kept securely in a locked, access restricted location e.g. locked cabinet
- Electronic data should password protected and encrypted
- Data should be anonymized as soon as it is practical to do so
- On all study-specific documents, other than the signed consent, the participant should be referred to by the study participant number/code, not by name
- Name and any other identifying details not included in any study data or electronic file including case report form (CRF)
- Access to the final data set should remain with the chief investigator
- All source data and study documentation should be available to external auditors if required.

Definitions

Case report form (CRF)
This is a document designed to record all the protocol-required information. It collects all the data relevant to the clinical trial. It is then sent for statistical or other analysis.

Source Documents
Source documents are original documents, data, and records from which participants' CRF data are obtained. This includes hospital records, clinical charts, laboratory, and pharmacy records, radiographs, and correspondence.

Investigator site folder (ISF)

This contains essential documents which demonstrate that the clinical trial site and investigator are following the regulatory requirements set out by GCP guidelines. It includes much of the information submitted as part of the information submitted to the HRA:

- Trial protocol
- Participant information sheet and consent forms
- Investigator brochure
- Regulatory documents, applications, and approvals
- Delegation logs (see next)
- Deviation from protocol log
- Safety reports
- Correspondence between delegated site staff and sponsor

Delegation log
- All research projects should have a delegation log
- The principal investigator at each site can delegate tasks to other people at the participating organization
- The PI must:
  - Complete the delegation log before tasks are carried out

- Confirm that people to whom tasks have been delegated have been appropriately trained to carry out those tasks before they perform them
- Keep the original log up-to-date according to the requirements of the sponsor

Data retention and archiving

- Archiving will be authorized by the sponsor following the site close-out visit which occurs when the study is closed or completed at the site
- Essential documents will be retained for a minimum of 5 years after the completion of the study. These documents will be retained for longer if required by the applicable regulatory requirements. This is normally around 25 years for CTIMPs
- The study protocol will state the archiving period. See Chapter 8, Information governance: Research governance

Publication

- All individuals who make substantial intellectual, scientific, and practical contributions to the study and the manuscript should, where possible, be credited as authors
- All individuals credited as authors should deserve that designation
- It is the responsibility of the CI, PI, and sponsors to ensure that these principles are upheld
- The status of manuscripts in preparation should be reviewed by the CI, sponsor, and funder if required
- In all cases where journal policies permit, all investigators who contribute patients to the study should be acknowledged

The results of the study should be reported and disseminated in:
- Peer-reviewed scientific journals
- Internal reports, where possible article on institute web pages (publicly accessible)
- Conference presentation(s)
- Written feedback to patient support groups

Study management

Sources of research funding

Funding available to researchers in the UK may be categorized as:
- Commercial funders, including industry and private companies
- Non-commercial funders such as government departments, research councils, and charities
- Charities include hospital charities, who fund research studies conducted by staff or larger charities part of the Association of Medical Research Charities (AMRC) such as Anthony Nolan or the British Heart Foundation

Researchers' local R&D Offices will often have a research grants team who can help identify possible sources of funding and will be able to create detailed costings for the proposed study.

The National Institute for Health and Care Research

The National Institute for Health and Care Research (NIHR) is funded by the Department of Health and Social Care. Its roles include:
- Commission and fund NHS, social care, and public health research
- Work in partnership with the NHS, universities, local government, other research funders, patients, and the public
- Improve the quality, relevance, and focus of research in the NHS and social care
- Distribute funds transparently after open competition and peer review

Role of delivery staff

Other than doctors/dentists and service support departments, other staff involved in research studies are referred to as delivery staff.

They include clinical research nurses, clinical trial practitioners, data managers, and allied health professionals.

Clinical research nurses (CRNs) are:
- Responsible for patient care and data collection
- They are registered nurses who have undertaken specialized training in clinical research
- A dental nurse can become a CRN with appropriate training

Clinical trial practitioners (CTPs):
- Support research teams with patient recruitment, regulatory compliance, and data collection
- They typically hold degrees in healthcare and receive additional relevant training
- Many CTPs undertake additional training such as phlebotomy

Data managers:
- Ensure data integrity
- Have a background in data management
- Require training in clinical research data standards and security

Allied health professionals (AHPs):
- Support research teams with patient recruitment, regulatory compliance, and data collection
- This includes dental hygienists/therapists, dental technicians

Patient and public involvement and engagement

Patient and public involvement and engagement (PPIE) is essential to clinical research, ensuring that the needs of the target patient audience are understood, and that research meets those needs.

Full consideration should be given to PPIE for each of the research stages. It is the role of the CI to ensure:

- Day-to-day support of patients and the public involved in research
- Physical and mental well-being of patients and public engaged in research
- Adequate training and information is provided to patients and the public involved in the project
- Early and ongoing communication between the patient and public members and the rest of the team
- That any recompense for involvement or expenses related to involvement are processed in a timely fashion

It is the role of the PI to ensure:

- Sufficient and meaningful PPIE is involved in all stages of the study
- PPIE for the study has been fully costed
- That all contracts and written agreements with patients and the public are understood and complete

The UK standards for public involvement in research are:

- Inclusive opportunities—Offer public involvement opportunities that are accessible and broadreaching
- Working together—Value all contributions and build mutually respectful and productive relationships
- Offer and promote learning—Support opportunities that build confidence and skills for public involvement in research
- Communications—Use plain language for well-timed and relevant communications, as part of involvement plans and activities
- Impact—Seek improvement by identifying and sharing the difference that public involvement makes to research
- Governance—Involve the public in research management, regulation, leadership, and decision-making

Future/intended developments in research governance

CRN has become RDN

From October 2024, the NIHR Clinical Research Network became the NIHR Research Delivery Network (RDN). The NIHR RDN will support the effective and efficient initiation and delivery of funded research across the health and care system in England.

The whole of England is supported through 12 NIHR regional research delivery networks. These work with the Research Delivery Network Coordinating Centre (RDNCC).

Commercial clinical trials

Lord O'Shaughnessy's report on commercial clinical trials in the UK was released in May 2023. It is likely that recommendations from the report regarding the set up and management of commercial research in the UK including review timelines will be implemented in 2025.

ICH E6 (R3) GCP

The third revision (R3) of ICH E6, which is the formal name for GCP is currently in draft and is expected to be released in 2025.

The main revisions apply the application of GCP to new trial designs, technological innovations, and increase the proportionate risk-based approach of GCP to clinical trials of medicines to support regulatory and healthcare decision-making.

Scenario—Research consent

You are a new registrar at a district general hospital. The team is undertaking a randomized control trial on a new surgical technique. You have noticed a variation in the consent process for the study.

What issues does this raise?
- Compromising the validity of the research study
- Informed consent
- Inappropriate delegation or training

What do you do?
- Although you are not directly involved in the study, you have a duty of care to patients as a clinician in the department
- Assumptions regarding proper conduct should not be made. There may be aspects of the study you do not know or understand, such as an established variation in the study protocol
- In the first instance, you should seek information to clarify the situation
- Speak to the registrar or consultants involved in the study and query the difference in protocol. This conversation should not be accusatory but framed in an enquiring or confirming manner

You are unsure who is involved or responsible for the study, how could you ascertain this?
- You can ask dental colleagues or nurses in the department
- The name of the PI/CI will be recorded in the PIS, if available to you. This would not be available routinely, as these would be kept in the ISF which is locked and accessible only to study investigators
- The study will be recorded/registered with the R&D Office, they can be contacted to determine the name of the investigator, the principal investigator, or chief investigator
- If the study is interventional, it should be registered on a publicly accessible database, these could also be searched for information, specifically to determine who the CI is

The study protocol is not being followed, what do you do?
You should raise concerns to the appropriate person, escalating if your concerns are not considered, in the following order:
- Principal investigator
- R&D office
- Chief investigator
- Sponsor
- If you feel unable to speak to these individuals, or you have spoken to them, and your concerns have not been considered fairly you may consider speaking with the trust Freedom to Speak Up Champion. Care should be taken if speaking to anyone external to the site, to prevent confidentiality agreements being breached

It transpires that a consultant (a sub-investigator but not the Principal Investigator) had asked his senior registrar to help with the study protocol as they were unable to attend the clinic.

Is this a problem, and why?

- Yes
- The senior registrar may not be adequately trained or may not have been able to answer questions appropriately. Informed and continuing consent to the study may not have been achieved
- Deviation from the consent process may be considered a serious breach of GCP
- The variation affects the robustness of the study, jeopardizes its internal/external validity and reliability
- It may prevent the publication of study results or lead to exclusion in systematic reviews/meta-analyses studies in the future. The participants have therefore been unnecessarily subjected to a study
- Harm to the participant may or may not have occurred

No harm has occurred to the participant as a result of this. What steps, if any should be taken?

- This should be reported to the principal investigator of the study
- They in turn will inform the R&D office who will liaise with the study CI and sponsor
- Any variation in the study should be recorded in the study 'deviation from protocol log'. This document is checked at established intervals by the study's monitor
- It would be appropriate in this example to inform them immediately so that remedial action can be taken, the serious breach of GCP reporting timelines are met and the study is not further compromised. If the incident is confirmed as a serious breach of GCP, then a DATIX must be raised
- The PI must also inform the affected participants in line with the site's duty of candour policy and either re-consent the participants or remove them from the study if that is their preference
- The deviation should be noted in any study report (publication, conference poster)
- Appropriate statistical methods to analyse the data may be undertaken to determine the effect of this variation on the outcome measures, e.g. exclusion, sensitivity analysis

You are the chief investigator of the study and a consultant. What would you do?

- Seek advice from the sponsor on how to proceed
- Determine whether this will happen again, and whether participants could be harmed (even if they were not harmed in this instance). If harm could occur, action should be taken to prevent this, such as pausing the enrolment of participants at this research site
- If consent was taken incorrectly, this is a serious breach of GCP and the REC must be informed within 7 days of becoming aware of the breach
- Determine a course of action to prevent this situation from occurring in this, or another research site. This may include:
  - Formal discussion with the consultant responsible to ascertain what happened and the likelihood of recurrence

- Further training for the consultant investigator to highlight the roles/ responsibilities they have as a researcher and who may undertake research roles
- Take preventative action and inform other sites of what has happened to ensure their respective PIs disseminate this information

The consultant is no longer able to attend the required clinics. How can this be managed?

- An additional investigator may be added to the study. This can be a member of the clinical team, such as another consultant, registrar, staff grade, dental core trainee, or clinical research nurse
- If there are no appropriate members of the team available or willing, the sponsor should be informed
- The individual should be appropriately trained: GCP training, with additional consent/paediatric consent modules if required
- The principal investigator should outline their role and utilize the delegation log to establish the investigator's responsibilities
- The study delegation log should be updated by the PI to reflect the end date of the consultant's participation in the study

Further reading

ARSAC portal. Available at: https://digitaltools.phe.org.uk/servicedesk/customer/portal/22/user/login?destination=portal%2F22

Medical Research Council. Do I need NHS REC review? Available at: https://www.hra-decisiontools.org.uk/ethics/

NHS Health Research Authority. Safety reporting. Available at: https://www.hra.nhs.uk/approvals-amendments/managing-your-approval/safety-reporting/

NHS Health Research Authority. Amending an approval. Available at: https://www.hra.nhs.uk/approvals-amendments/amending-approval/

Research Data Scotland. Available at: https://www.researchdata.scot/accessing-data/initial-enquiry-form/

Chapter 11

Managing a dental laboratory

Roles and responsibilities

Maxillofacial and dental laboratories are an integral part of various clinical services within National Health Service (NHS) hospitals. They provide a diverse range of complex fixed and removable custom-made medical devices, including prototype medical devices for research purposes, in association with various medical and dental specialities (see Table 11.1). They also interact with non-clinical services within the hospital, such as biomedical engineering, IT, human resources, learning and development, and occupational health.

Laboratory manager

The most senior staff member will usually be the laboratory manager. They are responsible for managing workflow and adjusting priorities to accommodate urgent or unexpected cases, quality control and procurement etc. They are also responsible for staff management, training and supervision, and recruitment. Maxillofacial and dental laboratories must be run in accordance with relevant legislation, national and local policies, and formulate operational policies in line with these.

Table 11.1 Services offered by a dental and maxillofacial laboratory

Speciality	Maxillofacial and dental laboratory services		
Plastic surgery	Auricular prosthesis	Auricular splint	Buccinator flap appliance
	Cranioplasty plate	Maxillary cover plate	Keloid splint
Oral and maxillofacial surgery			Orthognathic surgery wafers
Orthodontics	Study Models	Diagnostic set up	
	Peer Assessment Rating (PAR) scoring	Space maintainer	Removable orthodontic appliance
	Functional appliances	Quad helix	Transpalatal arch (TPA)
	Removable retainer with pontic	Fixed retainer	Removable retainer
Prosthodontics and restorative dentistry		Crown	Bridge
	Denture	Inlay	Onlay
Speech and language therapy	Speech lift appliance	Speech prosthesis	Obturator
			Electropalatography plate

Health and safety

Maxillofacial and dental laboratory managers must ensure that materials and equipment are used safely and correctly. Laboratories must be run in accordance with:

- Health and Safety at Work Act 1974
- Management of Health and Safety at Work Regulations 1999
- The trust's health and safety policy

Materials used to produce medical devices must be managed in accordance with the Control of Substances Hazardous to Health (COSHH) legislation. These cover both chemical and biological substance exposure. In addition to examining material data sheets, documented thorough risk assessments are mandatory. For dental technicians, respiratory and skin symptoms can be related to occupational exposures, and particular care needs to be taken when methyl methacrylate is being used, which has a Work Exposure Limit (WEL). It is likely that most dental technicians will require regular health surveillance to monitor their health and reinforce their understanding of their exposures at work.

Laboratories must minimize the risk of infection and comply with:

- Infection and microbial contamination requirements under medical device legislation
- Code of Practice for the Prevention and Control of Health Care Associated Infections as set out in the Health and Social Care Act 2008
- Hospital trust's infection prevention and control policy

Audit

Laboratory staff may also partake in clinical audits and monitor orthodontic treatment efficiency. Where orthodontic treatment is carried out under an NHS contract, all cases must be examined using the PAR index.

- It is best practice for those assessing such cases to be calibrated in the index; laboratory staff may attain this calibration and monitor the orthodontic treatment outcomes
- Those who have attained PAR index calibration are registered in the British Orthodontic Society directory of calibrated PAR scorers
- Where this treatment is delivered under a cleft lip and palate (including non-cleft velopharyngeal dysfunction) contract, these outcomes need to be provided annually to the national specialized services quality dashboards (SSQD)

General Dental Council requirements

Maxillofacial and dental laboratories are usually staffed by dental technicians. Dental technicians working in the United Kingdom (UK) must maintain registration with the General Dental Council (GDC) and remain compliant with the necessary requirements, which include:

- Following the *Standards for the Dental Team*
- Undertaking continuous professional development (CPD)
- Having a personal development plan (PDP) in place
- Working within their scope of practice

Maxillofacial and dental laboratory managers should ensure that their staff remain compliant with these requirements.

Student dental technicians in training are exempt from the CPD and PDP requirements but must follow the GDC student professionalism and fitness to practice guidelines and have evidence that they are working towards a GDC registerable qualification.

While custom-made devices will usually be constructed by dental technicians, all dental professionals can have roles in providing these appliances under the GDC Scope of Practice, provided they are trained, competent, and indemnified (see Table 11.2).

Table 11.2 GDC scope of practice for custom-made device provision

GDC registrant group	Examples of procedures pertaining to custom-made device provision that may be carried out
Orthodontic therapists	Repair the acrylic component part of orthodontic appliances
Dental nurses	Construct bleaching trays, mouthguards, and vacuum formed retainers to the prescription of a dentist
Dental hygienists	Pour, cast, and trim study models
Dental therapists	
Dental technicians	Construct custom-made devices
Clinical dental technicians	Provide complete dentures direct to patients and other custom-made devices on prescription from a dentist
Dentists	Prescribe and construct custom-made devices

Medical device regulations

Most laboratory appliances are classified as custom-made medical devices and are subject to medical device legislation.

Custom-made devices

Custom-made devices are defined as those:

- Manufactured specifically in accordance with a written prescription from a registered medical practitioner, or other person authorized to write such a prescription by virtue of their professional qualification (such as a dentist), which gives under their responsibility, specific characteristics as to its design
- Intended for the sole use of a particular patient, but does not include a mass-produced product which comprises a medical device and medicinal product forming a single integral product which needs to be adapted to meet the specific requirements of the medical practitioner or professional user

The manufacturer of a custom-made device must meet the particular requirements of the UK MDR 2002.

Medical Device Directive/Medical Devices Regulations 2002

Until 26 May 2021, custom-made devices manufactured within the European Union (EU) were subject to the Medical Device Directive (MDD), which was transposed into UK law in the Medical Devices Regulations 2002 (UK MDR 2002).

Under these regulations, device manufacturers are required to:
- Inform the competent authority in their member state. In the UK, this means registering with the Medicines and Healthcare products Regulatory Agency (MHRA)
- Comply with the relevant Annex I Essential Requirements
- Prepare documentation, indicating manufacturing site(s) and allowing an understanding of the design, manufacture, and performance
- Draw up the statement that must be supplied with custom-made devices
- Retain a copy of this documentation for five years
- Review and document post-production experience
- Report serious incidents and field safety corrective actions, via the MHRA's Manufacturer's On-line Reporting Environment in the UK

Medical devices that are manufactured within a health institution for a patient within that establishment are known as in-house manufacture.

There are no regulatory requirements for such devices as they are not considered to have been placed on the market. Under this health institution exemption (HIE), manufacturers are still required to comply with the relevant Annex I Essential Requirements, prepare technical documentation and comply with the post-production requirements but they are not required to register with the MHRA or supply/retain a copy of the statement.

The labels on a custom-made device must include:
- The name or trade name and address of the manufacturer or, for devices imported into the United Kingdom, the name and address of the UK responsible person

- The details strictly necessary for the healthcare professional to identify the device and the contents of the packaging (e.g. patient name/description of device)
- The words 'custom-made device'

EU Medical Device Regulation

In the EU, the MDD has been replaced by the EU Medical Device Regulation (EU MDR).

Manufacturers of medical devices in Northern Ireland are required to follow the EU MDR under the terms of the protocol on Ireland/Northern Ireland.

The requirements for manufacturers of custom-made devices under the EU MDR are as follows:

- Register with the competent authority (MHRA in the UK)
- Appoint a person responsible for regulatory compliance (a new requirement similar to the 'qualified person' in pharmaceuticals)
- Establish, document, implement, maintain, keep up to date and continually improve a quality management system (another new requirement which can be mapped to parts of the ISO [International Organization for Standardization] standard ISO 13485 Medical devices—Quality management systems—Requirements for regulatory purposes)
- Comply with the General Safety and Performance Requirements set out in EU MDR Annex I. These obligations are comparable with the MDD Annex I requirements but the risk management requirements are more well-defined and in alignment with ISO 14971 Medical devices—Application of risk management to medical devices
- Follow the procedure in EU MDR Annex XIII, which provides the statement, documentation, and post-production obligations (broadly equivalent with MDD Annex VIII)
- Review and document post-production experience
- Report serious incidents and field safety corrective actions

Health institutions that wish to maintain an HIE must now satisfy the conditions set out in EU MDR Article 5(5).

Further reading

British Orthodontic Society. Quality Assurance in NHS Primary Care Orthodontics. Available at: ⅏ https://www.bos.org.uk/Professionals-Members/Research-Audit/Quality-Assurance-in-Orthodontics/Quality-Assurance-in-NHS-Primary-Care-Orthodontics

Control of Substances Hazardous to Health Regulations 2002 (Statutory Instrument 2002/2677). Available at: ⅏ https://www.legislation.gov.uk/uksi/2002/2677/pdfs/uksi_20022677_en.pdf

Department of Health. The Health and Social Care Act 2008: code of practice on the prevention and control of infections and related guidance. 2015. Available at: ⅏ https://assets.publishing.service.gov.uk/government/uploads/system/uploads/attachment_data/file/449049/Code_of_practice_280715_acc.pdf

Health and Safety at Work Act 1974. Available at: ⅏ https://www.legislation.gov.uk/ukpga/1974/37/pdfs/ukpga_19740037_en.pdf

International Organization for Standardization (ISO). ISO 13485 Medical devices—Quality management systems—requirements for regulatory purposes. Available at: ⅏ https://www.iso.org/standard/59752.html

International Organization for Standardization (ISO). ISO 14971 Medical devices—Application of risk management to medical devices. Available at: ⅏ https://www.iso.org/obp/ui#iso:std:iso:14971:ed-3:v1:en

Management of Health and Safety at Work Regulations 1999 (Statutory Instrument 1999/3242). Available at: ℘ https://www.legislation.gov.uk/uksi/1999/3242/pdfs/uksi_19993242_en.pdf

Medicines and Healthcare products Regulatory Agency. In-house manufacture of medical devices in Great Britain. 2020. Available at: ℘ https://www.gov.uk/government/publications/in-house-manufacture-of-medical-devices/in-house-manufacture-of-medical-devices

NHS England. Specialised Services Quality Dashboards—Women and Children metric definitions for 2020/21: Cleft Lip and or Palate Services including Non-cleft Velopharyngeal Dysfunction (VPD) (All Ages) 2020/21. Available at: ℘ https://www.england.nhs.uk/wp-content/uploads/2020/07/women-ssqd-cleft-lip-and-or-palate-services-including-non-cleft-velopharyngeal-dysfunction-all-ages-20-21.pdf

Regulation (EU) 2017/745 of the European Parliament and of the Council of 5 April 2017 on medical devices, amending Directive 2001/83/EC, Regulation (EC) No 178/2002 and Regulation (EC) No 1223/2009 and repealing Council Directives 90/385/EEC and 93/42/EEC. Available at: ℘ https://eur-lex.europa.eu/legal-content/EN/TXT/PDF/?uri=CELEX:32017R0745

The Medical Devices Regulations 2002 (UK) (Statutory Instrument 2002/618). Available at: ℘ https://www.legislation.gov.uk/uksi/2002/618/pdfs/uksi_20020618_en.pdf

Approaching scenarios

How to approach scenario questions

There are myriad of different types of scenarios that could be asked in an interview or examination and it would not be possible to prepare each one in advance! Nor should you try to. Throughout the book, we have outlined possible approaches to answering some scenarios. All of the scenarios are fictional and any resemblance to real life is through coincidence. You will see that despite the questions varying significantly, the answers always centre around key themes.

If you have a strong understanding of a finite number of core topics, then you will be able to confidently approach any scenario, in the real world or simulated. You need to be able to recognize what issues a particular scenario may cause and then you will see how the same core topics are central to managing the scenarios and how much overlap there will be in answering them.

As a trainee, obtain as much experience as possible, by:
- Organizing local training and attending courses
- Attend consultant and trust board meetings
- Meet with clinical and non-clinical staff, e.g. general managers and waiting list managers
- Ask to sit in on meetings responding to incidents, complaints, etc.
- Actively involve yourself in local management projects
- Shadow senior staff, e.g. general manager or medical director
- Read trust and NHS policies and publications
- Keep abreast of developments/topical issues in healthcare delivery at local and national levels

Key themes to prepare

The themes listed here centre around various aspects of clinical governance. Linking a scenario to the correct theme/themes aids its appropriate management and provides the basis of a well-structured and comprehensive answer/response.

- Patient safety and how to prioritize it
- Duty of candour
- Conduct and capability
- Disciplinary pathway/ grievance management
- Escalation pathway for concerns in a hospital, whether about a patient, a staff member, a procedure, criminal activity
- Complaints management
- Whistleblowing
- Supporting staff—training, appraisal, occupational health
- Equality and diversity
- Safeguarding children and adults
- Improving, developing or setting up a service, including a business case for new equipment/staff appointments
- Management of healthcare services, e.g. waiting lists, referrals
- Finance related—managing a reduced budget, improving efficiency
- Justification of a service and continuing provision
- Data protection
- Health and safety/incident at work, e.g. needlestick injury

The Intercollegiate Speciality Fellowship Examination's syllabus lists the following:

- Evidence-based practice, clinical guidelines, and outcomes
- Teaching/training/assessment/CPD
- Medicolegal responsibilities, jurisprudence, ethics
- Clinical effectiveness/audit
- Appraisal/performance/peer review
- Clinical risk management/complaints
- Health services management, administration, and use of resources
- Confidentiality/freedom of information/data protection

Candidates at more junior levels might not need knowledge of all of these topics (e.g. service provision, financial management of a department), more so an awareness that they exist within the trust and the most appropriate person or department to approach as needed.

Formulating your answer

Most scenario-based exams will allow candidates some time to prepare prior to questions being asked.

- Use this time to identify the key themes that the scenario raises and the likely stakeholders involved (see Table 12.1)
- Acronyms may help guide preparation for a scenario answer, particularly in an exam setting which may be stressful (see Table 12.2 and Table 12.3)
- Don't worry if you do not immediately come up with the final solution or cannot predict the direction in which the questions will go; the examiners will guide you in delivering your answers and you will collect marks along the way in answering
- You do not need to know and remember everything possible about the scenario when you are reading it

You are also not required to memorize all the policies which your hospital has, but rather to be aware of their existence, recognize which policies may be relevant and have an understanding of the implication of said policy and how events are likely to unfold.

Hospital policies vary in detail but the overall management approach will be similar, therefore do not get hung up on the minor details but rather, the process. For example, it is a bonus if you can remember how many days it will take for an employee to be notified following a disciplinary hearing or how many days they have to appeal, but if not, having a robust understanding of the actual process will suffice.

When you first begin to approach the scenario, it may be helpful to outline the issues that the scenario raises and the related policies +/—any relevant government publications. For example, in an exam situation, you could say 'this scenario raises a concern for safeguarding children and staff disciplinary action and so I would review those hospital policies'. This is a confident start to your answer, will settle your nerves, and helps to focus you and your answer in the correct direction. It instantly reassures the examiners that you have correctly identified the theme and most appropriate first steps.

Table 12.1 Considerations when structuring scenario answers

Issue	What is the fundamental issue?
Information	What information do you need to manage it?
People	Who would need to be involved?
Records	What records are needed?
Policy	What policies/regulations are relevant?
Feedback	Who needs feedback and how can this be obtained?
Evaluation	How will the information be processed/assessed?
Support	Who needs support and how can this be provided?
Escalate	How and when does the issue need to be escalated?

Once you have identified the key themes, then start thinking about your management of the situation, divided into immediate, medium, and long term and have a structure to your answer.

Immediate management

- Always consider patient safety as your first management concern
- Does the treatment need to be stopped/a doctor removed from clinical practice/additional staff members called upon to assist
- Consider how to de-escalate a situation in that immediate moment—you may need to remove people from a clinical area, take family or parents to a quiet room, relieve staff from their clinical duty to resolve an immediate conflict
- Contingency plan for immediate management—if you suddenly have to manage an escalating situation, ask for help from a senior colleague, clinical team, or colleagues to assist with treatment you may have been carrying out or delegate tasks. If you are the most senior person in the department, seek help laterally if needed from consultants in other related departments
- Reassure and support the patient or person involved in the scenario

Medium-term management

This should cover the main details of how you would solve the issue. Once the immediate situation is taken care of, you should investigate and respond to the situation and escalate as required.

- Completing an incident report allows senior clinicians and support teams to be aware of the situation
- While a junior member of staff would escalate to a consultant, knowledge of what will happen is required. If you are at consultant level, you need an understanding of what that investigation is likely to involve and possible repercussions
- Information should be gathered to establish the details of the situation This may involve:
  - Speaking to members of the team who may have witnessed or been involved in the situation including nurses and other support staff
  - Establish whether the behaviour represents a pattern or is a one-off incident by speaking with those who may be aware of other instances. This would be their line manager: consultant, clinical lead, lead nurse or educational supervisor
  - An audit or service evaluation may provide objective information on clinical activity, clinical outcomes, or possible harms
- It may be necessary to involve other teams such as human resources, occupational health, audit team, PALS, risk management team, clinical governance team, and higher management if the issue is serious
- The responsible consultant or clinical lead is the first step, but you can escalate a concern straight to medical director level if the concern is serious
- Demonstrate you are escalating the situation through the correct channels while retaining ownership of the situation—supporting the staff involved (see Chapter 7, Staff management), ensuring contingency measures for ongoing high quality patient care and having the foresight to plan ahead depending on how the situation may unfold

- It may be necessary to carry out an internal enquiry and so an investigating officer may need to be appointed. This will depend on the nature of the concern. Consider a root-cause analysis
- Any changes or objectives should be SMART—specific, measurable, achievable, relevant, and time-bound
- It is always best (where safe and appropriate) to resolve a situation locally or informally by speaking to the individual concerned. There should still be a record of this
- Examples of dental patient safety issues and mitigations are given in Chapter 6, Patient safety and risk management

Long-term management

- Not all scenarios will require significant long-term management although all situations should be used as opportunities for learning
- Where changes have been made in the short/medium term, these should be monitored through audit and service evaluation
- Escalate concerns internally/external (whistleblowing) if they are not being resolved
- Support staff and patients
- Follow up with duty of candour
- Learn from events—audit, team meetings, feedback sessions, highlight teaching and learning objectives, refresher training
- Identify changes to protocols that may be required, or the need to devise LocSSIPS, SOPs, new guidelines, or a change in practice
- Link to appraisal and revalidation

Table 12.2 Useful acronym for staff management scenario

S	Seek information
P	Patient safety
I	Initiative
E	Escalate
S	Support

Table 12.3 Useful acronym for complaints scenario

E	Explanation
A	Apology
S	Solution
Y	Do it yesterday

Additional sample scenarios

The following are additional scenario examples highlighting the key themes and a loose outline of steps to consider. This is the outline a candidate might devise when in an examination setting and preparing their answer. These should be read in conjunction with appropriate chapter(s) and scenario(s).

Scenarios relating to 'poor performing colleagues', such as a colleague whose techniques are out of date, not sharing the workload equally, unwilling to participate in clinical governance activities

- Legislative framework: GDC/GMC Standards for Professionals, RCS England 'Good Surgical Practice', conduct and capability policy, raising concerns in the workplace, NCAS (National Clinical Assessment Service)
- Patient safety is the priority in this situation. Immediate management should consider this
- Consider this from a conduct, capability, and/or disciplinary aspect
- Consider the medium-term management: resource implications on you/team, managing patient workload, supporting the staff member while they retrain and reporting concerns or whistleblowing
- Long term: consider how to prevent this situation in future, encouraging active participation in clinical governance, impact on appraisal and revalidation, learning from events

Scenarios relating to complaints from a patient or an angry patient/parent

- Documents to consider: complaints policy, bullying and harassment, grievance, and conflict policy
- Themes of complaints can include: issues regarding compassion, communication, delay/poor coordination of care, missed opportunities to act on information, treatment provided
- Immediate management: calm the patient/parent, de-escalate the situation, consider other patients and the clinic workload, enlist help from your colleagues, apologize as appropriate, inform PALS
- Immediate local resolution is the goal
- Medium-term management: involve PALS (if not already aware), carry out an investigation as per the complaints policy protocol. Handling and closing of the complaint
- Long term: consider lessons learned, discuss with the team about handling of the event and how to prevent future occurrences, identify training requirements

Transfer of patient care that is not progressing well/there are clinical issues of which the patient is unaware

- Frameworks to consider: GMC/GDC standards of professional care, duty of candour, whistleblowing, training
- Immediate management: patient safety. Inform the patient, outline concerns. Consider advice from your indemnity provider. Support the patient in halting treatment/reassure about next steps
- Medium term: obtain information from the previous clinician, don't assume incompetence as there may be other clinical reasons for the suboptimal outcome
- Thorough note keeping and discuss with colleagues if required

- Establish a plan of action for progressing forward with the patient—possible solutions/need to change treatment goals
- Long term: whistleblowing if required, report to GMC/GDC if there are grave concerns
- Learning from the event for you and your team—how to prevent in future

Index

For the benefit of digital users, indexed terms that span two pages (e.g., 52–53) may, on occasion, appear on only one of those pages.

Note: Tables, figures, and boxes are indicated by an italic *t*, *f*, and *b* following the page number.